Frontiers in Anti-Infective Drug Discovery

(Volume 8)

Edited by

Atta-ur-Rahman, *FRS*

Kings College
University of Cambridge
Cambridge
UK

&

M. Iqbal Choudhary

H.E.J. Research Institute of Chemistry,
International Center for Chemical and Biological Sciences,
University of Karachi, Karachi,
Pakistan

Frontiers in Anti-Infective Drug Discovery

Volume # 8

Editors: Atta-ur-Rahman, *FRS* and M. Iqbal Choudhary

ISSN (Online): 1879-663X

ISSN (Print): 2451-9162

ISBN (Online): 978-981-14-1238-7

ISBN (Print): 978-981-14-1237-0

ISBN (Paperback): 978-981-14-7005-9

need for a court order if at any point you breach any terms of this License Agreement. In no event will any delay or failure by Bentham Science Publishers in enforcing your compliance with this License Agreement constitute a waiver of any of its rights.

3. You acknowledge that you have read this License Agreement, and agree to be bound by its terms and conditions. To the extent that any other terms and conditions presented on any website of Bentham Science Publishers conflict with, or are inconsistent with, the terms and conditions set out in this License Agreement, you acknowledge that the terms and conditions set out in this License Agreement shall prevail.

Bentham Science Publishers Pte. Ltd.
80 Robinson Road #02-00
Singapore 068898
Singapore
Email: subscriptions@benthamscience.net

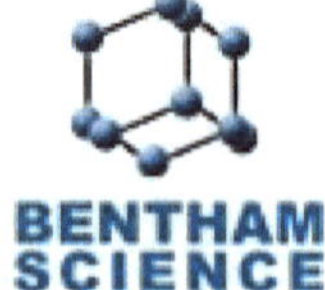

CONTENTS

*Pankaj Satapathy, Aishwarya S, Rashmi M Shetty, Akshaya Simha N, Dhanapal G,
Aishwarya Shree R, Antara Biswas, Kounaina K, Anirudh G. Patil, Avinash MG,
Aishwarya T Devi, Shubha Gopal, Nagendra Prasad MN, Veena SM, Hudeda SP,
Muthuchelian K, Sunil S. More, Govindappa Melappa* and *Farhan Zameer*

PREFACE

The recent COVID-19 pandemic has further highlighted our human incapacity to control infections. Pathogens of all forms and types are fast learners, and their mutations, spread and virulence can overwhelm the entire health care system within weeks. The COVID-19 pandemic has also exposed our inability to quickly come up with treatment and prevention regimes, despite the tremendous progress in pharmaceutical and biomedical sciences. In the post COVID-19 world major attention to the surveillance, prevention, and treatment of infections of all kinds is expected. Research on infections and anti-infectious drug discovery is already truly interdisciplinary in nature, and is published in journals of diverse disciplines, such as microbiology, molecular and structural biology, genomics, immunology, epidemiology, *etc*. It is imperative that the most exciting discoveries in this field are compiled as critically written reviews in frontier areas.

The aim of the book series *"Frontiers in Anti-infectious Drug Discovery"* is to focus on recent important developments. Experts in various important aspects of anti-infectious drug discovery have therefore contributed review articles on the most recent advancements. Volume 8, like the previous volumes, of this well received book series, comprises eight (8) scholarly written review articles on certain key aspects. These include genomic based identification of new drug targets and metagenomics for antimicrobials; fragment-based approach for drug designing, and of various types of antimicrobials ranging from synthetic analogs against coronaviruses, to bacterial phages against infections, nanoparticle based agents, as well as aptamers.

The chapter contributed by Gisbert and McNicholl focuses on the key advantages of concomitant non-bismuth quadruple therapy for a range of infections caused by Helicobactor pylori. Silva-Junior *et al* have presented an interesting review on the discovery and development of bioactive drug leads against the recent pandemic caused by SARS-CoV-2, based on analogs developed during the past SARS and MERS epidemics. Advances and challenges in fragment-based designing of new antibiotics is the key focus of the article by Kwan *et al*, supported by numerous examples. Foodborne bacterial infections are widespread. Ilyina *et al* review the recent applications of phage therapies as alternatives to antimicrobials for the treatment of food borne bacterial infections. Amjad *et al* have contributed a chapter on the applications of subtractive genomics to identify essential genes involved in crucial metabolic pathways of pathogens, and validating their protein products as novel drug targets. Metagonomics has emerged as a key technique for the discovery of novel antibiotics from yet uncultured microbes. The tremendous pool of new antimicrobials in unexplored microbial flora is the focus of the review by Chopra *et al*. Zameer has contributed a chapter on the use of nanoparticles as drug careers of synthetic and natural antimicrobial agents. In the last chapter, Syed *et al* have touched upon an important new field of the use of aptamers (oligonucleotides or peptide molecules) as novel diagnostic and anti-infective agents.

We would to express our sincere thanks eminent to all the authors for their excellent contributions in this vibrant, and exciting field of biomedical and pharmaceutical research. The efforts of Ms. Fariya Zulfiqar (Manager Publications) and the excellent management of Mr. Mahmood Alam (Director Publications) are also gratefully acknowledged.

<table>
<tr><td>

Prof. Dr. Atta-ur-Rahman, *FRS*
Honorary Life Fellow
Kings College
University of Cambridge Cambridge
UK

</td><td align="center">

Prof. Dr. M. Iqbal Choudhary
H.E.J. Research Institute of Chemistry
International Center for Chemical and Biological Sciences
University of Karachi
Karachi
Pakistan

</td></tr>
</table>

LIST OF CONTRIBUTORS

A. Ilyina	Nanobioscience Research Group, University of Coahuila, Coahuila, Mexico
Adrian G. McNicholl	Department of Gastroenterology, Hospital Universitario de La Princesa, Instituto de Investigación Sanitaria Princesa (IIS-IP), Universidad Autonoma de Madrid (UAM), Madrid, Spain
Ammar Ahmed	Department of Medical Laboratory Sciences, University of Lahore, Islamabad, Pakistan
Amjad Ali	Atta-ur-Rahman School of Applied Biosciences (ASAB), National University of Sciences and Technology (NUST), Islamabad, Pakistan
Ann H. Kwan	School of Life and Environmental Sciences, University of Sydney, Sydney, Australia
A.C. Flores-Gallegos	Research Group in Molecular Biology, University of Coahuila, Coahuila, Mexico
Aishwarya T. Devi	Department of Biotechnology, JSS Science and Technology University, Karnataka, India
Anirudh G. Patil	Department of Biological Sciences, Dayananda Sagar University, Karnataka, India
Antara Biswas	Department of Biological Sciences, Dayananda Sagar University, Karnataka, India
Azeddine Chaiba	Department of industrial Engineering, University of Khenchela, Algeria
Bushra Jamil	Department of Medical Laboratory Sciences, University of Lahore, Islamabad, Pakistan
Chirag Chopra	School of Bioengineering and Biosciences, Lovely Professional University, Phagwara, India
Daljeet Singh Dhanjal	School of Bioengineering and Biosciences, Lovely Professional University, Phagwara, India
Edeildo Ferreira da Silva-Júnior	Chemistry and Biotechnology Institute, Federal University of Alagoas, Maceió, Brazil Laboratory of Medicinal Chemistry, Pharmaceutical Sciences Institute, Federal University of Alagoas, Maceió, Brazil
E.P. Segura-Ceniceros	Nanobioscience Research Group, University of Coahuila, Coahuila, Mexico
Fayssal Amrane	LAS Research Laboratory Department of Electrical Engineering, University of Setif-1, Setif, Algeria
Fatima Shahid	Atta-ur-Rahman School of Applied Biosciences (ASAB), National University of Sciences and Technology (NUST), Islamabad, Pakistan
Farhan Zameer	Department of Biological Sciences, Dayananda Sagar University, Karnataka, India
G. Dhanapal	Department of Biological Sciences, Dayananda Sagar University, Karnataka, India

Govindappa Melappa	Department of Botany, Davangere University, Karnataka, India
N. Akshaya Simha	Department of Biological Sciences, Dayananda Sagar University, Karnataka, India
Igor José dos Santos Nascimento	Chemistry and Biotechnology Institute, Federal University of Alagoas, Maceió, Brazil
João Xavier de Araújo-Júnior	Laboratory of Medicinal Chemistry, Pharmaceutical Sciences Institute, Federal University of Alagoas, Maceió, Brazil
Javier P. Gisbert	Department of Gastroenterology, Hospital Universitario de La Princesa, Instituto de Investigación Sanitaria Princesa (IIS-IP), Universidad Autonoma de Madrid (UAM), Madrid, Spain
K. Muthuchelian	Department of Biological Sciences, Dayananda Sagar University, Karnataka, India
K. Kounaina	Department of Dravyaguna, JSS Ayurvedic Medical College, Karnataka, India
Lorna Wilkinson-White	Sydney Analytical Core Research Facility, University of Sydney, Sydney, Australia
M.G. Avinash	Department of Studies in Microbiology, University of Mysore, Karnataka, India
M.L Chávez González	Nanobioscience Research Group, University of Coahuila, Coahuila, Mexico
Muhammad Ali Syed	Department of Microbiology, The University of Haripur, Haripur, Pakistan
Muhammad Shehroz	Atta-ur-Rahman School of Applied Biosciences (ASAB), National University of Sciences and Technology (NUST), Islamabad, Pakistan
M.N. Nagendra Prasad	Department of Biotechnology, JSS Science and Technology University, Karnataka, India
Nayab Ali	Department of Microbiology, The University of Haripur, Haripur, Pakistan
Pankaj Satapathy	Department of Biological Sciences, Dayananda Sagar University, Karnataka, India
Paulo Fernando da Silva Santos-Júnior	Chemistry and Biotechnology Institute, Federal University of Alagoas, Maceió, Brazil
R. Aishwarya Shree	Department of Biological Sciences, Dayananda Sagar University, Karnataka, India
R. Rodríguez-Herrera	Research Group in Molecular Biology, University of Coahuila, Coahuila, Mexico
R. Ramos-González	Faculty of Chemical Sciences of the Autonomous, University of Coahuila, Coahuila, Mexico
Reena Singh	School of Bioengineering and Biosciences, Lovely Professional University, Phagwara, India
Rashmi M. Shetty	Department of Biological Sciences, Dayananda Sagar University, Karnataka, India

S. Aishwarya	Department of Biological Sciences, Dayananda Sagar University, Karnataka, India
S. Pacios-Michelena	Research Group in Molecular Biology, University of Coahuila, Coahuila, Mexico Nanobioscience Research Group, University of Coahuila, Coahuila, Mexico
S.P. Hudeda	Department of Dravyaguna, JSS Ayurvedic Medical College, Karnataka, India
Sanjay Yapabandara	School of Life and Environmental Sciences, University of Sydney, Sydney, Australia
Sandro Ataide	School of Life and Environmental Sciences, University of Sydney, Sydney, Australia
Shubha Gopal	Department of Studies in Microbiology, University of Mysore, Karnataka, India
Sunil S. More	Department of Biological Sciences, Dayananda Sagar University, Karnataka, India
Tahreem Zaheer	Atta-ur-Rahman School of Applied Biosciences (ASAB), National University of Sciences and Technology (NUST), Islamabad, Pakistan
S.M. Veena	Department of Biotechnology, Sapthagiri Engineering College, Karnataka, India
Thiago Mendonça de Aquino	Chemistry and Biotechnology Institute, Federal University of Alagoas, Maceió, Brazil

CHAPTER 1

Eradication of *Helicobacter pylori* Infection with Non-Bismuth Quadruple Concomitant Therapy

Javier P. Gisbert[*] and **Adrian G. McNicholl**

Department of Gastroenterology, Hospital Universitario de La Princesa, Instituto de Investigación Sanitaria Princesa (IIS-IP), Universidad Autonoma de Madrid (UAM), and Centro de Investigación Biomédica en Red de Enfermedades Hepáticas y Digestivas (CIBEREHD), Madrid, Spain

Abstract: Background: The main recommended regimens to eradicate *Helicobacter pylori* infection fail in ≥20% of the cases. Several substitutes for triple therapies have been proposed, and non-bismuth quadruple therapy is one of the most widely used.

Aim: To systematically review the efficacy of non-bismuth quadruple regimen (proton pump inhibitor, clarithromycin, amoxicillin and a nitroimidazole) in the eradication of *H. pylori* infection.

Methods: Bibliographical searches were performed in MEDLINE/EMBASE and relevant congresses. We pooled studies evaluating the concomitant regimen, and of the randomized controlled trials comparing concomitant *vs.* standard triple therapy, and concomitant *vs.* sequential therapy.

Results: Fifty-five studies were included (6,906 patients). The meta-analysis showed that concomitant regimen offers an overall eradication rate of 87%. A sub-analysis of studies comparing one-to-one concomitant and triple therapies showed an *odds ratio* of 2.14 (95% CI=1.51-3.04) towards higher efficacy with concomitant regimen. This figure increased up to 2.41 (95% CI=1.80-3.24; 85% *vs.* 72%) when comparing arms lasting the same number of days. We also sub-analyzed the comparative efficacy between non-bismuth quadruple concomitant and sequential treatments, and concomitant achieved an *odds ratio* of 1.49 (95% CI=1.21-1.85) towards higher eradication results than sequential regimen.

Conclusions: Non-bismuth quadruple (concomitant) therapy achieves high efficacy in *H. pylori* eradication, superior to standard triple and sequential therapy. Concomitant may be more appropriate than sequential therapy for patients with clarithromycin and/or metronidazole resistance. Higher acid suppression and/or longer duration are optimizations that can increase even more its efficacy.

---

[*] **Corresponding author Javier P. Gisbert:** Department of Gastroenterology, Hospital Universitario de La Princesa, Instituto de Investigación Sanitaria Princesa (IIS-IP), Universidad Autonoma de Madrid (UAM), Madrid, Spain; Tel.: 34-913093911; Fax: 34-915204013, E-mail: javier.p.gisbert@gmail.com

Atta-ur-Rahman and M. Iqbal Choudhary (Eds.)

Keywords: Amoxicillin, Clarithromycin, Concomitant therapy, *Helicobacter pylori*, Metronidazole, Non-bismuth quadruple, Proton pump inhibitor, Resistance, Sequential therapy, Treatment.

INTRODUCTION

Approximately fifty percent of the world population is infected by *Helicobacter pylori*, a bacterium linked to a broad range of upper gastrointestinal conditions such as gastritis, peptic ulcer disease, and gastric cancer [1]. The most commonly used therapy for the eradication of *H. pylori*, traditionally recommended by international consensus, is the proton pump inhibitor (PPI)–based, standard triple therapy, adding two antibiotics (clarithromycin plus amoxicillin or metronidazole) to a PPI [2 - 6]. However, the eradication rates with this regimen have fallen considerably [7, 8]. Previous meta-analyses (with more than 53,000 included patients) showed an efficacy below 80% [9, 10]. Therefore, recent debate has been raised regarding how ethical it is to continue using standard triple therapy, and alternative approaches have been recommended [11]. Although, efforts to improve eradication prolonging triple therapy's duration have been tested, data have not consistently provided significant benefits [12, 13]. Consequently, new combinations to improve treatment of naïve patients remain as an urgent need.

Sequential treatment involving a dual regimen with a PPI plus amoxicillin for the first 5 days followed by a triple regimen including a PPI, clarithromycin, and a nitroimidazole for the following 5 days, was proposed as an alternative [14]. Several randomized clinical trials and meta-analyses have shown that the sequential regimen was more effective than the standard triple [15 - 19]. Therefore, some consensus conferences suggested sequential regimen as a substitute to standard triple for the first-line eradication of *H. pylori* [20]. Nevertheless, results obtained by a meta-analysis by the Cochrane Collaboration [21] concluded that sequential regimen outcomes were heterogeneous, and that many of the latest manuscripts were unable to show any benefit from sequential over standard triple therapy. The conclusions of the meta-analysis were clear even though the pooled eradication rate was 85%, and a potential trend towards reduced efficacy was observed in the last years [21].

Sequential treatment faced another relevant issue, whether sequential administration was really necessary or if the 4 drugs could be given concurrently [14, 22, 23]. Questions were raised regarding the risk of failure to comply with the treatment due to regimen complexity [11, 24] Moreover, the combination of amoxicillin, clarithromycin and a nitroimidazole with a PPI has previously been evaluated as a concomitant regimen in 1998: two research teams, one in Japan and the other in Germany, recommended that this drug combination should be prescribed as a concomitant 4-drug, 3-antibiotic, known as non–bismuth quadruple therapy [25, 26], providing high efficacy even in short durations (>90% by intention-to-treat in 5-day regimens).

This "non-bismuth quadruple concomitant" regimen has regained presence in recent years [27]. It is easy to convert the standard triple therapy (PPI-clarithromycin-amoxicillin) to concomitant therapy by adding of 500 mg of metronidazole (or tinidazole) twice daily [28]. Beware that "concomitant" (taking all drugs all together) may cause confusion; this term is actually a misnomer, as all *H. pylori* treatments, except sequential therapy, could be called concomitant therapies. Nonetheless, this will be the name used hereafter as it has been the most common denomination in the literature.

OBJECTIVE

The aim of the present chapter is to perform a critical review of published evidence on the efficacy and safety of concomitant therapy in the eradication of *H. pylori* infection. We will review the following aspects: 1) Efficacy of the concomitant regimen; 2) Comparison between the concomitant regimen and standard triple therapy; 3) Comparison between the concomitant and the sequential therapies; 4) Effects of different variables on the efficacy of concomitant therapy; 5) How could we increase the efficacy of the concomitant treatment? and finally; 6) What are the results with the concomitant treatment in clinical practice? (the experience of the European registry on *H. pylori* management).

BIBLIOGRAPHICAL SEARCHES

Bibliographical searches were performed in MEDLINE and ENDBASE using the following keywords (all fields): ((concomitant OR quadruple OR concurrent OR ((amoxicillin OR amoxycillin) AND (metronidazole OR tinidazole OR nitroimidazole) AND clarithromycin) AND ("*Helicobacter pylori*" OR "*H. pylori*"). No language restriction was applied. Bibliography from selected manuscripts and reviews were hand-searched to identify further relevant studies. Authors conducted a hand-search of communications from the American *Digestive Disease Week,* the *International Workshop of the European Helicobacter Study Group,* and the *United European Gastroenterology Week.* Summaries of the manuscripts selected in the different searches were reviewed, and screened for exclusion and inclusion criteria. In cases of duplicate reporting of studies or evidently based on overlapping study population, the latest valid report was considered.

EFFICACY OF THE CONCOMITANT REGIMEN

A summary of studies evaluating concomitant regimen's efficacy is shown in Table **1** [25, 26, 29 - 80]. Concomitant combinations were prescribed homogenously, with only minimal alterations: the nitroimidazole (tinidazole or metronidazole) and the PPI (omeprazole, lansoprazole, rabeprazole, or esomeprazole) and. However, there was a wide duration range between three and fourteen days. The analysis of the 55 studies (6,906 patients) showed a pooled eradication percentage by intention-to-treat of 87%, with a 95% confidence interval (95% CI) ranging from 86 to 89% (Fig. **1**). The data were pooled using the generic inverse variance method, which involves a weighted average of the effect estimates from the included studies. The weight for each study equals one divided by the square of the standard error (inverse of the variance) of the effect estimate. As population and regimens lengths were heterogeneous, a random effects model (DerSimonian and Laird) was applied to perform the meta-analysis (using Review Manager 5.0.25, developed by the Cochrane Collaboration).

Table 1. Studies evaluating the efficacy of non-bismuth quadruple (concomitant) regimen for the treatment of *Helicobacter pylori* infection.

Author	Country	Publication Year	Study Design	Disease Type	Therapy Regimen	Days ¶	No. of Patients	Eradication Rate (%) (ITT)	Eradication Rate (%) (PP)
Ang *et al.* [80]	Singapore	2015	RCT	-	O 20 mg bd + A 1 g bid + C 500 mg bid + M 400 mg bid	10	153	125/153 (82)	125/131 (95)
Apostolopoulos *et al.* [29]	Greece	2013	RCT	-	P 40 mg od + A 1 g bid + C 500 mg bid + M 500 mg bid	10	33	29/33 (88)	29/30 (97)
Calvet *et al.* [30]	Spain	2000	NC	PUD	O 20 mg bid + A 1 g bid + C 500 mg bid + T 500 mg bid	4	56	49/56 (87)	49/54 (91)

(Table 1) cont.....

Author	Country	Publication Year	Study Design	Disease Type	Therapy Regimen	Days ¶	No. of Patients	Eradication Rate (%) (ITT)	Eradication Rate (%) (PP)
Catalano *et al.* [31]	Italy	2000	RCT	PUD	O 40 mg od + A 1 g bid + C 500 mg bid + M 500 mg bid	3	56	50/56 (89)	50/54 (93)
Chan *et al.* [32]†	China	2001	NC	PUD, NUD, others	O 20 mg bid + A 20 mg/kg tid + C 7.5 mg/kg tid + M 7.5 mg/kg 5 times a day	7	33	31/33 (94)	31/33 (94)
Choi *et al.* [34]	Korea	2011	NC	-	R 20 mg bid + A 1 g bid + C 500 mg bid + M 500 mg tid	14	38	24/38 (63)	24/38 (63)
Choi *et al.* [79]	Korea	2012	RCT	-	R 20 mg bid + A 1 g bid + C 500 mg bid + M 500 mg tid	14	36	32/36 (89)	31/35 (89)
De Francesco *et al.* (a) [36]	Italy	2014	RCT	PUD, NUD	O 20 mg bid + A 1 g bid + C 500 mg bid + T 500 mg bid	5	110	86/110 (78)	86/101 (85)
De Francesco *et al.* (b) [36]	Italy	2014	RCT	PUD, NUD	O 20 mg bid + A 1 g bid + C 500 mg bid + T 500 mg bid	14	110	95/110 (86)	95/100 (95)

(Table 1) cont.....

Author	Country	Publication Year	Study Design	Disease Type	Therapy Regimen	Days ¶	No. of Patients	Eradication Rate (%) (ITT)	Eradication Rate (%) (PP)
Georgopoulos *et al.* [37]	Greece	2011	NC	PUD, NUD	E 40 mg bid + A 1 g bid + C 500 mg bid + M 500 mg bid	10	131	120/131 (92)	120/127 (94)
Georgopoulos *et al.* (a) [38]	Greece	2013	NC	PUD, NUD	E 40 mg bid + A 1 g bid + C 500 mg bid + M 500 mg bid	10	165	151/165 (91)	151/159 (95)
Georgopoulos *et al.* (b) [39]	Greece	2013	RCT	PUD, NUD	E 40 mg bid + A 1 g bid + C 500 mg bid + M 500 mg bid	10	127	115/127 (90)	111/119 (93)
Georgopoulos *et al.* [40]	Greece	2014	RCT	-	E 40 mg bid + A 1 g bid + C 500 mg bid + M 500 mg bid	10	110	98/110 (89)	98/105 (93)
Greenberg *et al.* [41]	Latin America	2011	RCT	PUD, NUD, others	L 30 mg bid + A 1 g bid + C 500 mg bid + M 500 mg bid	5	488	360/489 (74)	348/442 (79)
Heo *et al.* (a) [77]	Korea	2014	RCT	-	L 30 mg bid + A 1 g bid + C 500 mg bid + M 500 mg bid	10	169	137/174 (79)	133/150 (89)
Heo *et al.* (b) [43]	Korea	2014	RCT	-	E 20 mg bid + A 1 g bid + C 500 mg bid + M 500 mg bid	10	238	187/238 (79)	176/196 (90)

(Table 1) cont.....

Author	Country	Publication Year	Study Design	Disease Type	Therapy Regimen	Days	No. of Patients	Eradication Rate (%) (ITT)	Eradication Rate (%) (PP)
Hsu *et al.* [76]	Taiwan	2014	RCT		P 40 mg bid + A 1 g bid + C 500 mg bid + M 500 mg bid	7	102	96/102 (94)	96/102 (94)
Huang *et al.* [44]	Taiwan	2012	RCT	PUD, NUD	L 30 mg bid + A 1 g bid + C 500 mg bid + M 500 mg bid	10	84	74/84 (88)	70/74 (95)
Kalapothakos *et al.* [45]	Greece	2013	RCT	-	O 20 mg bid + A 1 g bid + C 500 mg bid + M 500 mg bid	10	95	88/102 (86)	88/95 (93)
Kao *et al.* [46]	Taiwan	2012	NC	PUD, NUD	P 40 mg bid + A 1 g bid + C 500 mg bid + M 500 mg bid	7	319	299/319 (94)	297/308 (96)
Kim *et al.* [47]	Korea	2013	RCT	PUD, NUD	L 30 mg bid + A 1 g bid + C 500 mg bid + M 500 mg bid	5	135	109/135 (81)	106/116 (91)
Kim *et al.* (a) [48]	Korea	2014	RCT	-	PPI 20 mg bid + A 1 g bid + C 500 mg bid + M 500 mg bid	10	65	52/65 (80)	50/52 (96)
Kim *et al.* (b) [78]	Korea	2014	NC	-	L 30 mg bid + A 1 g bid + C 500 mg bid + M 500 mg bid	10	68	118/125 (94)	108/116 (93)

(Table 1) cont.....

Author	Country	Publication Year	Study Design	Disease Type	Therapy Regimen	Days ¶	No. of Patients	Eradication Rate (%) (ITT)	Eradication Rate (%) (PP)
Kongchayanun *et al.* (a) [50]	Thailand	2012	RCT	NUD	R 20 mg bid + A 1 g bid + C* 1 g od + M 500 mg tid	5	55	49/55 (89)	49/55 (89)
Kongchayanun *et al.* (b) [50]	Thailand	2012	RCT	NUD	R 20 mg bid + A 1 g bid + C* 1 g od + M 500 mg tid	10	55	53/55 (96)	53/55 (96)
Kwon *et al.* (a) [51]	Korea	2011	RCT	-	L 30 mg bid + A 1 g bid + C 500 mg bid + M 500 mg bid	5	48	42/48 (87)	42/48 (87)
Kwon *et al.* (b) [51]	Korea	2011	RCT	-	L 30 mg bid + A 1 g bid + C 500 mg bid + M 500 mg bid	7	49	44/49 (90)	44/49 (90)
Lee *et al.* [75]	Korea	2015	RCT	PUD-NUD	R 20 mg bid + A 1 g bid + C 500 mg bid + M 500 mg bid	7	170	135/170 (79)	135/143 (94)
Lim *et al.* [52]	Korea	2013	RCT	PUD, NUD	R 20 mg bid + A 1 g bid + C 500 mg bid + M 500 mg bid	14	78	63/78 (81)	61/75 (81)
McNicholl *et al.* (a) [53]	Spain	2014	RCT	PUD, NUD	O 20 mg bid + A 1 g bid + C 500 mg bid + M 500 mg bid	10	168	146/168 (87)	125/137 (91)

(Table 1) cont.....

Author	Country	Publication Year	Study Design	Disease Type	Therapy Regimen	Days	No. of Patients	Eradication Rate (%) (ITT)	Eradication Rate (%) (PP)
McNicholl *et al.* (b1) [54]	Spain	2014	NC	PUD, NUD	E 40 mg bid + A 1 g bid + C 500 mg bid + M 500 mg bid	14	471	427/471 (91)	401/432 (93)
McNicholl *et al.* (b2) [54]	Spain	2014	NC	PUD, NUD	O 20 mg bid + A 1 g bid + C 500 mg bid + M 500 mg bid	10	356	305/356 (86)	282/329 (86)
Molina-Infante *et al.* [55]	Spain	2012	NC	PUD, NUD	PPI bid + A 1 g bid + C 500 mg bid + M 500 mg bid	10	182	182/209 (87)	180/203 (89)
Molina-Infante *et al.* [56]	Spain	2013	RCT	PUD, NUD	O 40 mg bid + A 1 g bid + C 500 mg bid + M 500 mg bid	14	170	156/170 (92)	150/156 (96)
Molina-Infante [57]	Spain	2014	NC	PUD, NUD	E 40 mg bid + A 1 g bid + C 500 mg bid + M 500 mg bid	14	298	272/298 (91)	272/290 (94)
Moon *et al.* [58]	Korea	2011	RCT	-	PPI bid + A 1 g bid + C 500 mg bid + M 500 mg bid	7	53	43/53 (81)	43/53 (81)
Moon *et al.* [59]	Korea	2014	NC	-	PPI bid + A 500 mg tid + C 500 mg bid + M 500 mg tid	7	106	81/106 (76)	81/101 (80)

(Table 1) cont.....

Author	Country	Publication Year	Study Design	Disease Type	Therapy Regimen	Days ¶	No. of Patients	Eradication Rate (%) (ITT)	Eradication Rate (%) (PP)
Nagahara *et al.* [60]	Japan	2000	RCT	PUD, NUD	R 10 mg bid + A 750 mg bid + C 200 mg bid + M 250 mg bid	5	55	52/55 (94)	52/53 (98)
Nagahara *et al.* [61]	Japan	2001	RCT	PUD, NUD	R 20 mg bid + A 750 mg bid + C 200 mg bid + M 250 mg bid	5	80	74/80 (92)	74/79 (94)
Neville *et al.* [62]	UK	1999	RCT	PUD, NUD, others	L 30 mg bid + A 1 g bid + C 250 mg bid + M 400 mg bid	5	56	49/56 (87)	49/54 (91)
Ntouli *et al.* [63]	Greece	2014	RCT	-	PPI bid + A 500 mg tid + C 500 mg bid + T 500 mg bid	10	108	98/108 (91)	98/108 (91)
Okada *et al.* [26]	Japan	1998	RCT	PUD, NUD, others	O 20 mg bid + A 500 mg tid + R 150 mg bid + M 250 mg tid	7	90	85/90 (94)	85/88 (97)
Okada *et al.* [64]	Japan	1999	RCT	PUD, NUD, others	O 20 mg bid + A 500 mg tid + R 150 mg bid + M 250 mg tid	7	169	155/169 (92)	155/163 (95)
Seo *et al.* [65]	Korea	2014	NC	-	R - + A - + C - + M -	7	210	194/210 (92)	-

(Table 1) cont.....

Author	Country	Publication Year	Study Design	Disease Type	Therapy Regimen	Days ¶	No. of Patients	Eradication Rate (%) (ITT)	Eradication Rate (%) (PP)
Sharara *et al*(a) [66]	Lebanon	2014	RCT	PUD, NUD	R 20 mg bid + A 1 g bid + C 500 mg bid + M 500 mg bid	7	100	78/100 (78)	78/95 (82)
Sharara *et al*(b) [66]	Lebanon	2014	RCT	PUD, NUD	R 20 mg od + A 1 g od + C 500 mg od + M 500 mg od	7	100	78/100 (78)	78/93 (84)
Tepes [68]	Slovenia	2014	RCT	-	E 20 mg bid + A 1 g bid + C 500 mg bid + M 500 mg bid	7	120	110/120 (92)	-
Toros *et al.* [69]	Turkey	2011	NC	NUD	L 30 mg bid + A 1 g bid + C 500 mg bid + M 500 mg tid	14	84	63/84 (75)	63/84 (75)
Treiber *et al* (a) [70]	Germany	2002	RCT	PUD, NUD, others	L 30 mg bid + A 1 g bid + C 250 mg bid + M 400 mg bid	3	80	65/80 (81)	65/76 (85)
Treiber *et al* (b) [70]	Germany	2002	RCT	PUD, NUD, others	L 30 mg bid + A 1 g bid + C 250 mg bid + M 400 mg bid	5	83	74/83 (89)	74/79 (94)
Treiber *et al.* [25]	Germany	1998	RCT	PUD, others	O 20 mg bid + A 1 g bid + C 250 mg bid + M 400 mg bid	5	46	42/46 (91)	42/44 (95)

(Table 1) cont.....

Author	Country	Publication Year	Study Design	Disease Type	Therapy Regimen	Days ¶	No. of Patients	Eradication Rate (%) (ITT)	Eradication Rate (%) (PP)
Wang *et al.* [71]	China	2014	RCT	-	E 20 mg bid + A 1 g bid + C 250 mg bid + T 500 mg bid	7	81	74/81 (91)	74/80 (92)
Wu *et al.* [72]	Taiwan	2010	RCT	PUD, NUD, others	E 40 mg bid + A 1 g bid + C 500 mg bid + M 500 mg bid	10	115	107/115 (93)	107/115 (93)
Yanai *et al.* [73]	Japan	2012	RCT	PUD, NUD	L 30 mg bid + A 750 mg bid + C 200 mg bid + M 250 mg bid	7	59	56/59 (95)	56/57 (98)
Zullo *et al.* [74]	Italy	2013	RCT	NUD	O 20 mg bid + A 1 g bid + C 500 mg bid + M 500 mg bid	5	90	77/90 (86)	77/84 (92)

ITT, intention-to-treat; PP, per-protocol.
RCT, randomized controlled trial. NC, non-controlled.
PUD, peptic ulcer disease; NUD, non-ulcer disease.
PPI, proton pump inhibitor (at standard dose); O, omeprazole; L, lansoprazole; R, rabeprazole; E, esomeprazole; A: amoxicillin; C, clarithromycin; M, metronidazole; T, tinidazole; R, roxithromycin.
od, once daily; bid: two times a day; tid: three times a day
¶Days of antibiotic treatment; †Pediatric patients; C*Sustained release clarithromycin.

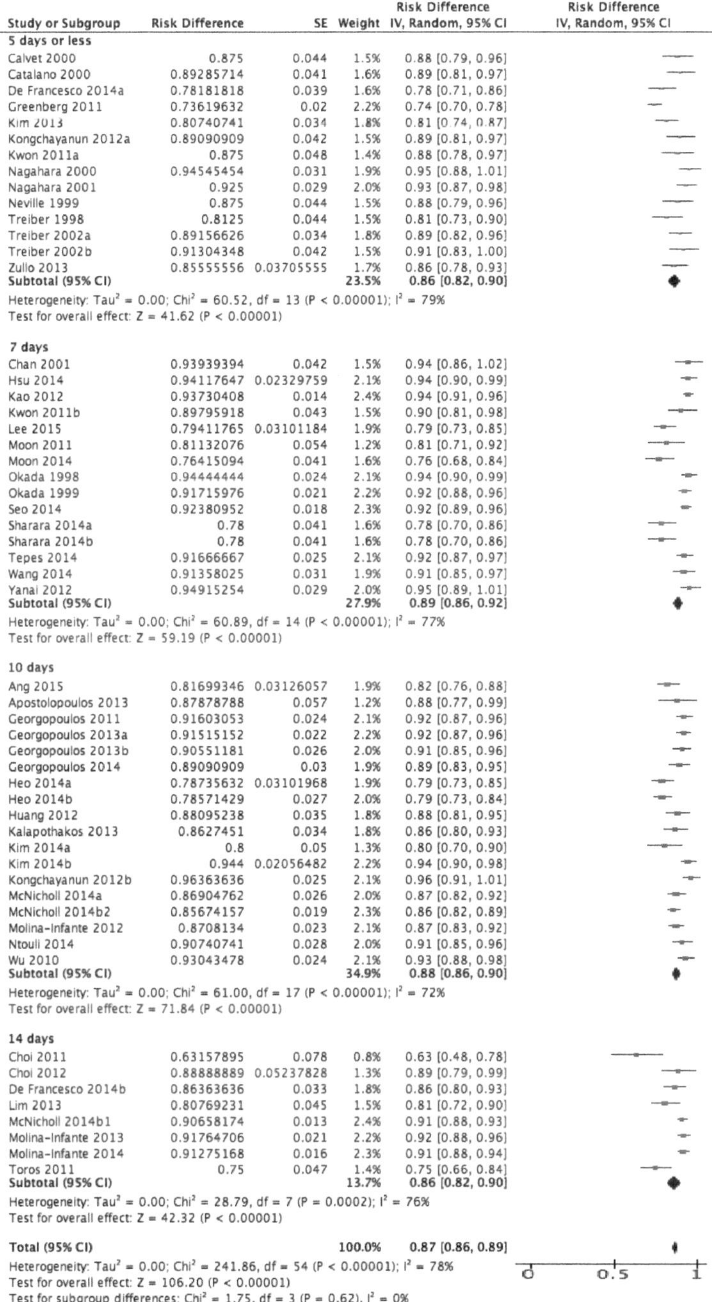

Fig. (1). Meta-analysis of efficacy (intention-to-treat) of studies evaluating the concomitant regimen for the treatment of *H. pylori* infection.

COMPARISON BETWEEN CONCOMITANT AND STANDARD TRIPLE REGIMEN

The superiority of concomitant therapy over standard triple therapy has been confirmed in several randomized trials. A recent meta-analysis [81] evaluated 9 prospective studies treating *H. pylori* with a concomitant regimen for up to 7 days. Prescribed regimens generally lasted 5 days (ranging from 4 in one study to 7 in another). Overall, concomitant therapy achieved 90% intention-to-treat eradication (93% per-protocol). Moreover, the estimates of the meta-analysis of the 5 randomized controlled trials demonstrated the superiority of concomitant regimen over standard triple therapy (*odds ratio* of 2.86; 95% CI, 1.73-4.73).

For this chapter, we have updated these meta-analytical evaluations with more recent studies and have updated it including the new trials that have compared these two treatments. Table **2** describes the studies comparing the *H. pylori* eradication rate of concomitant regimen with that of standard triple therapy by intention-to-treat [25, 31, 39, 41, 42, 47, 48, 58, 60 - 62, 67, 68, 71, 73].

Table 2. Studies comparing the efficacy (intention-to-treat) of the concomitant regimen with that of standard triple therapy for the eradication of *H. pylori* infection.

Author	Standard Triple Therapy	Days ¶	Eradication Rate (%) (ITT)	Concomitant Therapy	Days ¶	Eradication Rate (%) (ITT)
Catalano *et al* [31]	O 40 mg od + A 1 g bid + C 500 mg bid	10	45/55 (82)	O 40 mg od + A 1 g bid + C 500 mg bid + M 500 mg bid	3	50/56 (89)
Georgopoulos *et al* [39]	E 40 mg bid + A 1 g bid + C 500 mg bid	10	96/130 (74)	E 40 mg bid + A 1 g bid + C 500 mg bid + M 500 mg bid	10	115/127 (90)
Greenberg *et al* [41]	L 30 mg bid + A 1 g bid + C 500 mg bid	14	401/488 (82)	L 30 mg bid + A 1 g bid + C 500 mg bid + M 500 mg bid	5	360/489 (74)
Hsu *et al*	P 40 mg bid + A 1 g bid + C 500 mg bid	7	84/102 (82)	P 40 mg bid + A 1 g bid + C 500 mg bid + M 500 mg bid	7	96/108 (94)
Heo *et al*	L 30 mg bid + A 1 g bid + C 500 mg bid	10	123/174 (71)	L 30 mg bid + A 1 g bid + C 500 mg bid + M 500 mg bid	10	137/174 (79)
Kim *et al* [47]	L 30 mg bid + A 1 g bid + C 500 mg bid	7	98/135 (72)	L 30 mg bid + A 1 g bid + C 500 mg bid + M 500 mg bid	5	109/135 (81)

(Table 2) cont.....

Author	Standard Triple Therapy	Days ¶	Eradication Rate (%) (ITT)	Concomitant Therapy	Days ¶	Eradication Rate (%) (ITT)
Kim *et al* [48]	PPI 20 mg bid + A 1 g bid + C 500 mg bid	10	47/79 (59)	PPI 20 mg bid + A 1 g bid + C 500 mg bid + M 500 mg bid	10	52/65 (80)
Lee *et al*	L 30 mg bid + A 1 g bid + C 500 mg bid	7	109/170 (64)	L 30 mg bid + A 1 g bid + C 500 mg bid + M 500 mg bid	7	135/170 (79)
	L 30 mg bid + A 1 g bid + M 500 mg bid	7	117/170 (69)			
Moon *et al* [58]	PPI bid + A 500 mg tid + C 500 mg bid	7	55/85 (65)	PPI bid + A 500 mg tid + C 500 mg bid + M 500 mg bid	7	43/53 (81)
Nagahara *et al* [60]	R 10 mg bid + A 750 mg bid + C 200 mg bid	5	40/50 (80)	R 10 mg bid + A 750 mg bid + C 200 mg bid + M 250 mg bid	5	52/55 (94)
Nagahara *et al* [61]	R 20 mg bid + A 750 mg bid + C 200 mg bid	7	65/80 (81)	R 20 mg bid + A 750 mg bid + C 200 mg bid + M 250 mg bid	5	74/80 (92)
Neville *et al* [62]	L 30 mg bid + A 1 g bid + C 250 mg bid	5	33/56 (59)	L 30 mg bid + A 1 g bid + C 250 mg bid + M 400 mg bid	5	49/56 (87)
Ang *et al* [67]	O 20mg bid + A 1 g bid + C 500 mg bid	10	129/155 (83)	O 20mg bid + A 500 mg bid + C 500 mg bid + M 400 mg bid	10	125/153 (82)
Tepes [68]	E 20 mg bid + A 1 g bid + C 500 mg bid	7	97/116 (77)	E 20 mg bid + A 1 g bid + C 500 mg bid + M 500 mg bid	7	110/120 (92)
Treiber *et al* [25]	O 20 mg bid + C 250 mg bid + M 400 mg bid	7	38/42 (90)	O 20 mg bid + A 1 g bid + C 250 mg bid + M 400 mg bid	5	42/46 (91)
Wang *et al* [71]	E 20 mg bid + A 1 g bid + C 250 mg bid	7	65/82 (79)	E 20 mg bid + A 1 g bid + C 250 mg bid + T 500 mg bid	7	74/81 (91)
Yanai *et al* [73]	L 30 mg bid + A 750 mg bid + C 200 mg bid	7	41/60 (68)	L 30 mg bid + A 750 mg bid + C 200 mg bid + M 250 mg bid	7	56/59 (95)

PPI, proton pump inhibitor (at standard dose); O, omeprazole; L, lansoprazole; R, rabeprazole; E, esomeprazole; A: amoxicillin; C, clarithromycin; M, metronidazole; T, tinidazole.
od, once daily; bid: two times a day; tid: three times a day
¶Days of antibiotic treatment.

As summarized in Fig. (**2**), 2, 059 patients received the concomitant regimen and 2,268 the standard triple regimen. The former was more effective than the latter: 81% *vs.* 74% in the intention-to-treat analysis. The *odds ratio* for this comparison was 2.14 (95% CI, 1.51-3.04) (Fig. **2A**). A sub-analysis was performed excluding those studies in which both treatments had different treatment durations between arms. This sub-analysis showed (Fig. **2B**) that, when comparing both concomitant and triple therapies lasting the same number of days, concomitant achieved an *odds ratio* of 2.41 (95% CI= 1.80-3.24; 85% *vs.* 72%). If we subdivide by length of both arms the differences in efficacy between both treatments were, as expected, smaller at longer regimens due to the rapid decrease in the efficacy of standard triple therapy at shorter regimens (Fig. **2B**).

Regarding tolerance, in a previously published meta-analysis [81], no severe side effects were reported in any of the manuscripts, except anaphylactic reactions to study drugs [26, 64, 70]. However, these antibiotic treatments do show a high rate of moderate or mild adverse events, in Essa *et al.* meta-analysis 27-51% of patients in the concomitant group suffered some discomfort with treatment (*vs.* 21-48% standard triple therapy group) [81], suggesting that a similar safety profile can be expected from concomitant and standard triple therapies.

COMPARISON BETWEEN CONCOMITANT AND SEQUENTIAL REGIMENS

As previously discussed, sequential therapy faces a limitation due to its complexity, as switching drugs in the middle of treatment may compromise compliance. In this situation, studies comparing sequential regiment with another regimen using the same combination of drugs but concomitantly were necessary. Such comparisons would determine whether the two phase administration of sequential regiment is actually helpful [24]. A one-to-one comparison of concomitant and sequential therapies would also answer which of these 2 candidates can eventually substitute triple therapies in first-line recommendations [82].

A)

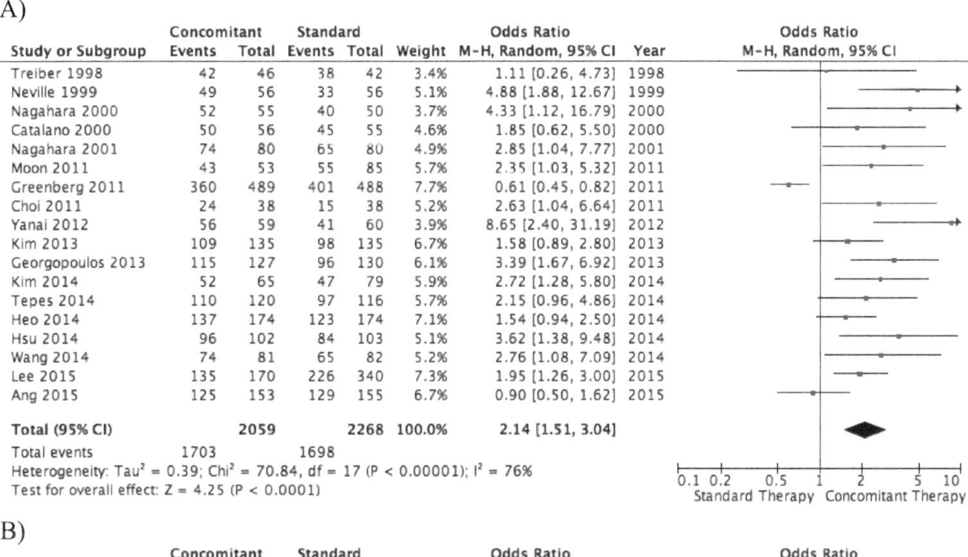

B)

Fig. (2). Meta-analysis comparing the efficacy (intention-to-treat) of the concomitant regimen with that of standard triple therapy for the eradication of *H. pylori* infection: **A)** overall; **B)** both arms with the same length of treatment.

Studies comparing the efficacy (intention-to-treat) of the concomitant regimen with that of sequential therapy for the eradication of *H. pylori* infection are summarized in Table **3** [29, 33, 34, 40, 44, 45, 48, 49, 52, 53, 63, 67, 72, 74 - 80]. Twelve studies (Fig. **3**) met the inclusion criteria (1,219 patients treated with concomitant and 1,226 with sequential), 7 of them were performed in Asia and 5 in Europe. Concomitant achieved an *odds ratio* of 1.49 (95% CI= 1.21-1.85; $I^2=$ 0%) towards higher eradication results than sequential; and a tendency towards increased differences at shorter treatment durations can be observed.

Table 3. Studies comparing the efficacy (intention-to-treat) of the concomitant regimen with that of sequential therapy for the eradication of *H. pylori* infection.

Author	Sequential Therapy	Days ¶	Eradication Rate (%) (ITT)	Concomitant Therapy	Days ¶	Eradication Rate (%) (ITT)
Apostolopoulos *et al* [29]	P 40 mg bid + A 1 g bid // P 40 mg bid + C 500 mg bid + M 500 mg bid	10	19/30 (63)	P 40 mg od + A 1 g bid + C 500 mg bid + M 500 mg bid	10	29/33 (88)
Choi *et al*	R 20 mg bid + A 1 g bid // R 20 mg bid + C 500 mg bid + M 500 mg bid	14	23/27 (85)	R 20 mg bid + A 1 g bid + C 500 mg bid + M 500 mg tid	10	32/36 (89)
Georgopoulos *et al* [40]	E 40 mg bid + A 1 g bid // E 40 bid + C 500 mg bid + M 500 mg bid	10	88/109 (82)	E 40 mg bid + A 1 g bid + C 500 mg bid + M 500 mg bid	10	98/110 (89)
Huang *et al* [44]	L 30 mg bid + A 1 g bid // L 30 mg bid + C 500 mg bid + M 500 mg bid	10	68/85 (80)	L 30 mg bid + A 1 g bid + C 500 mg bid + M 500 mg bid	10	74/84 (88)
Kalapothakos *et al* [45]	O 20 mg bid + A 1 g bid // O 20 mg bid + C 500 mg bid + M 500 mg bid	10	87/102 (85)	O 20 mg bid + A 1 g bid + C 500 mg bid + M 500 mg bid	10	88/102 (86)
Kim *et al* [48]	PPI bid + A 1 g bid // PPI bid + C 500 mg bid + M 500 mg bid	10	52/65 (80)	PPI bid + A 1 g bid + C 500 mg bid + M 500 mg bid	10	49/72 (68)

(Table 3) cont.....

Author	Sequential Therapy	Days [¶]	Eradication Rate (%) (ITT)	Concomitant Therapy	Days [¶]	Eradication Rate (%) (ITT)
Lim *et al* [52]	R 20 mg bid + A 1 g bid // R 20 mg bid + C 500 mg bid + M 500 mg bid	14	65/86 (76)	R 20 mg bid + A 1 g bid + C 500 mg bid + M 500 mg bid	14	63/78 (81)
McNicholl *et al*(a) [53]	O 20 mg bid + A 1 g bid // O 20 mg bid + C 500 mg bid + M 500 mg bid	10	138/170 (81)	O 20 mg bid + A 1 g bid + C 500 mg bid + M 500 mg bid	10	146/168 (87)
Ntouli *et al* [63]	PPI bid + A 1 g bid // PPI bid + C 500 mg bid + M 500 mg bid	10	87/104 (84)	PPI bid + A 500 mg tid + C 500 mg bid + T 500 mg bid	10	98/108 (91)
Ang *et al* [67]	O 20 mg bid + A 1 g bid // O 20 mg bid + C 500 mg bid + M 400 mg bid	10	119/135 (88)	PPI bid + A 1 g bid + C 500 mg bid + M 400 mg bid	10	125/153 (82)
Wu *et al* [72]	O 20 mg bid + A 1 g bid // O 20 mg bid + C 500 mg bid + M 500 mg bid	10	130/154 (84)	E 40 mg bid + A 1 g bid + C 500 mg bid + M 500 mg bid	10	107/115 (93)

PPI, proton pump inhibitor (at standard dose); O, omeprazole; L, lansoprazole; R, rabeprazole; E, esomeprazole; A: amoxicillin; C, clarithromycin; M, metronidazole; T, tinidazole.
od, once daily; bid: two times a day; tid: three times a day
[¶]Days of antibiotic treatment.

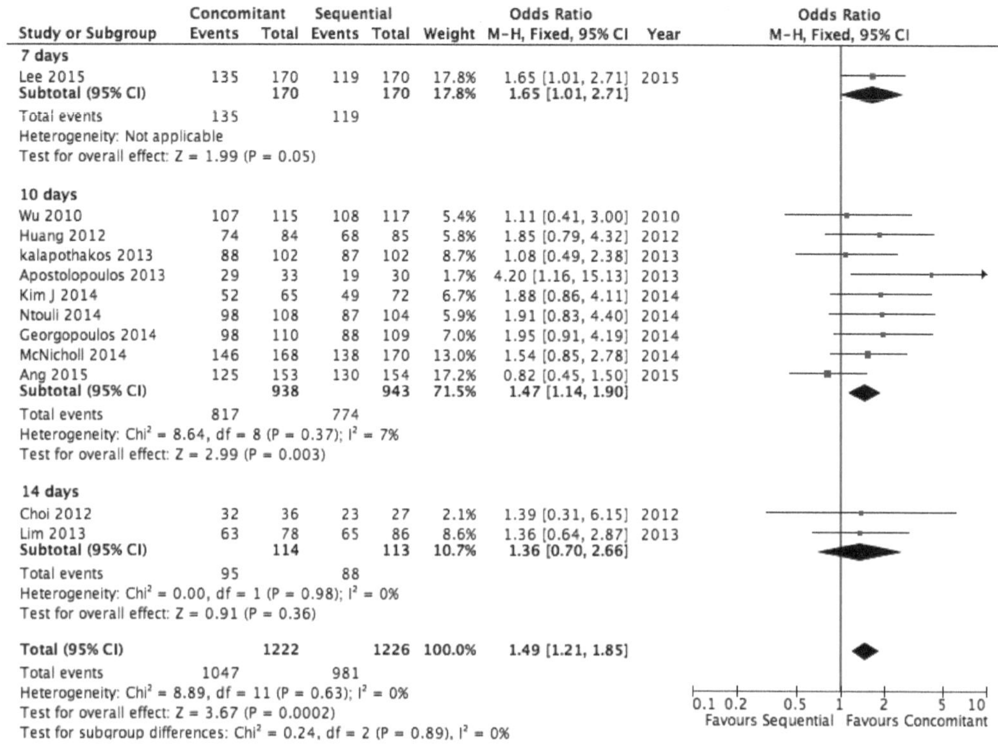

Fig. (3). Meta-analysis comparing the efficacy (intention-to-treat) of the concomitant regimen with that of sequential therapy for the eradication of *H. pylori* infection.

The alleged superiority of concomitant therapy –compared to sequential therapy – may be due to the longer period of time each antibiotic is prescribed (10 days in the concomitant and 5 in the sequential treatments), or the expected lower impact of antibiotic resistance when the 3 antibiotics are administered concurrently, favoring synergistic effects.

EFFECTS OF DIFFERENT VARIABLES ON THE EFFICACY OF CONCOMITANT THERAPY

The eradication rate achieved with the concomitant treatment is affected by multiple factors.

Clarithromycin Resistance

Antimicrobial resistance is largely responsible for the poor eradication rates with standard triple therapy [83 - 85]. One meta-analysis identified an approximate 60% reduction in efficacy with standard triple therapy if strains were clarithromycin resistant [83, 86]. Taking this in consideration, the prescription of standard triple therapies may be acceptable only in regions where the rate of resistance to clarithromycin is below 15-20% [2]. Clarithromycin resistance impacts the success rate of sequential regimen, although not as markedly as in triple therapy [14, 16 - 19, 87 - 89].

The potential benefits of sequential therapy regarding resistance seem to be also applicable to concomitant regimen. The effect of *H. pylori* antibiotic resistance on the efficacy of first-line treatments was determined in an early meta-analysis. The data clearly identified that quadruple combinations (especially those containing both clarithromycin and metronidazole) could cure clarithromycin or metronidazole resistance [85]. That meta-analysis showed that clarithromycin resistance's effect on concomitant regimens was minor, with 95% cure-rate in patients with clarithromycin-sensitive strains, and 96% in resistant [85].

Table **4** summarizes the studies that, up to now, have evaluated the efficacy of clarithromycin resistance on the concomitant regimen [38, 44, 55, 56, 62, 64, 70, 72]. From these data, a mean eradication rate of 83% was calculated in patients with clarithromycin resistant strains. If only studies including in the same protocol both non-bismuth quadruple regimens were considered [44, 55, 72], the eradication rate in patients with clarithromycin-resistant strains was 62% for the sequential treatment and 92% for the concomitant one.

Table 4. Studies evaluating the efficacy of clarithromycin resistance (in patients with metronidazole-susceptible strains) on the concomitant regimen.

Author	Sequential n/N (%)	Concomitant n/N (%)	Treatment Duration (days)
Huang *et al* [44]	3/5 (60%)	3/3 (100%)	10
Georgopoulos *et al* [38]	-	13/15 (85%)	10
Molina-Infante *et al* [55]	3/4 (75%)	5/5 (100%)	10
Molina-Infante *et al* [56]	-	5/5 (100%)	14
Neville *et al* [62]	-	17/20 (85%)	5
Okada *et al* [64]	-	25/27 (93%)	7
Treiber *et al* [70]	-	8/16 (50%)	5
Wu *et al* [72]	4/7 (57%)	3/4 (75%)	10
n - patients cured, N – patients evaluated, % efficacy by ITT.			

Nitroimidazole Resistance

Experience with concomitant therapy in patients with metronidazole-resistant strains is still limited, but seems to be encouraging. Table **5** summarizes the studies that, up to now, have evaluated the efficacy of metronidazole resistance on the concomitant regimen [40, 44, 55, 56, 72]. From these data, a mean eradication rate of 98% was calculated in patients with nitroimidazole resistant strains. If only studies including in the same protocol both non-bismuth quadruple regimens were considered [40, 44, 72], the eradication rate in patients with metronidazole-resistant strains was 82% for the sequential treatment and 97% for the concomitant one.

Table 5. Studies evaluating the efficacy of metronidazole resistance (in patients with clarithromycin-susceptible strains) on the concomitant regimen.

Author	Sequential n/N (%)	Concomitant n/N (%)	Treatment Duration (days)
Georgopoulos *et al* [38]	-	25/25 (100%)	10
Georgopoulos *et al* [40]	21/28 (75%)	21/21 (100%)	10
Huang *et al* [44]	14/18 (78%)	16/16 (100%)	10
Molina-Infante *et al* [55]	-	8/8 (100%)	10
Molina-Infante *et al* [56]	-	8/8 (100%)	14
Wu *et al* [72]	27/30 (90%)	24/26 (92%)	10
n - patients cured, N – patients evaluated, % efficacy by ITT.			

Dual Clarithromycin and Metronidazole Resistance

Table **6** summarizes the studies that, up to now, have evaluated the efficacy of both clarithromycin and metronidazole resistance on the concomitant regimen [38, 40, 44, 55, 56, 64, 70, 72]. From these data, a mean eradication rate of 79% was calculated in patients with dual clarithromycin and nitroimidazole resistant strains. If only studies including in the same protocol both non-bismuth quadruple regimens were considered [40, 44, 55, 72], the eradication rate in patients with both clarithromycin and metronidazole-resistant strains was 47% for the sequential treatment and 79% for the concomitant one. Therefore, sequential regimen does not qualify as a good therapeutic when the prevalence of dual –clarithromycin plus metronidazole– resistant strains is greater than 5% [90]. The lower effect of antibiotic resistance on the eradication rate with concomitant therapy than with sequential therapy may be due to the longer duration of therapy with one or all of the components of the concomitant therapy.

Based on aforementioned data, it may be concluded that the main limitation of concomitant therapy is this dual resistance to metronidazole–clarithromycin [90]. Although isolated clarithromycin or metronidazole resistances by themselves did not significantly impair concomitant therapy, it is expected that dual resistance rates over 15% may cause the efficacy to fall below 90% [91]. Therefore, concomitant therapy may be the recommended therapy of choice in areas and patient groups with low risk of dual resistance, but it cannot be recommended as a first-line empirical regimen in populations expected to have high dual resistance rates (*i.e.* after clarithromycin or metronidazole treatment failures) or in situations when metronidazole resistance reaches 60%, such as China, the Islamic Republic of Iran, India, or Central and South America [91]. As expected from these recommendations, good/excellent reported outcomes have been published in Southern Europe and some Asian countries with relatively low metronidazole resistance regardless of the clarithromycin resistance rate (even at 40% resistance prevalence); and poor results were obtained in areas with high prevalence of clarithromycin or, specially, metronidazole resistances.

Table 6. Studies evaluating the efficacy of dual clarithromycin and metronidazole resistance on the concomitant regimen.

Author	Sequential n/N (%)	Concomitant n/N (%)	Treatment Duration (days)
Georgopoulos *et al* [40]	2/5 (40%)	7/9 (78%)	10
Georgopoulos *et al* [38]	-	7/10 (70%)	10
Huang *et al* [44]	2/4 (50%)	2/2 (100%)	10
Molina-Infante *et al* [55]	3/5 (60%)	3/4 (75%)	10
Molina-Infante *et al* [56]	-	3/3 (100%)	14
Okada *et al* [64]	-	3/4 (75%)	7
Treiber *et al* [70]	-	2/2 (50%)	5
Wu *et al* [72]	1/3 (33%)	3/4 (75%)	10
n - patients cured, N – patients evaluated, % efficacy by ITT.			

In summary, there is clear and abundant evidence pointing towards the superiority of concomitant over sequential therapy, even more in populations expected to have moderate to high dual resistances (>15%).

Duration of Treatment

The first meta-analysis including 9 manuscripts, Essa *et al* [81] identified that concomitant regimen achieved excellent results, even in very short treatment durations. The results of the studies included in Table **1** and in Fig. (**1**) have not been able to show a clear higher eradication results with longer treatments. However, several randomized controlled trials have compared, in the same study and with the same protocol, two different durations of the concomitant therapy, and have demonstrated that the longer duration is more effective, when comparing 3 *vs.* 5 days (81% *vs.* 89% [70], 5 *vs.* 7 days (87% *vs.* 90%) [51], 5 *vs.* 10 days (89% *vs.* 96%) [50], or 5 *vs.* 14 days (78% *vs.* 86%) [36].

HOW COULD WE EVEN INCREASE THE EFFICACY OF THE CONCOMITANT TREATMENT?

It has been pointed out that we should look for "good" or even "excellent" treatments, with eradication rates higher than 90% [93]. A recent study has compared the efficacy and tolerability of the standard and the so called "optimized" concomitant regimen (using new generation PPIs at high doses and longer treatment duration) [54]. Thus, in a prospective multicenter study, *H. pylori*-infected patients were consecutively treated with one of these two treatments: in a first phase, 356 patients received a standard concomitant therapy with omeprazole 20 mg, amoxicillin 1 g, clarithromycin 500 mg and metronidazole 500 mg for 10 days b.i.d.; in a second phase, 471 patients received the same regimen but with esomeprazole 40 mg b.i.d. and lasting 14 days. Compliance with treatment was 94% and 95%, respectively (non-statistically significant differences). Per-protocol eradication rates with standard concomitant and the optimized concomitant treatments were 86% and 93% (p<0.01). Respective intention-to-treat cure rates were 86% and 91% (p<0.01). Adverse effects (mostly mild) were reported in 32% of patients in the standard concomitant group and in 44% in optimized one (p<0.05), the most common being metallic taste, diarrhea, nausea and abdominal pain. Therefore, the authors concluded that an optimized (fourteen-day and high-dose esomeprazole) non-bismuth quadruple concomitant regimen for the eradication of *H. pylori* is more effective than the standard concomitant one, and achieves over 90% cure rate (and also concluded that although the incidence of adverse events is higher with the optimized treatment, these are mostly mild, and do not negatively impact the compliance). However, this study does not allow drawing conclusions regarding what percentage of that improvement is due to the longer regimen or to the high acid inhibition. Different meta-analyses have proved these beneficial effects (separately for each variable) on other anti-*H. pylori* treatments such as triple therapies [12, 94 - 96]; however, only a head to head randomized trial with the different concomitant regimens (*e.g.*, 10 *vs.* 14 days; and standard dose *vs.* high dose PPI) would be able to answer this question.

In another multicenter study −the OPTRICON Study [97], the authors compared the effectiveness and safety of two "optimized" triple and concomitant therapies. This was a prospective study performed in 16 Spanish centers using triple therapy in clinical practice. In a 3-month two-phase fashion, the first 402 patients received an optimized triple therapy [esomeprazole (40 mg b.i.d.), amoxicillin (1 g b.i.d) and clarithromycin (500 mg b.i.d) for 14 days] and the last 375 patients received an optimized concomitant treatment [optimized triple therapy plus metronidazole (500 mg b.i.d)]. The optimized concomitant therapy achieved significantly higher eradication rates in the per protocol (82.3% *vs.* 93.8%; P<0.001) and intention-t--treat analysis (81.3% *vs.* 90.4%; P<0.001]. Adverse events (97.2% mild/moderate) were significantly more common with optimized concomitant therapy (39% *vs.* 47%, P<0.05), but full compliance with therapy was similar between groups. In the multivariate analysis, optimized concomitant therapy was the only significant predictor of successful eradication. Therefore, the authors concluded that empiric optimized concomitant therapy achieves significantly higher cure rates (>90%) compared to optimized triple therapy; and that addition of metronidazole to optimized concomitant therapy increased eradication rates by 10%, resulting in more mild adverse effects, but without impairing compliance with therapy.

WHAT ARE THE RESULTS WITH THE CONCOMITANT TREATMENT IN CLINICAL PRACTICE? THE EXPERIENCE OF THE EUROPEAN REGISTRY ON *H. PYLORI* MANAGEMENT

Aiming to evaluate the results from the clinical practice of European gastroenterologists regarding the management of *H. pylori*, the European Helicobacter Study Group organized a project to register the daily clinical practice of 300 researchers from 30 European Countries: The European Registry on *H. pylori* Management (Hp-EuReg). This project has been ongoing for less than two years but it has already included 10.000 patients, and it is expected to last for 10 years. The results from clinical practice presented during the International Workshop on Helicobacter (Rome, 2014) [98] correlate with the meta-analytical estimation: for example the overall eradication rate estimated for concomitant regimen is 87% while the observed efficacy in the Registry for the standard commonly used concomitant treatment is also 87%, although the coadjuvation with esomeprazole and lengthening the regimen to 14 days is able to increase the efficacy up to 92%.

The Hp-EuReg also includes data on other treatment options such as standard triple therapies, bismuth quadruple and sequential, all of them both in regular and optimized regimens (longer and double dose PPIs). The registry shows a clear superiority of concomitant regimen over standard triple therapies (76%). However, so far it has not been able to obtain statistically significant differences between concomitant, sequential and bismuth quadruple (at identical durations). The discordance with the meta-analytical estimation when comparing concomitant and sequential in the registry may be explained to the fact that many of the sequential prescriptions have used esomeprazole and probiotic coadjuvation, which may have indirectly increased the efficacy of sequential treatment.

The preliminary results presented in Rome in 2014 concluded that the use of standard triple therapies (still the most frequently prescribed) offers sub-optimal results in Europe, and that quadruple therapies achieved higher eradication rates, especially in longer treatment durations and/or with the coadjuvation of esomeprazole.

CONCLUSIONS

Standard triple therapy is still the most widely used treatment in clinical practice in many countries. However, the prevalence of clarithromycin resistance has increased substantially in recent years, and there has been a corresponding decrease in the eradication rate for *H. pylori* infection. Eradication rates are at their lowest levels since a decade ago and are likely to fall further as antimicrobial resistance becomes more prevalent worldwide [92]. It is clear that alternative treatment regimens are urgently needed, particularly for patients with clarithromycin-resistant strains of *H. pylori* [99].

In the present chapter, we have critically reviewed the evidence on the role of non-bismuth quadruple –concomitant– therapy in the treatment of *H. pylori* infection. Our meta-analysis of the 55 studies (including 6,906 patients) that up to now have evaluated the efficacy of the concomitant treatment revealed a mean *H. pylori* cure rate (intention-to-treat) of approximately 90%. In addition, based on the results of several randomized controlled trials comparing concomitant *vs.* standard triple therapy, we have performed a meta-analysis which demonstrates that the first therapy is more effective than the second. Finally, our meta-analysis of randomized controlled trials comparing sequential and concomitant regimens concluded that the concomitant regimen is more effective.

The efficacy of concomitant therapy was not significantly impaired by either clarithromycin or metronidazole isolated resistance, but it is expected to fall below 90% when the prevalence of dual clarithromycin–metronidazole-resistant strains is greater than 15%.

In summary, non-bismuth quadruple concomitant therapy has shown to be an effective, and well-tolerated substitute to standard triple therapy and being more effective and less complex than sequential therapy. Therefore, this regimen has valid use in situations where the efficacy of triple therapy is unacceptably low. In addition, concomitant therapy represents a valid alternative to bismuth quadruple regimen when its implementation is troublesome. Concomitant therapy may be more suitable than sequential therapy for patients with clarithromycin or metronidazole resistance, and mainly with dual resistance. However, the main limitation of concomitant therapy is dual metronidazole–clarithromycin resistance.

CONSENT FOR PUBLICATION

Not applicable.

CONFLICT OF INTEREST

Dr. Gisbert has served as a speaker, a consultant and advisory member for or has received research funding from MSD, Abbvie, Hospira, Pfizer, Kern Pharma, Biogen, Takeda, Janssen, Roche, Sandoz, Celgene, Ferring, Faes Farma, Shire Pharmaceuticals, Dr. Falk Pharma, Tillotts Pharma, Chiesi, Casen Fleet, Gebro Pharma, Otsuka Pharmaceutical, Vifor Pharma, Casen Recordati, Mayoly, Allergan, Advia, Diasorin. Dr. McNicholl has received honoraria for educative actions for Allergan, Takeda, and Mayoly, and is a member of an advisory board for Mayoly.

ACKNOWLEDGEMENTS

Declared none.

REFERENCES

[1]   McColl KE. Clinical practice. *Helicobacter pylori* infection. N Engl J Med 2010; 362(17): 1597-604.
        [http://dx.doi.org/10.1056/NEJMcp1001110] [PMID: 20427808]

[2]   Malfertheiner P, Megraud F, O'Morain C, *et al.* Current concepts in the management of *Helicobacter pylori* infection: the Maastricht III Consensus Report. Gut 2007; 56(6): 772-81.
        [http://dx.doi.org/10.1136/gut.2006.101634] [PMID: 17170018]

[3]   Chey WD, Wong BC. American College of Gastroenterology guideline on the management of *Helicobacter pylori* infection. Am J Gastroenterol 2007; 102(8): 1808-25.
        [http://dx.doi.org/10.1111/j.1572-0241.2007.01393.x] [PMID: 17608775]

[4]   Lam SK, Talley NJ. Report of the 1997 Asia Pacific Consensus Conference on the management of *Helicobacter pylori* infection. J Gastroenterol Hepatol 1998; 13(1): 1-12.
        [http://dx.doi.org/10.1111/j.1440-1746.1998.tb00537.x] [PMID: 9737564]

[5]   Coelho LG, León-Barúa R, Quigley EM. Latin-American Consensus Conference on *Helicobacter pylori* infection. Latin-American National Gastroenterological Societies affiliated with the Inter-American Association of Gastroenterology (AIGE). Am J Gastroenterol 2000; 95(10): 2688-91.
        [http://dx.doi.org/10.1111/j.1572-0241.2000.03174.x] [PMID: 11051336]

[6]   Gisbert JP, Calvet X, Gomollón F, Monés J. Eradication treatment of *Helicobacter pylori*. Recommendations of the II Spanish Consensus Conference. Med Clin (Barc) 2005; 125(8): 301-16.
        [http://dx.doi.org/10.1157/13078424] [PMID: 16159556]

[7]   Graham DY, Lu H, Yamaoka Y. A report card to grade *Helicobacter pylori* therapy. Helicobacter 2007; 12(4): 275-8.
        [http://dx.doi.org/10.1111/j.1523-5378.2007.00518.x] [PMID: 17669098]

[8]   Sasaki M, Ogasawara N, Utsumi K, *et al.* Changes in 12-Year First-Line Eradication Rate of *Helicobacter pylori* Based on Triple Therapy with Proton Pump Inhibitor, Amoxicillin and Clarithromycin. J Clin Biochem Nutr 2010; 47(1): 53-8.
[http://dx.doi.org/10.3164/jcbn.10-10] [PMID: 20664731]

[9]   Janssen MJ, Van Oijen AH, Verbeek AL, Jansen JB, De Boer WA. A systematic comparison of triple therapies for treatment of *Helicobacter pylori* infection with proton pump inhibitor/ ranitidine bismuth citrate plus clarithromycin and either amoxicillin or a nitroimidazole. Aliment Pharmacol Ther 2001; 15(5): 613-24.
[http://dx.doi.org/10.1046/j.1365-2036.2001.00974.x] [PMID: 11328254]

[10]   Laheij RJ, Rossum LG, Jansen JB, Straatman H, Verbeek AL. Evaluation of treatment regimens to cure *Helicobacter pylori* infection--a meta-analysis. Aliment Pharmacol Ther 1999; 13(7): 857-64.
[http://dx.doi.org/10.1046/j.1365-2036.1999.00542.x] [PMID: 10383518]

[11]   Graham DY, Lu H, Yamaoka Y. Therapy for *Helicobacter pylori* infection can be improved: sequential therapy and beyond. Drugs 2008; 68(6): 725-36.
[http://dx.doi.org/10.2165/00003495-200868060-00001] [PMID: 18416582]

[12]   Calvet X, García N, López T, Gisbert JP, Gené E, Roque M. A meta-analysis of short *versus* long therapy with a proton pump inhibitor, clarithromycin and either metronidazole or amoxycillin for treating *Helicobacter pylori* infection. Aliment Pharmacol Ther 2000; 14(5): 603-9.
[http://dx.doi.org/10.1046/j.1365-2036.2000.00744.x] [PMID: 10792124]

[13]   Fuccio L, Minardi ME, Zagari RM, Grilli D, Magrini N, Bazzoli F. Meta-analysis: duration of first-line proton-pump inhibitor based triple therapy for *Helicobacter pylori* eradication. Ann Intern Med 2007; 147(8): 553-62.
[http://dx.doi.org/10.7326/0003-4819-147-8-200710160-00008] [PMID: 17938394]

[14]   Gisbert JP, Calvet X, O'Connor A, Mégraud F, O'Morain CA. Sequential therapy for *Helicobacter pylori* eradication: a critical review. J Clin Gastroenterol 2010; 44(5): 313-25.
[http://dx.doi.org/10.1097/MCG.0b013e3181c8a1a3] [PMID: 20054285]

[15]   Moayyedi P. Sequential regimens for *Helicobacter pylori* eradication. Lancet 2007; 370(9592): 1010-2.
[http://dx.doi.org/10.1016/S0140-6736(07)61455-X] [PMID: 17889226]

[16]   Zullo A, De Francesco V, Hassan C, Morini S, Vaira D. The sequential therapy regimen for *Helicobacter pylori* eradication: a pooled-data analysis. Gut 2007; 56(10): 1353-7.
[http://dx.doi.org/10.1136/gut.2007.125658] [PMID: 17566020]

[17]   Jafri NS, Hornung CA, Howden CW. Meta-analysis: sequential therapy appears superior to standard therapy for *Helicobacter pylori* infection in patients naive to treatment. Ann Intern Med 2008; 148(12): 923-31.
[http://dx.doi.org/10.7326/0003-4819-148-12-200806170-00226] [PMID: 18490667]

[18]   Tong JL, Ran ZH, Shen J, Xiao SD. Sequential therapy *vs.* standard triple therapies for *Helicobacter pylori* infection: a meta-analysis. J Clin Pharm Ther 2009; 34(1): 41-53.
[http://dx.doi.org/10.1111/j.1365-2710.2008.00969.x] [PMID: 19125902]

[19]   Gatta L, Vakil N, Leandro G, Di Mario F, Vaira D. Sequential therapy or triple therapy for *Helicobacter pylori* infection: systematic review and meta-analysis of randomized controlled trials in adults and children. Am J Gastroenterol 2009; 104(12): 3069-79.
[http://dx.doi.org/10.1038/ajg.2009.555] [PMID: 19844205]

[20]   Caselli M, Zullo A, Maconi G, *et al.* "Cervia II Working Group Report 2006": guidelines on diagnosis and treatment of *Helicobacter pylori* infection in Italy. Dig Liver Dis 2007; 39(8): 782-9.
[http://dx.doi.org/10.1016/j.dld.2007.05.016] [PMID: 17606419]

[21]   Nyssen OP, McNicholl AG, Megraud F, *et al.* Meta-Analysis of Sequential *vs.* Standard Triple Therapy for *Helicobacter pylori* Eradication: Final Results of a Cochrane Systematic Review.

Gastroenterology 2014; 146 (Suppl. 5): S-393.
[http://dx.doi.org/10.1016/S0016-5085(14)61413-X]

[22]   Zullo A, De Francesco V, Hassan C. Sequential or concomitant therapy for *Helicobacter pylori*
        eradication? J Clin Gastroenterol 2010; 44(9): 658-9.
        [http://dx.doi.org/10.1097/MCG.0b013e3181d6b543] [PMID: 20308919]

[23]   Vakil N. *Helicobacter pylori* treatment: is sequential or quadruple therapy the answer? Rev
        Gastroenterol Disord 2008; 8(2): 77-82.
        [PMID: 18641590]

[24]   Graham DY, Lu H. Is there a role for sequential in sequential anti-*H. pylori* therapy? Gastroenterology
        2006; 130(6): 1930-1.
        [http://dx.doi.org/10.1053/j.gastro.2006.03.037] [PMID: 16697763]

[25]   Treiber G, Ammon S, Schneider E, Klotz U. Amoxicillin/metronidazole/omeprazole/clarithromycin: a
        new, short quadruple therapy for *Helicobacter pylori* eradication. Helicobacter 1998; 3(1): 54-8.
        [http://dx.doi.org/10.1046/j.1523-5378.1998.08019.x] [PMID: 9546119]

[26]   Okada M, Oki K, Shirotani T, *et al.* A new quadruple therapy for the eradication of *Helicobacter
        pylori*. Effect of pretreatment with omeprazole on the cure rate. J Gastroenterol 1998; 33(5): 640-5.
        [http://dx.doi.org/10.1007/s005350050150] [PMID: 9773927]

[27]   Gisbert JP, Calvet X. Review article: non-bismuth quadruple (concomitant) therapy for eradication of
        Helicobater pylori. Aliment Pharmacol Ther 2011; 34(6): 604-17.
        [http://dx.doi.org/10.1111/j.1365-2036.2011.04770.x] [PMID: 21745241]

[28]   Graham DY, Shiotani A. New concepts of resistance in the treatment of *Helicobacter pylori*
        infections. Nat Clin Pract Gastroenterol Hepatol 2008; 5(6): 321-31.
        [http://dx.doi.org/10.1038/ncpgasthep1138] [PMID: 18446147]

[29]   Apostolopoulos P, Koumoutsos I, Tsibouris P, *et al.* Sequential *vs.* concomitant therapy for the first-
        line *Helicobacter pylori* eradication treatment. UEG Journal 2013; 1(1S): A423.

[30]   Calvet X, Titó L, Comet R, García N, Campo R, Brullet E. Four-day, twice daily, quadruple therapy
        with amoxicillin, clarithromycin, tinidazole and omeprazole to cure *Helicobacter pylori* infection: a
        pilot study. Helicobacter 2000; 5(1): 52-6.
        [http://dx.doi.org/10.1046/j.1523-5378.2000.00007.x] [PMID: 10672052]

[31]   Catalano F, Branciforte G, Catanzaro R, Cipolla R, Bentivegna C, Brogna A. *Helicobacter pylori*-
        positive duodenal ulcer: three-day antibiotic eradication regimen. Aliment Pharmacol Ther 2000;
        14(10): 1329-34.
        [http://dx.doi.org/10.1046/j.1365-2036.2000.00839.x] [PMID: 11012478]

[32]   Chan KL, Zhou H, Ng DK, Tam PK. A prospective study of a one-week nonbismuth quadruple
        therapy for childhood *Helicobacter pylori* infection. J Pediatr Surg 2001; 36(7): 1008-11.
        [http://dx.doi.org/10.1053/jpsu.2001.24726] [PMID: 11431766]

[33]   Cheung D, Kim H, Seo J, *et al.* The comparison of Helicobacter eradication rates of three regimens:
        concomitant therapy *vs.* sequential therapy *vs.* standard triple therapy. Helicobacter 2014; 19(suppl. 1):
        P11.29.

[34]   Choi C, Lee D, Chon I, *et al.* Concomitant therapy was more effective than ppi-base triple therapy in
        Korea: a preliminary report. Helicobacter 2011; 16(suppl. 1).

[35]   Chung J, Chung J, Kim K, *et al.* Ten-days concomitant therapy is superior to sequential therapy for
        Helicobacter pylori eradication. Helicobacter 2014; 19(suppl. 1): P11.30.

[36]   De Francesco V, Hassan C, Ridola L, Giorgio F, Ierardi E, Zullo A. Sequential, concomitant and
        hybrid first-line therapies for *Helicobacter pylori* eradication: a prospective randomized study. J Med
        Microbiol 2014; 63(Pt 5): 748-52.
        [http://dx.doi.org/10.1099/jmm.0.072322-0] [PMID: 24586031]

[37]   Georgopoulos S, Papastergiou V, Xirouchakis E, *et al.* Evaluation of a four-drug, three-antibiotic, nonbismuth-containing "concomitant" therapy as first-line *Helicobacter pylori* eradication regimen in Greece. Helicobacter 2012; 17(1): 49-53.
[http://dx.doi.org/10.1111/j.1523-5378.2011.00911.x] [PMID: 22221616]

[38]   Georgopoulos SD, Xirouchakis E, Martinez-Gonzalez B, *et al.* Clinical evaluation of a ten-day regimen with esomeprazole, metronidazole, amoxicillin, and clarithromycin for the eradication of *Helicobacter pylori* in a high clarithromycin resistance area. Helicobacter 2013; 18(6): 459-67.
[http://dx.doi.org/10.1111/hel.12062] [PMID: 23714140]

[39]   Georgopoulos S, Papastergiou V, Xirouchakis E, *et al.* Nonbismuth quadruple "concomitant" therapy *versus* standard triple therapy, both of the duration of 10 days, for first-line *H. pylori* eradication: a randomized trial. J Clin Gastroenterol 2013; 47(3): 228-32.
[http://dx.doi.org/10.1097/MCG.0b013e31826015b0] [PMID: 22858517]

[40]   Georgopoulos SD, Xirouchakis E, Zampeli E, *et al.* A randomised study comparing 10 days concomitant and sequential treatments for the eradication of *Helicobacter pylori*, in a high clarithromycin resistance area. Helicobacter 2014; 19(suppl.1): W2.4.
[http://dx.doi.org/10.1016/S0016-5085(14)61432-3]

[41]   Greenberg ER, Anderson GL, Morgan DR, *et al.* 14-day triple, 5-day concomitant, and 10-day sequential therapies for *Helicobacter pylori* infection in seven Latin American sites: a randomised trial. Lancet 2011; 378(9790): 507-14.
[http://dx.doi.org/10.1016/S0140-6736(11)60825-8] [PMID: 21777974]

[42]   Heo J, Jeon S, Cho C, *et al.* Randomised, Multicenter Clinical Trial: Comparison of 10-Day Standard Triple Therapy and Non-Bismuth-Containing Concomitant Therapy for *Helicobacter pylori* Infection in Korea (Interim Result). Gastroenterology 2014; 146(supl.1).

[43]   Heo J, Jeon S, Lee L, *et al.* Randomized clinical trial: Comparison of concomitant therapy with hybrid therapy for *Helicobacter pylori* eradication. Helicobacter 2014; 19(suppl. 1): P13.03.

[44]   Huang YK, Wu MC, Wang SS, *et al.* Lansoprazole-based sequential and concomitant therapy for the first-line *Helicobacter pylori* eradication. J Dig Dis 2012; 13(4): 232-8.
[http://dx.doi.org/10.1111/j.1751-2980.2012.00575.x] [PMID: 22435509]

[45]   Kalapothakos P, Georgakila E, Georgantas P, Bizanias M, Spiliades C. Initial empirical treatment for *Helicobacter pylori* eradicaton in routine clinical practice. Non bismuth sequential or concomitant regimen? A preliminary prospective comparative study in Sparta Greece. UEG Journal 2013; 1(1S): A272.

[46]   Kao SS, Chen WC, Hsu PI, *et al.* 7-Day Nonbismuth-Containing Concomitant Therapy Achieves a High Eradication Rate for *Helicobacter pylori* in Taiwan. Gastroenterol Res Pract 2012; 2012: 463985.
[http://dx.doi.org/10.1155/2012/463985] [PMID: 22888337]

[47]   Kim SY, Lee SW, Hyun JJ, *et al.* Comparative study of *Helicobacter pylori* eradication rates with 5-day quadruple "concomitant" therapy and 7-day standard triple therapy. J Clin Gastroenterol 2013; 47(1): 21-4.
[http://dx.doi.org/10.1097/MCG.0b013e3182548ad4] [PMID: 22647826]

[48]   Kim J, Kim J, Kim B, *et al.* Triple therapy, sequential therapy, and concomitant therapy for *Helicobacter pylori* infection in Korea: a multicenter, randomized controlled trial. Helicobacter 2014; 19(suppl. 1): W2.6.

[49]   Kim SY, Lee J, Chung SY, *et al. Helicobacter pylori* Eradication Rates with 10-day Non-bismuth Quadruple Therapy and 10-day Sequential Therapy in Korea. Helicobacter 2014; 19(suppl. 1): P11.10.

[50]   Kongchayanun C, Vilaichone RK, Pornthisarn B, Amornsawadwattana S, Mahachai V. Pilot studies to identify the optimum duration of concomitant *Helicobacter pylori* eradication therapy in Thailand. Helicobacter 2012; 17(4): 282-5.

[http://dx.doi.org/10.1111/j.1523-5378.2012.00953.x] [PMID: 22759328]

[51]　Kwon BS, Park EB, Lee DH, *et al.* Effectiveness of 5-day and 7 day quadruple "concomitant" therapy regimen for *Helicobacter pylori* infection in Korea. Helicobacter 2011; 16 (Suppl. 1): 135.

[52]　Lim JH, Lee DH, Choi C, *et al.* Clinical outcomes of two-week sequential and concomitant therapies for *Helicobacter pylori* eradication: a randomized pilot study. Helicobacter 2013; 18(3): 180-6.
　　　[http://dx.doi.org/10.1111/hel.12034] [PMID: 23305083]

[53]　McNicholl AG, Marin AC, Molina-Infante J, *et al.* Randomised clinical trial comparing sequential and concomitant therapies for *Helicobacter pylori* eradication in routine clinical practice. Gut 2014; 63(2): 244-9.
　　　[http://dx.doi.org/10.1136/gutjnl-2013-304820] [PMID: 23665990]

[54]　McNicholl A, Molina-Infante J, Bermejo F, *et al.* Non-bismuth quadruple concomitant therapies in the eradication of *Helicobacter pylori*: standard *vs.* optimized (14 days, high-dose PPI) regimens in clinical practice. Helicobacter 2014; 19(suppl. 1): P11.11.

[55]　Molina-Infante J, Pazos-Pacheco C, Vinagre-Rodriguez G, *et al.* Nonbismuth quadruple (concomitant) therapy: empirical and tailored efficacy *versus* standard triple therapy for clarithromycin-susceptible *Helicobacter pylori* and *versus* sequential therapy for clarithromycin-resistant strains. Helicobacter 2012; 17(4): 269-76.
　　　[http://dx.doi.org/10.1111/j.1523-5378.2012.00947.x] [PMID: 22759326]

[56]　Molina-Infante J, Romano M, Fernandez-Bermejo M, *et al.* Optimized nonbismuth quadruple therapies cure most patients with *Helicobacter pylori* infection in populations with high rates of antibiotic resistance. Gastroenterology 2013; 145: 121-128 e1.
　　　[http://dx.doi.org/10.1053/j.gastro.2013.03.050]

[57]　Molina-Infante J, Lucendo AJ, Angueira T, *et al.* Optimized empiric triple and concomitant therapy for *Helicobacter pylori* eradication in clinical practice: the OPTRICON study. Helicobacter 2014; 19(suppl. 1): P11.13.

[58]　Moon B, Lim H, Lee S, Han K, Chung J, Lee Y. Efficacy of concomitant nonbithmuth-based quadruple therapy as first-line treatment for eradication of *Helicobacter pylori*. Helicobacter 2011; 16 (Suppl. 1): 131.

[59]　Moon BS. Comparison of the efficacy of 10 day-triple therapy-based, bismuth-containing quadruple therapy with sequential therapy and concomitant therapy of *Helicobacter pylori*. Helicobacter 2014; 19 (Suppl. 1): P11.17.

[60]　Nagahara A, Miwa H, Ogawa K, *et al.* Addition of metronidazole to rabeprazole-amoxicilli--clarithromycin regimen for *Helicobacter pylori* infection provides an excellent cure rate with five-day therapy. Helicobacter 2000; 5(2): 88-93.
　　　[http://dx.doi.org/10.1046/j.1523-5378.2000.00013.x] [PMID: 10849057]

[61]　Nagahara A, Miwa H, Yamada T, Kurosawa A, Ohkura R, Sato N. Five-day proton pump inhibitor-based quadruple therapy regimen is more effective than 7-day triple therapy regimen for *Helicobacter pylori* infection. Aliment Pharmacol Ther 2001; 15(3): 417-21.
　　　[http://dx.doi.org/10.1046/j.1365-2036.2001.00929.x] [PMID: 11207518]

[62]　Neville PM, Everett S, Langworthy H, *et al.* The optimal antibiotic combination in a 5-day *Helicobacter pylori* eradication regimen. Aliment Pharmacol Ther 1999; 13(4): 497-501.
　　　[http://dx.doi.org/10.1046/j.1365-2036.1999.00493.x] [PMID: 10215734]

[63]　Ntouli V, Vrakas S, Charalampopoulos S, *et al.* Sequential *versus* concomitant treatment against H.Pylori study in a Greek Population. Helicobacter 2014; 19(suppl. 1): P11.22.

[64]　Okada M, Nishimura H, Kawashima M, *et al.* A new quadruple therapy for *Helicobacter pylori*: influence of resistant strains on treatment outcome. Aliment Pharmacol Ther 1999; 13(6): 769-74.
　　　[http://dx.doi.org/10.1046/j.1365-2036.1999.00551.x] [PMID: 10383506]

[65]　Seo J, Cheung D, Kim S, Kim J, Park S. Comparison of *Helicobacter pylori* eradication rate among

concomitant, tailored, and sequential therapy. Helicobacter 2014; 19(suppl. 1): P11.32.

[66]   Sharara AI, Sarkis FS, El-Halabi MM, *et al.* Challenging the dogma: a randomized trial of standard *vs.* half-dose concomitant nonbismuth quadruple therapy for *Helicobacter pylori* infection. United European Gastroenterol J 2014; 2(3): 179-88.
       [http://dx.doi.org/10.1177/2050640614530919] [PMID: 25360301]

[67]   Song M, Leong Ang T, Ming Fock K. An Update: A Randomized Controlled Trial of Triple Therapy *Versus* Sequential Therapy *Versus* Concomitant Therapy As First Line Treatment for *H. pylori* Infection in Singapore. Gastroenterology 2014; 146 (Suppl. 1): S-104-5.
       [http://dx.doi.org/10.1016/S0016-5085(14)60376-0]

[68]   Tepes B, Vujasinovič M, Šeruga M, Stefanovič M, Forte A, Jeverica S. Triple, sequential and concomitant treatment of *Helicobacter pylori* infection -prospective randomized study. Helicobacter 2014; 19(suppl. 1): P11.20.

[69]   Toros AB, Ince AT, Kesici B, Saglam M, Polat Z, Uygun A. A new modified concomitant therapy for *Helicobacter pylori* eradication in Turkey. Helicobacter 2011; 16(3): 225-8.
       [http://dx.doi.org/10.1111/j.1523-5378.2011.00823.x] [PMID: 21585608]

[70]   Treiber G, Wittig J, Ammon S, Walker S, van Doorn LJ, Klotz U. Clinical outcome and influencing factors of a new short-term quadruple therapy for *Helicobacter pylori* eradication: a randomized controlled trial (MACLOR study). Arch Intern Med 2002; 162(2): 153-60.
       [http://dx.doi.org/10.1001/archinte.162.2.153] [PMID: 11802748]

[71]   Wang S, Wang W, Chu Y, Teng G, Hu F. Non-bismuth quadruple therapy *versus* standard triple therapy for *Helicobacter pylori* eradication: a randomized controlled study. Zhonghua Yi Xue Za Zhi 2014; 94(8): 576-9.
       [PMID: 24762684]

[72]   Wu DC, Hsu PI, Wu JY, *et al.* Sequential and concomitant therapy with four drugs is equally effective for eradication of *H pylori* infection. Clin Gastroenterol Hepatol 2010; 8(1): 36-41.e1.
       [http://dx.doi.org/10.1016/j.cgh.2009.09.030] [PMID: 19804842]

[73]   Yanai A, Sakamoto K, Akanuma M, Ogura K, Maeda S. Non-bismuth quadruple therapy for first-line *Helicobacter pylori* eradication: A randomized study in Japan. World J Gastrointest Pharmacol Ther 2012; 3(1): 1-6.
       [http://dx.doi.org/10.4292/wjgpt.v3.i1.1] [PMID: 22408744]

[74]   Zullo A, Scaccianoce G, De Francesco V, *et al.* Concomitant, sequential, and hybrid therapy for *H. pylori* eradication: a pilot study. Clin Res Hepatol Gastroenterol 2013; 37(6): 647-50.
       [http://dx.doi.org/10.1016/j.clinre.2013.04.003] [PMID: 23747131]

[75]   Lee HJ, Kim JI, Lee JS, *et al.* Concomitant therapy achieved the best eradication rate for *Helicobacter pylori* among various treatment strategies. World J Gastroenterol 2015; 21(1): 351-9.
       [http://dx.doi.org/10.3748/wjg.v21.i1.351] [PMID: 25574111]

[76]   Hsu PI, Wu DC, Chen WC, *et al.* Randomized controlled trial comparing 7-day triple, 10-day sequential, and 7-day concomitant therapies for *Helicobacter pylori* infection. Antimicrob Agents Chemother 2014; 58(10): 5936-42.
       [http://dx.doi.org/10.1128/AAC.02922-14] [PMID: 25070099]

[77]   Heo J, Jeon SW, Jung JT, *et al.* A randomised clinical trial of 10-day concomitant therapy and standard triple therapy for *Helicobacter pylori* eradication. Dig Liver Dis 2014; 46(11): 980-4.
       [http://dx.doi.org/10.1016/j.dld.2014.07.018] [PMID: 25132282]

[78]   Kim SY, Park DK, Kwon KA, Kim KO, Kim YJ, Chung JW. Ten day concomitant therapy is superior to ten day sequential therapy for *Helicobacter pylori* eradication. Korean J Gastroenterol 2014; 64(5): 260-7.
       [http://dx.doi.org/10.4166/kjg.2014.64.5.260] [PMID: 25420735]

[79]   Choi C, Lee D, Chon I, Park H. The two weeks sequential therapy and the concomitant therapy for

Helicobacter pylori eradication were effective as a first line therapy in Korea: A preliminary report Digestive Disease Week; 2012: Gastroenterology. 2012. p. S-740 AGa.
[http://dx.doi.org/10.1016/S0016-5085(12)62872-8]

[80]   Ang TL, Fock KM, Song M, *et al.* Ten-day triple therapy *versus* sequential therapy *versus* concomitant therapy as first-line treatment for *Helicobacter pylori* infection. J Gastroenterol Hepatol 2015; 30(7): 1134-9.
[http://dx.doi.org/10.1111/jgh.12892] [PMID: 25639278]

[81]   Essa AS, Kramer JR, Graham DY, Treiber G. Meta-analysis: four-drug, three-antibiotic, non-bismut--containing "concomitant therapy" *versus* triple therapy for *Helicobacter pylori* eradication. Helicobacter 2009; 14(2): 109-18.
[http://dx.doi.org/10.1111/j.1523-5378.2009.00671.x] [PMID: 19298338]

[82]   de Boer WA, Kuipers EJ, Kusters JG. Sequential therapy; a new treatment for *Helicobacter pylori* infection. But is it ready for general use? Dig Liver Dis 2004; 36(5): 311-4.
[http://dx.doi.org/10.1016/j.dld.2004.01.016] [PMID: 15191198]

[83]   Mégraud F. *H pylori* antibiotic resistance: prevalence, importance, and advances in testing. Gut 2004; 53(9): 1374-84.
[http://dx.doi.org/10.1136/gut.2003.022111] [PMID: 15306603]

[84]   Megraud F. *Helicobacter pylori* and antibiotic resistance. Gut 2007; 56(11): 1502.
[http://dx.doi.org/10.1136/gut.2007.132514] [PMID: 17938430]

[85]   Fischbach L, Evans EL. Meta-analysis: the effect of antibiotic resistance status on the efficacy of triple and quadruple first-line therapies for *Helicobacter pylori*. Aliment Pharmacol Ther 2007; 26(3): 343-57.
[http://dx.doi.org/10.1111/j.1365-2036.2007.03386.x] [PMID: 17635369]

[86]   Houben MH, van de Beek D, Hensen EF, de Craen AJ, Rauws EA, Tytgat GN. A systematic review of *Helicobacter pylori* eradication therapy--the impact of antimicrobial resistance on eradication rates. Aliment Pharmacol Ther 1999; 13(8): 1047-55.
[http://dx.doi.org/10.1046/j.1365-2036.1999.00555.x] [PMID: 10468680]

[87]   Zullo A, Vaira D, Vakil N, *et al.* High eradication rates of *Helicobacter pylori* with a new sequential treatment. Aliment Pharmacol Ther 2003; 17(5): 719-26.
[http://dx.doi.org/10.1046/j.1365-2036.2003.01461.x] [PMID: 12641522]

[88]   Vaira D, Zullo A, Vakil N, *et al.* Sequential therapy *versus* standard triple-drug therapy for *Helicobacter pylori* eradication: a randomized trial. Ann Intern Med 2007; 146(8): 556-63.
[http://dx.doi.org/10.7326/0003-4819-146-8-200704170-00006] [PMID: 17438314]

[89]   Gatta L, Vakil N, Vaira D, Scarpignato C. Global eradication rates for *Helicobacter pylori* infection: systematic review and meta-analysis of sequential therapy. BMJ 2013; 347: f4587.
[http://dx.doi.org/10.1136/bmj.f4587] [PMID: 23926315]

[90]   Molina-Infante J, Gisbert JP. Optimizing clarithromycin-containing therapy for *Helicobacter pylori* in the era of antibiotic resistance. World J Gastroenterol 2014; 20(30): 10338-47.
[http://dx.doi.org/10.3748/wjg.v20.i30.10338] [PMID: 25132750]

[91]   Graham DY, Lee YC, Wu MS. Rational *Helicobacter pylori* therapy: evidence-based medicine rather than medicine-based evidence. Clin Gastroenterol Hepatol 2014; 12: 17-86. e3; Discussion e12-3
[http://dx.doi.org/10.1016/j.cgh.2013.05.028]

[92]   Vakil N. *H. pylori* treatment: new wine in old bottles? Am J Gastroenterol 2009; 104(1): 26-30.
[http://dx.doi.org/10.1038/ajg.2008.91] [PMID: 19098845]

[93]   Graham DY. Efficient identification and evaluation of effective *Helicobacter pylori* therapies. Clin Gastroenterol Hepatol 2009; 7(2): 145-8.
[http://dx.doi.org/10.1016/j.cgh.2008.10.024] [PMID: 19026766]

[94]   McNicholl AG, Linares PM, Nyssen OP, Calvet X, Gisbert JP. Meta-analysis: esomeprazole or

rabeprazole *vs.* first-generation pump inhibitors in the treatment of *Helicobacter pylori* infection. Aliment Pharmacol Ther 2012; 36(5): 414-25.
[http://dx.doi.org/10.1111/j.1365-2036.2012.05211.x] [PMID: 22803691]

[95]   Villoria A, Garcia P, Calvet X, Gisbert JP, Vergara M. Meta-analysis: high-dose proton pump inhibitors *vs.* standard dose in triple therapy for *Helicobacter pylori* eradication. Aliment Pharmacol Ther 2008; 28(7): 868-77.
[PMID: 18644011]

[96]   Hsu PI, Wu DC, Wu JY, Graham DY. Is there a benefit to extending the duration of *Helicobacter pylori* sequential therapy to 14 days? Helicobacter 2011; 16(2): 146-52.
[http://dx.doi.org/10.1111/j.1523-5378.2011.00829.x] [PMID: 21435093]

[97]   Molina-Infante J, Lucendo AJ, Angueira T, *et al.* Optimized empiric triple and concomitant therapy for *Helicobacter pylori* eradication in clinical practice: the OPTRICON study. Aliment Pharmacol Ther 2015; 41(6): 581-9.

[98]   McNicholl AG, Gasbarrini A, Tepes B, *et al.* Pan-European Registry on *H. pylori* Management (Hp-EuReg): Interim Analysis of 5,792 Patients. Helicobacter. 2014; p. 69.

[99]   Gisbert JP. Rescue therapy after *Helicobacter pylori* eradication failure. Gastroenterol Hepatol 2011; 34(2): 89-99.
[http://dx.doi.org/10.1016/j.gastrohep.2010.10.013] [PMID: 21371619]

CHAPTER 2

Drug Discovery Strategies Against Emerging Coronaviruses: A Global Threat

Paulo Fernando da Silva Santos-Júnior[1], Igor José dos Santos Nascimento[1], Thiago Mendonça de Aquino[1], João Xavier de Araújo-Júnior[2] and Edeildo Ferreira da Silva-Júnior[1,2,*]

[1] *Chemistry and Biotechnology Institute, Federal University of Alagoas, Maceió, Brazil*

[2] *Laboratory of Medicinal Chemistry, Pharmaceutical Sciences Institute, Federal University of Alagoas, Maceió, Brazil*

Abstract: After the discovery of the infectious bronchitis virus (IBV) in 1932, *Coronaviridae* emerged as a family of viruses constituted of a positive-sense single-stranded RNA ((+)ssRNA) genome. Recently, the Coronavirus disease-2019 (COVID-19), which is caused by a new virus called SARS-CoV-2 (provisionally titled 2019-nCoV), was declared pandemic since it reached global levels of infection. In comparison, this disease spread globally more quickly than previously reported SARS- and MERS-CoV outbreaks. The impacts on global health systems (as well as the world economy, estimated to cost US\$ 1 trillion) highlighted the urgent need to search for efficient pharmacotherapy targeting potential macromolecules from SARS-CoV-2 since there are no licensed vaccines or approved drugs until today. In this chapter, we will demonstrate all strategies that have been used to discover and design bioactive molecules against this viral infection, compiling from classical to computer-aided drug design, including also the drug repurposing. This last, it is based on analogs produced for past outbreaks related to SARS- and MERS-CoV. Finally, we aim to provide valuable information that could be applied for designing new safe, low cost, and selective lead-compounds against these emerging viruses.

Keywords: Coronaviruses, Drug Design, MERS-CoV, SARS-CoV, SARS-CoV-2, HCoV.

INTRODUCTION

Coronaviridae term refers to the viruses family known as Coronavirus (CoV), which is potentially contagious to humans and causes severe infection in the res-

* **Corresponding author Edeildo Ferreira da Silva-Júnior:** Chemistry and Biotechnology Institute, Federal University of Alagoas, Maceió, Brazil; Tel: (+55)-87-9-9610-8311; E-mail: edeildo.junior@esenfar.ufal.br

piratory tract [1, 2]. Previously, CoV was responsible for the MERS-CoV outbreak in the Arabian Peninsula, with 2,123 cases and 740 deaths, leading to a high fatality rate of 35%. Furthermore, between the 2002-2003 SARS-CoV outbreaks in Guangdong province (China) infected 8,500 people, causing 800 deaths [3, 4].

On March 11th, 2020, WHO declared the so-called new Coronavirus (SARS-CoV-2) as a pandemic virus [5], in which it was first reported on December 8th, 2019, in Wuhan, Hubei, China. SARS-CoV-2 is an emerging and severe respiratory infection that causes severe pneumonia. Nowadays, more than 1,8 million individuals have been affected by 215 territories, leading to more than 116,000 deaths. Among these, 3,341 deaths were reported only in China [6 - 9].

The economic impact has reached global and catastrophic proportions, considering that China's production represents about 17% of the world. By comparison, in the past SARS 2003 outbreak, Chinese production represented 4% of the world [10]. Besides, the fact that China is the largest manufacturer and importer of crude oil, has led economists to reduce the annual expectation of global growth [11, 12].

Recently, several works have compiled targets and drugs with activity against Human-Coronaviruses (HCoV) to provide promising alternative treatments, such as potential vaccines, peptides, monoclonal antibodies, and small-molecules [13 - 15]. Also, the publication of the first crystal structure of the main protease (3CL^{pro}, also named as 3C or M^{pro}) from SARS-CoV-2 obtained by X-ray crystallography (PDB ID: 6LU7, ref [16].) will potentially contribute for developing selective inhibitors against this viral target.

Despite considerable recent advances, there are no approved treatments or selective antiviral agents against HCoV, even after the first global 2002 SARS outbreak [17, 18]. Thus, current therapy includes supplemental oxygen and maintenance of body fluids. Moreover, hygienic precautions and mask utilization can reduce the risks of virus transmission [19 - 21].

Considering that a new therapy may take months or even years to become available, this chapter summarizes the methods and strategies used for discovering active molecules targeting SARS-CoV, MERS-CoV, and SARS-CoV-2. In this context, we aim to demonstrate the targets studied and the most active compounds, whether from synthetic or natural sources, to contribute to developing novel antiviral drugs that could be more selective and effective, reducing costs and time in the drug-race against this emerging global threat.

BIOLOGICAL ASPECTS, SIGNS/SYMPTOMS AND DIAGNOSIS FOR MERS-COV, SARS-COV, AND SARS-COV-2

Coronaviruses are known to cause severe respiratory, enteric, as well as systemic infection, which can affect humans, swine, camels, horses, cats, rodents, dogs, bats, among several other hosts, facilitating the global spread [22, 23].

Similarly, SARS-CoV, MERS-CoV, and SARS-CoV-2 encode structural proteins, such as spike glycoproteins (S protein), membrane (M protein), nucleocapsid (N protein), and envelope (E protein) proteins. Additionally, non-structural proteins, such as RNA-dependent RNA polymerase (RdRp), 3-chymotrypsin-like protease (3CL^{pro}), helicase (Hel), and papain-like protease (PL^{pro}) are promising targets for bioactive molecules that could lead to the development of an unprecedented drug against these severe infections (Fig. **1**) [24, 25].

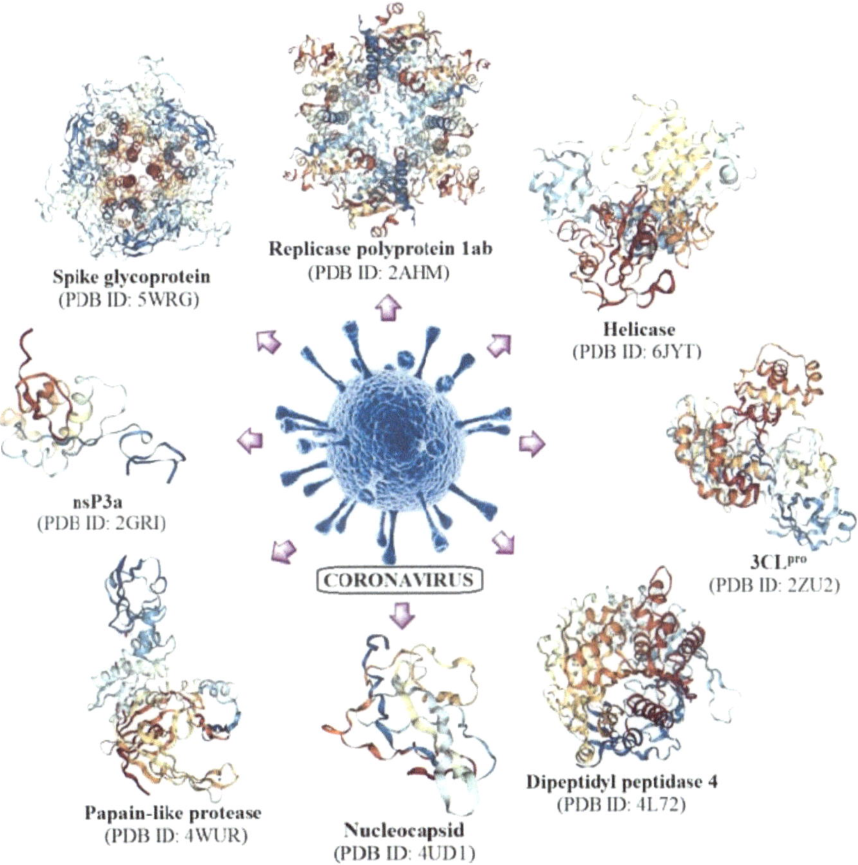

Fig. (1). Potential drug targets from Coronavirus.

Normally, in infected individuals with CoV are observed fever, dry cough, and tiredness, as clinical symptoms. In some cases, body pain, diarrhea or sore throat, runny nose, and nasal congestion can also be observed in patients [26 - 28].

However, it is important to realize that the clinical fever aspect can be differentiated between HCoV infections, being mild to moderate for SARS-Co--2, high for SARS-CoV and finally higher for MERS-CoV infections [29, 30]. Furthermore, infected patients by HCoV show similar incubation periods, such as 3-6 days for SARS-CoV-2, and 5 days for SARS-CoV and MERS-CoV [12, 31].

In general, bats act as natural hosts for CoV, in which the SARS-CoV comes from bats belonging to the *Hipposideridae* family [32]. Among infected humans, the transmission occurs through contact with droplets by sneezing or coughing, even in patients who are asymptomatic [27, 33]. In this context, contact with hands, mouth, and nose of infected individuals, as well as the habit of do not frequently wash hands facilitates HCoV dissemination, characterizing a crucial point for preventing these emerging infections [34, 35].

The diagnosis of SARS-CoV-2 is based on the patient's history, identifying previous HCoV and clinical infections on it, to verify if the patient presents persistent fever and cough, as well as if this patient resides or has been in endemic locations. Laboratory tests will be required, these include CT-scan, C-reactive protein, lactate dehydrogenase, ELISA, and creatinine have been also employed to confirm infection cases [12, 36]. However, nucleic acid detection using real-time quantitative polymerase chain reaction (RT-qPCR) and high-throughput sequencing of the viral genome have proved to be very effective, direct and low-cost methods for HCoV detection [37, 38]. Finally, hemoculture (although the virus isolation has not been recommended by the CDC, ref [39].) and high-throughput sequencing have been considered as official methods for HCoV diagnosis today [40, 41].

STRATEGIES USED FOR DISCOVERING NEW POTENTIAL DRUGS

Natural Source

Traditional Chinese herbs have been used for over 2000 years for various types of diseases, especially against viral infections such as HIV, Ebola virus (EBOV), and Coronaviruses [42 - 44], demonstrating recognized structural diversity and effectiveness in discovering active natural products [45]. From this perspective, one of the first studies associated with the activity of natural products against Coronaviruses was reported by Cinati and coworkers [46], shortly after the 2002-2003 SARS-CoV outbreak, where the authors demonstrated that the isolated natural product Glycyrrhizin **(1)**, a triterpenoid saponin glycoside from *Glycyrrhiza uralensis* (Liquorice) exhibited a promising antiviral activity (Fig. **2**). The authors analyzed its anti-SARS-CoV activity against a strain isolated from patients of the Clinical Center at the Frankfurt University (Germany), obtaining an EC_{50} value of 300 mg/L. Also, the compound **(1)** also presented good safety, exhibiting cellular toxicity over 20000 mg/L concentration. Finally, the authors were not able to completely elucidate its mechanism of action, although it was verified that the compound **(1)** induces nitrous oxide synthase (NOSs), inhibiting the viral replication in host cells.

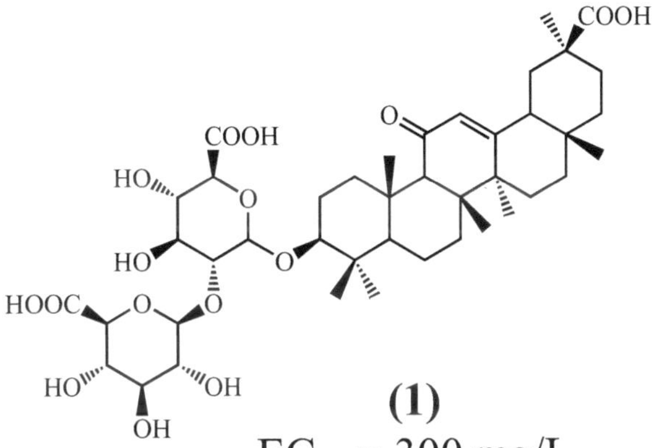

$$\textbf{(1)}$$
$$EC_{50} = 300 \text{ mg/L}$$
$$CC_{50} > 20000 \text{ mg/L}$$

Fig. (2). Glycyrrhizin extracted from *Glycyrrhiza urolensis* (Liquorice).

Posteriorly, Chen and colleagues (2004) that the isolated the natural product Baicalin **(2)** (Fig. **3**) obtained from a traditional Chinese medicinal herb, *Scutellaria baicalensis* (Huang Qin) [47]. This flavone glycoside represents a potential anti-SARS-CoV agent, with EC_{50} and CC_{50} values of 12.5 and > 100 µg/mL, respectively. Baicalin is normally used as 1500 mg tablets, in which these have an approximated half-life of 3 hours, in humans. However, the authors recommended a dose of 600 mg.

Performing a prospective study for an antiviral natural-derived from Chinese herbs, Li and collaborators (2005) selected different 200 extracts with reported SARS-CoV activity, using the virus-induced cytopathic effect (CPE) assay [48]. Thus, only ethanol extracts from *Lycoris radiata, Artemisia annua, Lindera aggregate,* and the chloroform extract from *Pyrrosia lingua* showed antiviral activity, with EC_{50} values ranging from 2.4 to 88.2 µg/mL (Table **1**). Besides, these extracts only exhibited cytotoxic effects in high concentrations toward host cells, ranging from 886.6 to 1374 µg/mL.

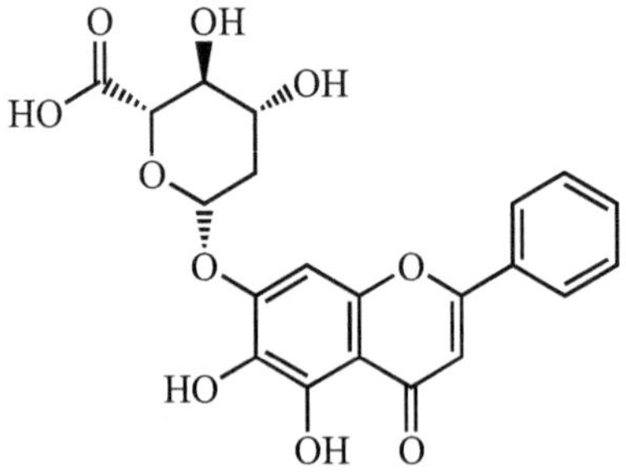

(2)

$$EC_{50} = 12.5 \ \mu g/mL$$
$$CC_{50} > 100 \ \mu g/mL$$

Fig. (3). Baicalin extracted from *Scutellaria baicalensis* (Huang Qin).

Table 1. Extracts screened against SARS-CoV by Li *et al.*, 2005.

Plant Extract	*Family*	*Part Used*	$CC_{50} \pm SD^a$	$EC_{50} - (BJ\text{-}001\ Viral\ Strain)$ $\pm SD^a$	SI^b
Lycoris radiata	*Amaryllis*	Stem cortex	886.6 ± 35	2.4 ± 0.2	370
Artemisia annua	*Compositae*	Whole plant	1053.0 ± 92.8	34.5 ± 2.6	31
Pyrrosia lingua	*Polypodiaceae*	Leaves	2378.0 ± 87.3	43.2 ± 14.1	55
Lindera aggregate	*Lauraceae*	Root	1374.0 ± 39	88.2 ± 7.7	16
Interferon alpha			$>100,000 \pm 710.1$	660.3 ± 119.1	>151

^{a}: values in $\mu g/mL \pm$ standard deviation. ^{b}: selectivity index.

Subsequently, the authors investigated the compound responsible for the antiviral activity observed in the extract from *Lycoris radiata*. Then, the alkaloid lycorine **(3)** (Fig. **4**) was isolated by RP-HPLC, using a MeOH:H_2O mixture (5:95). Finally, this alkaloid displayed EC_{50}, CC_{50}, and SI values of 15.7 ± 1.2 nM, $14980.0 \pm 912.0 \ \mu g/mL$, and 954, respectively. Finally, the authors suggested that the compound **(3)** represents a highly promising natural derivative to support other studies targeting CoV inhibitors.

(3)

$$EC_{50} = 15.7 \text{ nM}$$
$$CC_{50} = 14980.0 \text{ μg/mL}$$
$$SI = 954$$

Fig. (4). Lycorine alkaloid isolated from *Lycoris radiata*.

Lectins correspond to proteins with great structural diversity that can reversibly bind with carbohydrates, where they have no enzymatic activity [49, 50]. These proteins are related to viruses and can inhibit the viral replication of these organisms since these interact with glycoproteins from the viral envelope (E protein). Also, these proteins have demonstrated activity against Chikungunya (CHIKV), HIV, and other viruses [51, 52].

Plant lectins as anti-viral agents were first described by Keyaerts and collaborators (2007) [53], constituting an innovative study related to natural products against SARS-CoV, presenting promising results, as shown in Table **2**.

Table 2. Plant lectins with anti-SARS-CoV activity described by Keyaerts *et al.*, 2007.

Plant Lectin	$EC_{50} \pm SD^a$	$CC_{50}{}^a$	SI^b
Mannose-specific agglutinins			
HHA	3.2 ± 2.8	>100	>31.3
GNA	6.2 ± 0.6	>100	>16.1
NPA	5.7 ± 4.4	>100	>17.5
APA	0.45 ± 0.08	>100	>222.2
CA	4.9 ± 0.8	>100	>20
LOA	2.2 ± 1.3	>100	>45.5
EHA	1.8 ± 0.3	>100	>55.5
Morniga M II	1.6 ± 0.5	>100	>62.5
GlcNAc-specific agglutinins			
Nictaba	1.7 ± 0.3	>100	>58.8
(GlcNAc)$_n$-specific agglutinins			

(Table 2) cont.....

Plant Lectin	$EC_{50} \pm SD^a$	$CC_{50}{}^a$	SI^b
UDA	1.3 ± 0.1	>100	>76.9
Gal/GalNAc specific agglutinins			
ML II	0.0015 ± 0.003	<0.16	n.a.
GalNAcα(1,3)Gal>GalNAc>Gal-specific agglutinins			
IRA	2.2 ± 0.9	50	22.7
IRA b	4.4 ± 3.1	36	8.2
IRA r	3.4 ± 2.0	55	16.2

GlcNAc: *N*-acetyl glucosamine, GalNAc: *N*-acetyl galactosamine, Gal: galactose, n.a.: no activity. [a]: values in µg/mL ± standard deviation. [b]: selectivity index.

According to Table **2**, it is observed that the lectins mannose-specific agglutinins have a greater spectrum of action against SARS-CoV, with values of EC_{50} ranging from 0.45 to 6.2 µg/mL. Moreover, all of these plant lectins demonstrated low cytotoxicity values, over 100 µg/mL concentration. The most promising antiviral lectin was Gal/GalNAc specific agglutinins (UDA), which displayed a potential activity of 0.0015 µg/mL against SARS-CoV. However, cytotoxicity was also quite high, presenting a lower CC_{50} value than 0.16 µg/mL concentration, which contributes to low security in the administration of this product. Finally, the authors suggest that the mechanisms of action of these lectins are related to the early stages of the viral replication.

In 2008, Kim and collaborators developed a study involving methanolic extracts not previously evaluated for their anti-CoV activities. In total, 22 plants from traditional Oriental medicine were screened against SARS-CoV MHV-A59 strain, as shown in Table **3** [54].

Table 3. Plant extracts screened against SARS-CoV MHV-A59 strain by Kim *et al.*, 2008.

Plant Extract	$EC_{50}{}^a$	$CC_{50}{}^a$	SI^b
Cimicifuga rhizoma	19.4 ± 7.0	239.0 ± 44.4	12.3
Meliae cortex	13.0 ± 1.4	334.3 ± 7.0	25.6
Coptidis rhizoma	2.0 ± 0.5	71.3 ± 7.2	34.9
Phellodendron cortex	10.4 ± 2.2	139.5 ± 81.3	13.4
Sophora subprostrata radix	27.5 ± 1.1	307.3 ± 6.6	11.1
Moutan cortex radicis	61.9 ± 6.1	598.7 ± 12.5	9.7

[a]: values in µg/mL ± standard deviation. [b]: selectivity index.

Thus, Table **3** summarizes the results of the most active methanolic extracts against SARS-CoV MHV-A59. Thus, it is observed that the extract from *Coptidis* *rhizoma* proved to be more promising among those studied since it presented an EC_{50} value of 2.0 µg/mL. However, it was also the most cytotoxic, presenting a CC_{50} value of 71.3 µg/mL, where the others proved to be safer, with CC_{50} values ranging from 139.5 to 598.7 µg/mL concentrations.

Among the studies involving natural products against CoV described so far, one of the first studies involving computational methods was performed by Ryu and collaborators (2010), where 12 biflavonoid isolated from ethanolic extract of leaves from *Torreya nucifera* were used in such study [55]. Besides, they were also the first to report an isolated product targeting a specific CoV macromolecule - in this case, inhibition of 3CL^{pro} from SARS-CoV. It is extremely important for the infection and viral replication processes. This macromolecule contains a catalytic dyad constituted by a cysteine (Cys^{141}) and histidine (His^{163}) residues, which generate a nucleophile ($Cys(S^-)/His(H^+)$ ion-pair) by an acid-base mechanism [56, 57]. This study culminated in the biflavonoid amentoflavone (**4**), which proved to be the most promising compound among the isolated molecules, with an IC_{50} value of 8.3 µM upon SARS-CoV 3CL^{pro}, being a non-competitive inhibitor (K_i = 13.8 µM). By using molecular docking studies, it was possible to suggest that compound (**4**) fits into the S1 pocket, interacting through hydrogen-bonding interactions with the nitrogen atom at the His^{163} amino acid residue (at a distance of 3.15 Å) and with the hydroxyl group at the Leu^{141} amino acid residue (at a distance of 2.96 Å), besides S2 pocket, in a similar mode, hydrogen-bonding interactions with Gln^{189} (at a distance of 3,03 Å), exhibiting affinity energy of - 11.42 kcal/mol (Fig. **5**).

Park and coworkers (2012) reported tanshinones (Fig. **6**) from *Salvia miltiorrhiza* as potential inhibitors against 3CL^{pro} and PL^{pro} enzymes from SARS-CoV [58]. Also, this was the first study to correlate natural products with deubiquitinating (DUB) enzyme inhibitory activity. In this context, the compounds (**5–10**) were isolated from the ethanol extract by using Sephadex$^®$ LH-20 and octadecyl-functionalized silica gel. These compounds were properly characterized as tanshinone IIA (**5**), tanshinone IIB (**6**), methyl tanshinonate (**7**), cryptotanshinone (**8**), tanshinone I (**9**) and dihydrotanshinone I (**10**) (Fig. **6**). Finally, these were found to be non-competitive inhibitors for both 3CL^{pro} and PL^{pro} enzymes.

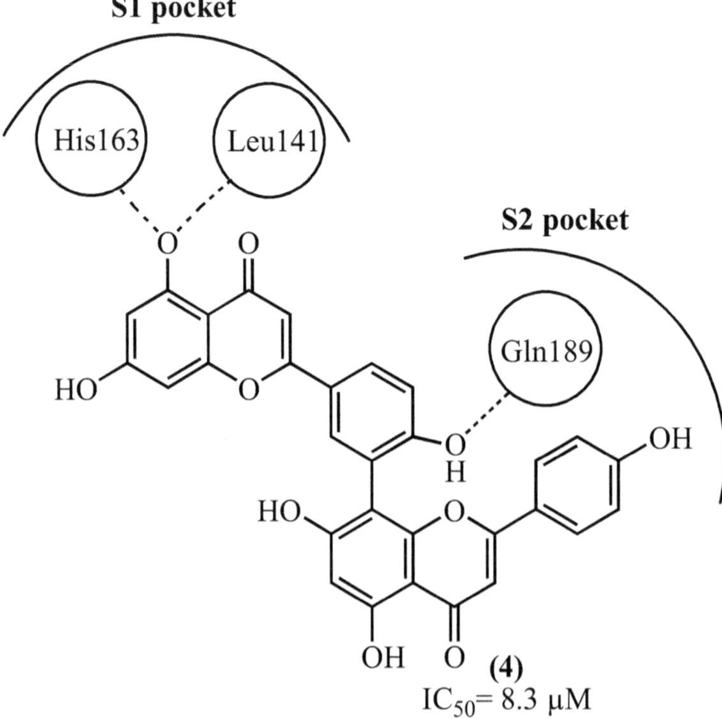

$IC_{50} = 8.3\ \mu M$

Fig. (5). Interactions of amentoflavone with 3CL[pro] from SARS-CoV.

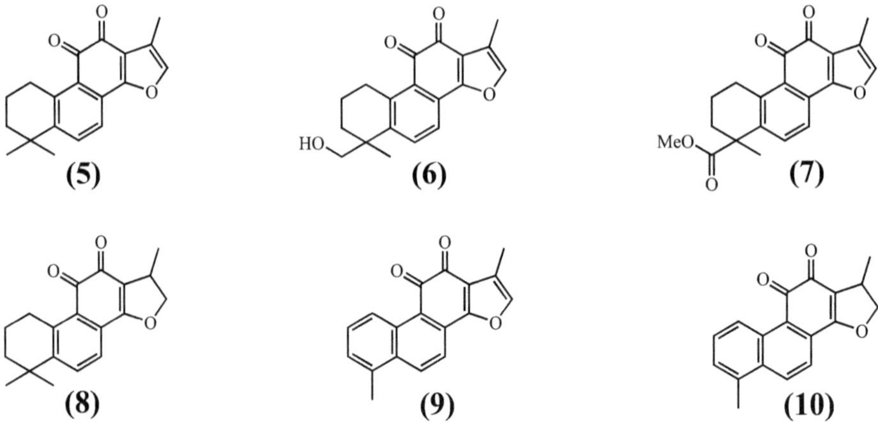

Fig. (6). Tanshinone compounds extracted from *Salvia miltiorrhiza* with activity against 3CL[pro] and PL[pro] enzymes from SARS-CoV.

These compounds were evaluated for their inhibitory activity against both SARS-CoV proteases, where it was verified that the compound **(10)** demonstrated the best value of IC_{50} towards 3CL[pro], corresponding to 14.4 µM. Concerning the PL[pro], the compound **(8)** presented an IC_{50} value of 0.8 µM, being the most promising inhibitor among the described compounds. Besides, the compound **(5)** showed very promising inhibition (IC_{50} value of 1.6 µM) upon the PL[pro] enzyme. Finally, compounds **(9)** and **(10)** demonstrated to be the best compounds for the inhibition of deubiquitinating (DUB) enzyme, in which their IC_{50} values were found to be 0.7 and 1.2 µM (Table **4**).

Table 4. Evaluation of the enzymatic inhibitory activity of tashinones by Young Park *et al.*, 2012.

		$IC_{50} \pm SD^a$	
Compound	*3CL^{pro}*	*PL^{pro}*	*DUB*
(5)	89.1 ± 5.2	1.6 ± 0.5	n.a.
(6)	24.8 ± 0.8	10.7 ± 1.7	52.0 ± 3.2
(7)	21.1 ± 0.8	9.2 ± 2.8	n.a.
(8)	226.7 ± 6.2	0.8 ± 0.2	87.6 ± 6.3
(9)	38.7 ± 8.2	8.8 ± 0.4	0.7 ± 0.2
(10)	14.4 ± 0.7	4.9 ± 1.2	1.2 ± 2.0

n.a. = not active at 200 µM concentration. [a]: values in µM ± standard deviation.

Following innovative studies involving inhibitors of 3CL[pro] from CoV, a study reported three anti-viral phlorotannins **(11-13)** (Fig. **7**) from edible brown algae *Ecklonia cava* [59].

(11)
IC_{50} = 2.7 µM
K_i = 2.4 µM

(12)
IC_{50} = 8.8 µM
K_i = 8.2 µM

(13)
IC_{50} = 13.3 µM
K_i = 24.0 µM

Fig. (7). Natural inhibitors of 3CL[pro] from SARS-CoV isolated from *Ecklonia cava*.

Among these, compounds **(11-13)** demonstrated to be the most active upon the $3CL^{pro}$ enzyme, with IC_{50} values of 2.7, 8.8, and 13.3 µM, respectively. All of these natural products displayed safely upon host cells, with CC_{50} values higher than 200 µM concentration. However, unlike the previous study, all isolated compounds were found to be competitive inhibitors, with K_i values of 2.4, 8.2, and 24.0 µM, respectively (see Fig. **7**). Moreover, the most promising compound, dieckol **(11)**, it is the unique compound among those studied that possess two eckol units bonded by a phenyl diether. Also, from *In silico* studies, it exhibited hydrogen bonding interactions with the catalytic dyad from $3CL^{pro}$ in S1 pocket, resulting in the lowest affinity energy among the isolated molecules (11.51 kcal/mol).

The latest study involving natural products active against HCoV-OC43 was reported by Kim and coworkers (2019) [60], also being the first to report alkaloids with such activity. The authors isolated the natural bis-benzylisoquinoline alkaloids tetrandrine (TET, **14**), fangchinoline (FAN, **15**), and cepharanthine (CEP, **16**) (Fig. **8**) from *Stephania tetrandra.* The *Stephania* genus (*Menispermaceae*) is native from Southeast Asia and is recognized for its great medicinal importance for providing natural products with several properties, such as antiviral, antibacterial, anti-inflammatory, antiparasitic, among others [61 - 63].

As exhibited in Fig. (**8**), bis-benzylisoquinoline alkaloids TET **(14)**, FAN **(15)**, and CEP **(16)** were potentially active against the HCoV-OC43 strain, where the compound **(14)** proved to be the most promising. Finally, the authors reported that the aforementioned compounds are active in the initial stage of infection, inhibiting the replication of the HCoV-OC43 lineage and viral protein expression.

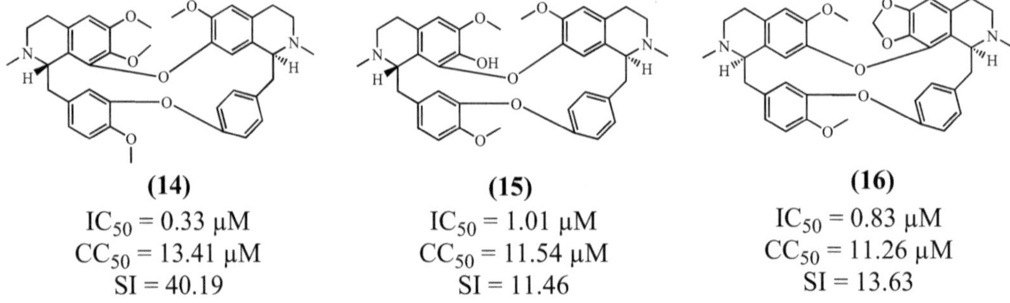

(14)
$IC_{50} = 0.33$ µM
$CC_{50} = 13.41$ µM
SI = 40.19

(15)
$IC_{50} = 1.01$ µM
$CC_{50} = 11.54$ µM
SI = 11.46

(16)
$IC_{50} = 0.83$ µM
$CC_{50} = 11.26$ µM
SI = 13.63

Fig. (8). Bis-benzylisoquinoline alkaloids active against HCoV-OC43.

Classical Methods Applied for Discovering New Antiviral Agents

The first study involving the design of inhibitors of viral RNA synthesis from

CoV was described by Keck and colleagues (1989) [64], in which the authors designed and screened five new 1-amino hydroxyguanidine tosylate derivatives (Fig. **9**) since guanidine had already been described as an inhibitor in a previously published study [65]. In this context, the authors added five aldehydes to the hydroxyguanidine tosylate, producing Schiff base-like structures.

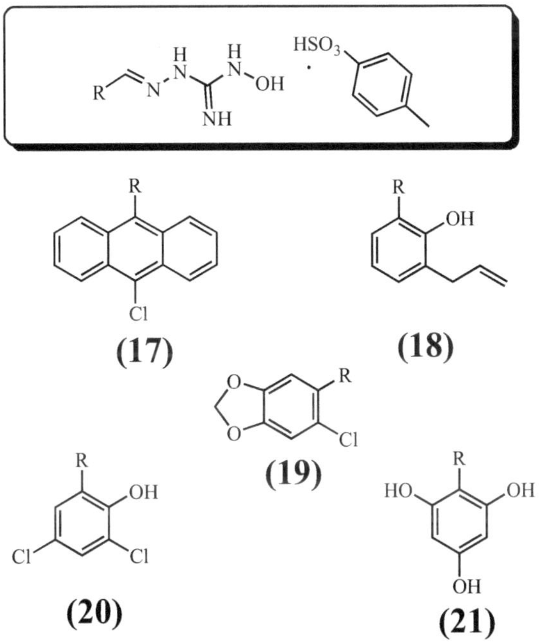

(17)   **(18)**

(19)

(20)   **(21)**

Fig. (**9**). 1-Amino hydroxyguanidine tosylate described as potential inhibitors of the RNA synthesis from CoV.

All the compounds (**17-21**) were evaluated as inhibitors and showed great results, with inhibition ranging from 86 to 95%, where all these derivatives were effective to inhibit the viral RNA synthesis (including negative-stranded RNA synthesis, mRNA transcription, and genome RNA replication). Besides, the compound (**20**) was found to be the most promising molecule from this series, showing inhibition of 95% of the viral RNA synthesis. However, the same derivative demonstrated 68% inhibition of human cellular RNA, conferring considerable toxicity. Even after this innovative study, over 15 years later, the design and synthesis of bioactive molecules against the HCoV were continued. Thus, Martina and collaborators (2005) [66] reported one of the first studies involving peptidomimetic analogs inhibiting the main SARS-CoV protease, 3CL^pro. The authors used the HPLC- and FRET-substrate-based screening techniques for screening 40 new electrophilic aziridinyl peptide analogs toward 3CL^pro (Table **5**). As a result, the first screening used the *VS* VNSTLQ|SGLRKMA amino acids sequence as a substrate and it was analyzed by HPLC. Then, the second screening was performed by using a fluorimetric assay, where FRET-pair labeled was used as the substrate for this technique.

Table 5. Aziridinyl electrophilic peptides screened by Martina *et al.*, 2005.

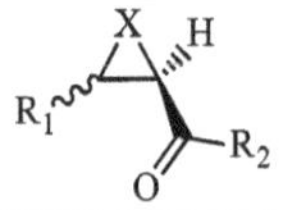

Compound	Configuration of the aziridine ring	R_1	R_2	X	Inhibition of SARS-CoV M^{pro} at 100 μM
(22)	*trans* (S,S)	EtO_2C	Gly-Gly-OBn	HN	$54 \pm 5^a / 75 \pm 7^b$
(23)[c]	(R + S)	H	OMe	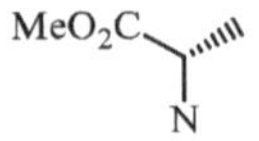 MeO_2C—N (aziridine)	39 ± 6^a
(24)[c]	(R + S)	H	OMe	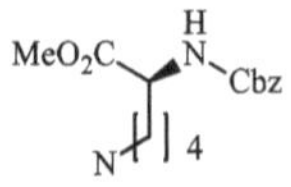 MeO_2C—N(H)-Cbz, N-(CH$_2$)$_4$	48 ± 6^a

[a] Percentage inhibition as obtained in the FRET-based assay, values are mean values of at least 2 independent assays. [b] Percentage inhibition as obtained in the HPLC assay, mean value of four independent assays. [c] Ratio of diastereomers.

It was observed that among 40 new analogs synthesized and screened, the compounds **(22-24)** were found to be the most promising analogs, with emphasis on the compound **(22)** which demonstrated inhibition of 54%, through FRET-based assay; while for HPLC assay, 75%. Thus, *In silico* studies revealed that the electrophilic region of the aziridine ring from the compound **(22)** is located close to the sulfur atom at the Cys[145] amino acid residue in S1 pocket, constituting valuable information for understanding about the mechanism of action of this analog.

Similarly, Chen and coworkers (2005) [67] developed 39 new peptidomimetic isatin-derived analogs, a recognized prototype inhibitor of 3CL^{pro} from *Rhinovirus*, where the active site of this protease is structurally similar to the SARS-CoV structure [68, 69]. Among all the compounds synthesized and screened by HPLC- and FRET-substrate-based techniques, the analogs **(25-28)** demonstrated potential inhibitory activity of 3CL^{pro} from SARS-CoV, with IC$_{50}$ values ranging from 0.98 to 4.82 μM (Fig. **11**). Besides, it was observed that among the best analogs (in comparison with isatin), the compound **(26)** has a bromine atom instead of a nitro group. In contrast, the compound **(28)** kept the nitro group conserved, however, there is a replacement of amide with iodine atom (Fig. **10**).

Fig. (10). Isatin analogs with inhibitory activity against 3CL^{pro} from SARS-CoV.

One of the first studies associated with thiopurine analogs as inhibitors of PL^{pro} from SARS-CoV was developed by Chou and collaborators (2008) [70]. This enzyme represents an essential factor for viral replication, constituting an excellent target for bioactive molecules [4]. Thus, the authors screened six new derivatives and categorized them as reversible, competitive, and selective inhibitors targeting PL^{pro} from SARS-CoV. Among the screened molecules, the 6-mercaptopurine derivative **(29)** and its active metabolite 6-thioguanine **(30)** (Fig. **11**) were considered the most promising compounds, where the thiocarbonyl group was found to be pharmacologically essential for this inhibitory action. Such compounds are used in current pharmacotherapy against lymphoblastic or myeloblastic leukemia, especially in children [71].

As noted in Fig. **(11)**, the 6-thioguanine **(30)** is a more potent inhibitor of PL^{pro} from SARS-CoV, with an IC$_{50}$ value of 5.0 μM. Thus, the structure–activity relationship (SAR) analysis and molecular docking simulations revealed that a primary amine is added between the nitrogens in the first ring, *via* metabolism, making this metabolite more active than its precursor. Also, both compounds interact *via* hydrogen bonding interaction between the thiocarbonyl group and Cys^{1651}, which can block the essential sulfhydryl group from the enzyme, preventing its action and consequently inhibiting it. Finally, it was verified that compounds **(29)** and **(30)** presented affinity energies of 8.2 and 14.7 kcal/mol, respectively.

Fig. (11). 6-Mercaptopurine (29) and its active metabolite 6-thioguanine (30) active against PL^{pro} from SARS-CoV.

After this study, Lee and coworkers (2009) [72] performed a study involving aryl diketoacids (Fig. **12**) as selective inhibitors of helicase duplex DNA-unwinding from SARS-CoV, based on the fact of this chemical class to be active against HIV-1 integrase and HCV RdRp enzymes. Also, the Hel is a potential target for bioactive drugs due to be fundamental for replication of the viral. Furthermore, this macromolecule has been targeted for other drugs against Herpes Simplex virus (HSV) and Hepatitis C virus (HCV) infections [73]. Thus, among the active analogs, the compound **(33)** demonstrated to be the most promising, with an IC_{50} value of 5.4 µM towards helicase duplex DNA-unwinding. It is observed that this derivative has a benzylamine group inserted at position 3 from the aromatic ring. Surprisingly, when a chlorine atom is inserted at position 4 of the benzylamine derivative **(34)** its activity practically decreases in half, with an IC_{50} value of 11 µM, indicating that electron-withdrawing groups at this position represent a not good strategy.

One year later, a study involving semi-synthesis of bioactive compounds against SARS-CoV was reported by Yang and collaborators (2009) [74]. From this, the authors identified phenanthroindolizine and phenanthroquinolizidine derivatives from the methanolic extract from *Tylophora indica* and *Tylophora ovata* species. These traditional Asian medicines are recognized suppliers of active alkaloids with antiviral activity [75, 76]. Thus, the compound tylophorine **(35)** was isolated through silica-gel open-column chromatography and HPLC. Subsequently, tylophorine-based compounds were synthesized, characterized **(36-39)**, and screened toward infected cells by SARS-CoV (Fig. **13**). All derivatives **(36-37)** were most promising than its natural precursor **(35)**, where the compound **(36)** was designed from the insertion of a methoxyl group at position 4. The biological evaluation of it revealed that this analog has EC_{50}, CC_{50}, and SI values of < 0.005, 0.5 µM, and > 100, respectively. In the analog **(37)**, the methoxyl group was removed from position 2, followed by the insertion of the hydroxyl group at position 14, resulting in an identical IC_{50} value (< 0.005 µM) observed for the compound **(36)**, but it is almost eight times less cytotoxic.

Fig. (12). Aryl diketoacid inhibitors of helicase duplex DNA-unwinding from SARS-CoV.

Fig. (13). Semi-synthetic analogs from tylophorine with anti-SARS-CoV activity.

This work contributed to the development of semi-synthetic analogs from natural bioactive molecules known from traditional Asian medicine, constituting new active molecules against this severe disease. In this context, pyrazolones are compounds with several activities reported in diverse studies, with emphasis on the edaravone which used in the treatment of brain and myocardial ischemia. Other pyrazolones have demonstrated antiviral activity against orthopoxvirus [77]. Based on these facts, Ramajayam and collaborators (2010) reported the synthesis of pyrazolone derivatives with inhibitory activity of 3CL^{pro} from SARS-CoV. This chemical class was identified by using a high-throughput screening assay [78]. Thus, 21 new pyrazolone derivatives were synthesized and screened, resulting in the three most active analogs **(40-42)** (Fig. **14**).

Fig. (14). Active pyrazolone analogs against SARS-CoV.

SAR analyses of these derivatives revealed that the compound **(40)** is the only one with a cyano group at position 4 of the pyrazolone nitrogen-fused phenyl ring. All three analogs have electron-withdrawing groups in this same position. Besides, docking studies suggest that the benzylidene group is placed into the S3 pocket from the 3CL^{pro}, and the carboxylic acid group interacts through a hydrogen bonding interaction with Gln^{192} amino acid residue.

Based on the study performed by Lee and coworkers in 2009 (as mentioned earlier in this chapter), Kim and colleagues (2011) [79] developed the other 10 aryl diketoacids by using classic bioisosterism and screened as NTPase/helicase inhibitors from SARS-CoV. As result, the compound **(43)** (Fig. **15**) was found to be a potent inhibitor of the NTPase and Hel enzymes from SARS-CoV, with an IC$_{50}$ value of 4 µM and 11 µM, respectively. Besides, this compound was shown to be safe, with a CC$_{50}$ value higher than 50 µM concentration. Finally, this study contributes to the design of new bioactive enzyme inhibitors against HCoV, supporting the discovery of multi-target antiviral drugs.

$$IC_{50} = 4.0\ \mu M \text{ and } 11.0\ \mu M$$

Fig. (15). 2,6-Bis-arylmethyloxy-5-hydroxychromones with anti-SARS-CoV activity.

Another study involving inhibitors of 3CL^{pro} from SARS-CoV was developed by Chuck and coworkers (2013) [80], in which it was one of the first works using the auto-cleavage sequence of SARS-CoV 3CL^{pro} (TSAVLQY) as a basis for designing peptidomimetic inhibitors. Besides, the study reports the insertion of a nitrile warhead as essential for inhibitory activity, since this group remains covalently bonded to the thiol group from the Cys^{145} amino acid residue from the catalytic dyad of 3CL^{pro}. Additionally, it was confirmed by crystal structures of enzyme-inhibitor complexes [81, 82]. Based on this, the authors synthesized four peptidomimetic analogs, where the derivative **(44)** was found to be the most promising inhibitor upon the 3CL^{pro} enzyme (Fig. **16**), displaying an IC$_{50}$ value of 4.6 μM. Also, it was observed that the Cbz protective group at the *N*-terminus increased the potency of this inhibitor about 10-times.

$$IC_{50} = 4.6\ \mu M$$

Fig. (16). Peptidomimetic with anti-SARS-CoV activity.

Considering the design of new inhibitors of 3CL^{pro} based on peptidomimetic compounds, Prior and colleagues (2013) evaluated a new class of analogs from tripeptidyl transition-state inhibitors, where it is compatible with the natural substrate of 3CL^{pro}, to provide better recognition and, consequently high inhibition

[83]. Based on this information, the general structure contains a glutamine residue (P1), a hydrophobic amino acid residue (P2) - in this case, leucine; and an arylalanine (P3), to facilitate cell absorption. Finally, it was added aldehydes, α-ketoamides, bisulfite adducts or α-hydroxyl phosphonates as warhead groups [81, 82]. Among these, the analogs **(45 and 46)** were the most promising derivatives identified in this study, where the aldehyde-containing analog **(45)** exhibited good activity, with an IC_{50} value of 0.23 μM against 3CL^{pro}. Also, the α-ketoamide-containing analog **(46)** was about 3-times less potent, with an IC_{50} value of 0.61 μM. Besides, both peptidomimetics showed safe cytotoxic profiles, with CC_{50} values of 87 and > 100 μM, respectively (Fig. **17**).

Fig. (17). Peptidomimetics inhibitors of 3CL^{pro} from SARS-CoV.

Fleximers process is a technique used for designing bioactive molecules from rigid analogs, with advantages such as increased affinity energy for the active site from enzymatic targets, as well as, ability to act on mutations [84]. Based on this information, Peters and collaborators (2015) developed three fleximers analogs from acyclovir (Fig. **18**), an antiviral drug nucleoside polymerase inhibitor used in pharmacotherapy against infections by Herpes Zoster virus (HZV) and HSV [85]. The derivative **(47)** demonstrated promising activity against the HCoV-NL63 strain, as well as MERS-CoV. It presented an IC_{50} value of 8.8 μM upon infected cells with HCoV-NL63 and CC_{50} value of 120 μM. Also, it towards cells with MERS-CoV exhibited IC_{50} and CC_{50} values of 23 and 71 μM.

Fig. (18). Fleximer analog from Acyclovir with anti-HCoV-NL63 activity.

Considering the drugs oseltamivir and zanamivir, neuraminidase (NA) inhibitors, Kumar and coworkers (2016) published a work reporting the screening of 19 analogs against 3CL^{pro} enzymes from SARS- and MERS-CoV [86]. All the synthesized compounds **(48-50)** exhibited promising activity against both SARS- and MERS-CoV 3CL^{pro} protease (Fig. **19**). Most of these compounds hydrophobically interact with Met^{49} and Gln^{189} amino acid residues, into S2 pocket. However, the analog **(51)**, which has a carboxylic acid group, preferentially interacts into pocket S1, through hydrogen bonding interactions.

Fig. (19). New pyrazolones analogs anti-3CL^{pro} from SARS- and MERS-CoV.

Virtual Screening and Computational Techniques for Designing New Antiviral Agents

The discovery of new drugs involves a long and complex process that includes diverse steps such as selection and validation of a biological target; screening of compounds from different libraries; and evaluation of resulting compounds *in vitro* and *in vivo* assays [87, 88]. In this context, computer modeling has gained more space in the field of medicinal chemistry, providing rapid screening in large compounds' libraries, making the process more economically viable and easy [89, 90]. Among the computational approaches in the search for new drugs, virtual screening is a fast and effective technique for identifying new *hits* compounds, as well as their optimized ones. Besides, it is divided into two categories: (*i*) structure-based drug design (SBDD), and (*ii*) ligand-based drug design (LBDD). In this context, the SBDD approach is described as the most effective, widely used in research laboratories worldwide. Based on this, it will be discussed in more detail in this chapter [90 - 92].

Computational modeling shows its importance not only in drug design but also in the development of vaccines, increasing the probability of new therapeutic alternatives to be developed [20, 33, 93].

The most attractive targets in the development of antiviral compounds against CoV are proteases, since they interfere in the viral replication and, consequently implicates in the maturation of viral replicases [13, 94]. The proteases PL^{pro} and 3CL^{pro} are critical for the pp1a and pp1b replicases [13]. Additionally, it is important to mention that the two proteins are cysteine proteases, and present a reactive thiol group responsible for attacking carbonyl groups at the peptide bonds, leading to the formation of proteins essential for the survival of the virus [73]. Some studies show that the SARS-CoV-2 PL^{pro} enzyme is highly homolog to the SARS- and MERS-CoV PL^{pro}. In this sense, it can be successfully used in molecular modeling studies for discovering new drugs to potentially treat the current outbreak [95, 96].

In this section, several compounds will also be shown (*e.g.,* ribavirin **(166)**, remdesivir **(170)**, and others) that are nucleotide or nucleoside analog compounds, presenting purine, pyrimidine, modified sugar portion in their structures, which also show promising inhibition of replication against the CoV [13, 97].

One of the first studies using computational techniques for developing new compounds against the CoV was carried out by Chou and collaborators (2003) [98]. The authors performed a molecular docking study of the compound KZ7088 **(53)**, an analog from AG7080 **(52)** developed by Pfizer, in which it is in clinical phase trials against rhinovirus. As shown in Fig. **(20)**, AG7080 **(52)** was modified by removing the methylene group from the side chain, generating KZ7080 **(53)**. Through docking simulations, it was possible to propose that the SARS-CoV 3CL^{pro} binding pocket consists of 23 amino acid residues, and the main interactions observed for the KZ7088 **(53)** are *via* hydrogen bonding interactions with Thr^{25}, Thr^{45}, Leu^{50}, Tyr^{54}, and Asp^{187} amino acid residues. The authors highlighted that this study has great importance for designing new drugs for the treatment of the CoV.

AG7088 (52)   KZ7088 (53)

Fig. (20). AG7088 (52) -based analog KZ7088 (53) with anti-SARS-CoV activity.

Molecular modeling studies have become a routine in the search for new molecules against the CoV. Accordingly, Niu and coworkers (2008) [99] considering the lead compound MAC-5576 **(54)**, synthesized a series of structurally related compounds (Fig. **21**), which were tested against SAR-CoV 3CL^{pro}. By using molecular docking, the main interactions of these molecules were proposed to obtain chemical information for designing new antiviral agents. Thus, it was shown that interactions with hydrophobic amino acids were related to these compounds. Also, it was verified that the 3-chloropyridine group has a strong affinity for pocket S1, showing that the amino acid residues in this cavity have a strong influence on the catalytic activity of the enzyme. Other important information obtained was that compounds **(55-66)** have a shorter distance between the ester group and Cys^{145}, which may suggest the formation of a covalent bond. Thus, the authors suggest that the ester bond can be replaced with another electrophilic group, which can increase the inhibitory activity. Finally, improvements in the side chain can increase interactions into S2 and S4 pockets, maximizing the interactions of these compounds.

With advances in the improvement of computational techniques, some researchers have started to use virtual screenings against the main targets from CoV. Thus, Mukherjee and colleagues (2008) performed a high-throughput virtual screening (HTS) in the Asinex Platinum database, containing approximately 120,000 compounds, consisting of about 500 exclusive scaffolding [100]. The screening protocol was applied to this set of molecules, resulting in 108 compounds that were evaluated against SARS-CoV 3CL^{pro}. Thus, compounds PJ07 **(67)** and PJ169 **(68)** (Fig. **22**) were the most active, with IC$_{50}$ values of 18.2 and 17.2 µM, respectively. Through molecular docking simulations, it was found that these compounds present interactions similar to that of the peptide substrate at the active site SARS-CoV 3CL^{pro}, with hydrogen bonding interactions (His^{163} and Glu^{166}) and hydrophobic interactions (Thr^{25}, Leu^{27}, Leu^{141}, and Asn^{142}). It was also identified that pocket S4 was not occupied by these molecules.

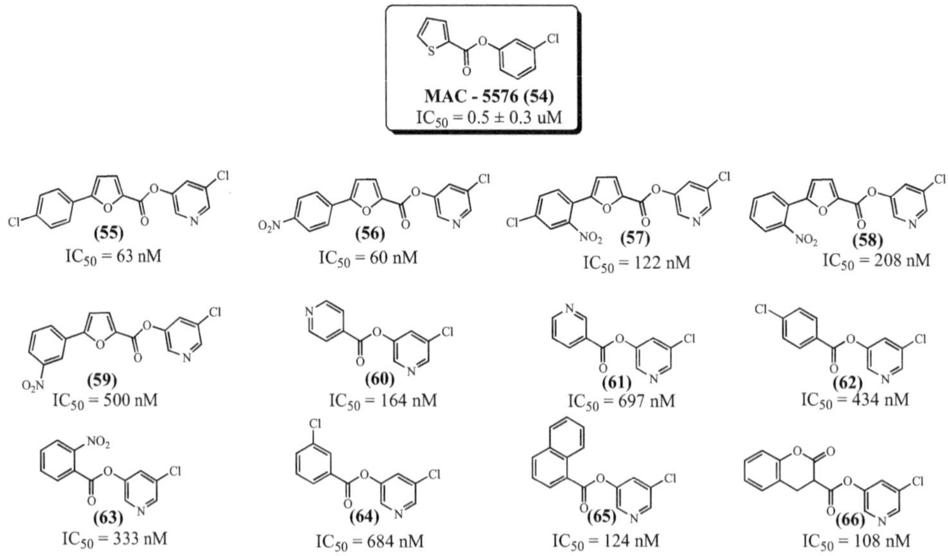

Fig. (21). SARS-CoV 3CL^{pro} inhibitors.

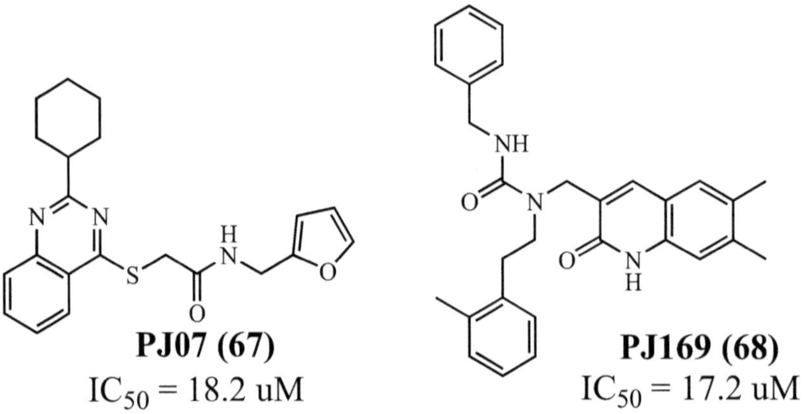

Fig. (22). SARS-CoV 3CL^{pro} inhibitors identified from the Asinex Platinum database.

Nguyen and collaborators (2011) carried out a virtual study by HTS against 3CL^{pro} involving 308,307 compounds from the ChemBridge database [101]. In their procedure, the compounds were initially ranked, resulting in 1468 molecules with affinity energy ranging from -14 to -17.09 kcal/mol. In total, 214 compounds were selected based on their hydrogen bonding interactions with the main amino acid residues. These compounds were categorized into 35 groups, where 53 compounds were selected for biological assays against 3CL^{pro}. In the sense, it was obtained IC$_{50}$ values ranging from 38.57 to 101.38 μM. After the docking studies, it was shown that these compounds are stabilized by hydrogen bonding interactions with catalytic residues and hydrophobic interactions in regions opposite the active site. Besides, K_i assays for compounds **(74)** and **(75)** (Fig. **23**) revealed that these molecules are competitive inhibitors, with values of 9.11 ± 1.61 and 9.93 ± 0.44 µM, respectively. Finally, the authors state that these compounds can serve as new scaffolds for discovering new compounds against the CoV.

(69)

IC_{50} = 58.35 ± 1.41 uM

(70)

IC_{50} = 62.79 ± 3.19 uM

(71)

IC_{50} = 101.38 ± 3.27 uM

(72)

IC_{50} = 77.09 ± 1.94 uM

(73)

IC_{50} = 90.72 ± 5.54 uM

(74)

IC_{50} = 38.57 ± 2.41 uM

(75)

IC_{50} = 41.39 ± 1.17 uM

Fig. (23). SARS-CoV 3CL^{pro} inhibitors identified from the ChemBridge database.

Zhu and coworkers (2011) carried out study kinetics of inhibition in the crystalline structure of the complex of six different peptide aldehydes (Fig. **24**) with the SARS-CoV 3CL^{pro} [102]. The authors showed the binding modes by X-ray crystallography for the compounds at the active site, displaying that peptide hydrophilic residues (Ser and Asp) of the P2 position are placed into the hydrophobic S2 pocket, and hydrophobic residue (Phe) in the P1 position is inserted into the hydrophilic S1 pocket S1. Also, the study showed that the specificity for these subsites can be canceled out by the presence of highly electrophilic chemical groups at P1 and P2 positions close to the aldehyde, which justifies the greater activity for the compound Cm-FF-H **(80)** (K_i = 2.24 ± 0.58

µM). Through these results, the authors suggest that these interactions should be explored for the discovery of new compounds against CoV.

Ac-ESTLQ-H (76)
SARS-CoV K_i = 8.27 ± 1.52 uM

Ac-NSTSQ-H (77)
SARS-CoV K_i = 40.98 ± 2.63 uM

Ac-DSFDQ-H (78)
SARS-CoV K_i = 41.24 ± 2.25 uM

Ac-NSFSQ-H (79)
SARS-CoV K_i = 72.73 ± 3.60 uM

Cm-FF-H (80)
SARS-CoV K_i = 2.24 ± 0.58 uM

Fig. (24). New SARS-CoV 3CL[pro] peptidomimetic inhibitors.

The study performed by Turlington and coworkers (2013) was developed based on compound **(81)** (IC_{50} = 6.2 µM against 3CL[pro] enzyme), where the interactions of the co-crystallized ligand with the enzyme were analyzed and used to propose structural modifications (Fig. **25**). However, the main interactions with the active site were maintained (Gly[163] and Glu[166]), leading to the synthesis of several compounds. From these, the compound ML300 **(82)** presented the best activity (IC_{50} = 4.11 ± 0.24 µM), showing that studies based on the structure of the targets (SBDD) could be extremely promising in the development of drugs against the Coronavirus [103].

Fig. (25). Benzotriazole inhibitors of SARS-CoV 3CL^{pro}.

Interestingly, Lee and collaborators (2014) combined *VS* techniques with enzymatic HTS in the search for new inhibitors of SARS-CoV 3CL^{pro} [104]. The *VS* protocol was applied to the ZINC database, containing approximately 621,000 compounds. In this context, only 68 were previously acquired and tested, obtaining eight compounds **(83-90)** with promising activity (Fig. **26**), with inhibition of over 50% and IC$_{50}$ values in the micromolar range. Based on the *VS* results, the authors conducted an HTS campaign on three databases, adding up to 40,000 compounds, where two compounds **(91-92)** (Fig. **26**) were promising in biological assays, with IC$_{50}$ values less than 50 μM. Thus, the authors concluded that the *VS* and HTS protocols could be considered as promising strategies for obtaining new scaffolding candidates for the optimization and design of new drugs anti-SARS-CoV.

Molecular modeling studies were used in the study performed by Wang and coworkers (2017) to determine the main interactions of the most active compounds, as well as to develop a QSAR model for the unsymmetrical aromatic disulfides derivatives synthesized and tested against the SARS-CoV 3CL^{pro} [105]. Then, the authors synthesized 40 very promising compounds (Fig. **27**), with IC$_{50}$ values ranging from 0.516 to 5.95 μM. The docking study for compound **(123)** (most promising) was carried out, suggesting that its activity is mainly due to hydrophobic interactions with Phe^{140}, Leu^{141}, His^{163}, Met^{165}, Glu^{166}, and His^{172}, as well as hydrogen bonding interactions with Asn^{142}, Gly^{143}, and Cys^{145}. Finally, the QSAR study obtained values of q^2 = 0.681 and r^2 = 0.916, showing that the steric contributions account with 43.6% for biological activity, and the electrostatic contributions, with 56.4%. Finally, the authors highlighted that these results are promising and could be used for developing compounds anti-SARS-CoV.

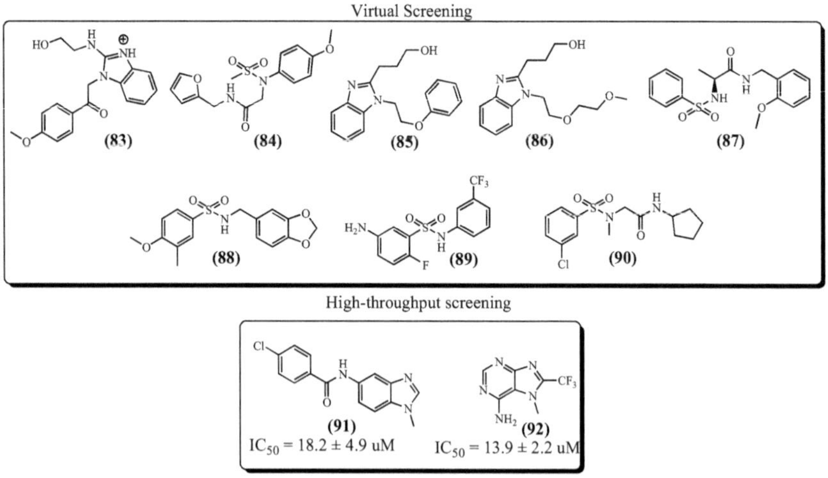

Fig. (26). <u>SARS-Cov 3CL^{pro} inhibitors</u> identified from the ZINC database.

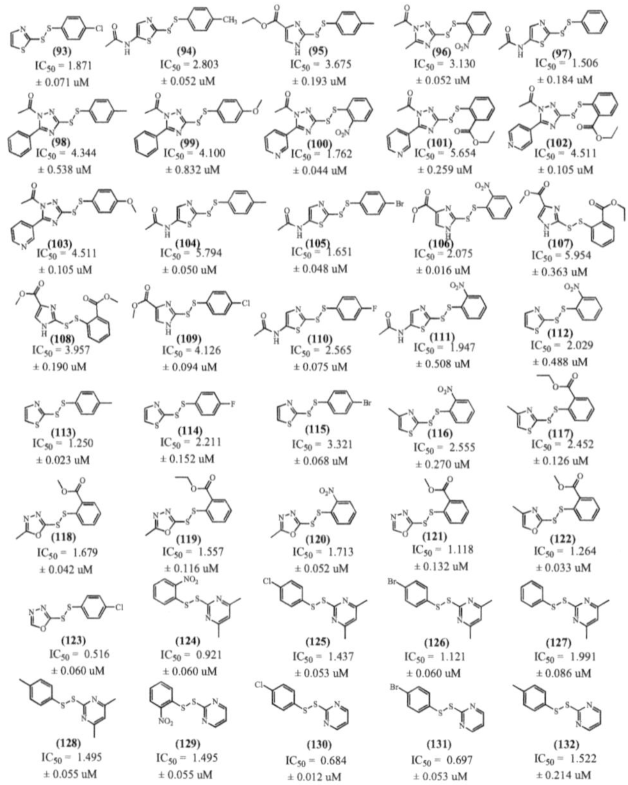

Fig. (27). SARS-CoV inhibitors synthesized by Wang *et al.* 2017.

In the study developed by Theerawatanasirikul and collaborators (2020), *VS* was carried out on a library of natural compounds with activity against feline infectious peritonitis virus (FIPV), a type of virus that also belongs to the *Coronaviridae* family [106]. The virtual campaign was developed against 3CL[pro]. In total, 8,338 natural compounds were found from searching on PubChem, Drugbank, ZINC, and NCI databases. When applying the protocol of molecular docking, the compounds were ranked and 64 were selected with the best results, in which only 15 compounds were selected for *in vitro* assays, where was observed a strong affinity to FIPV 3CL[pro]. Among these compounds, 7 **(133-139)** were more promising (Fig. **28**), with IC$_{50}$ values ranging from 6.36 to 78.40 µM, and K$_i$ values ranging from 3.69 to 48.84 µM. The molecular docking studies showed that an important factor for the biological activity of these compounds is the presence of an acyl group, which may suffer an attack by the reactive cysteine residue present in 3CL[pro] active site, as well as interactions with His[41] Cys[144] amino acid residues and other binding pocket's residues.

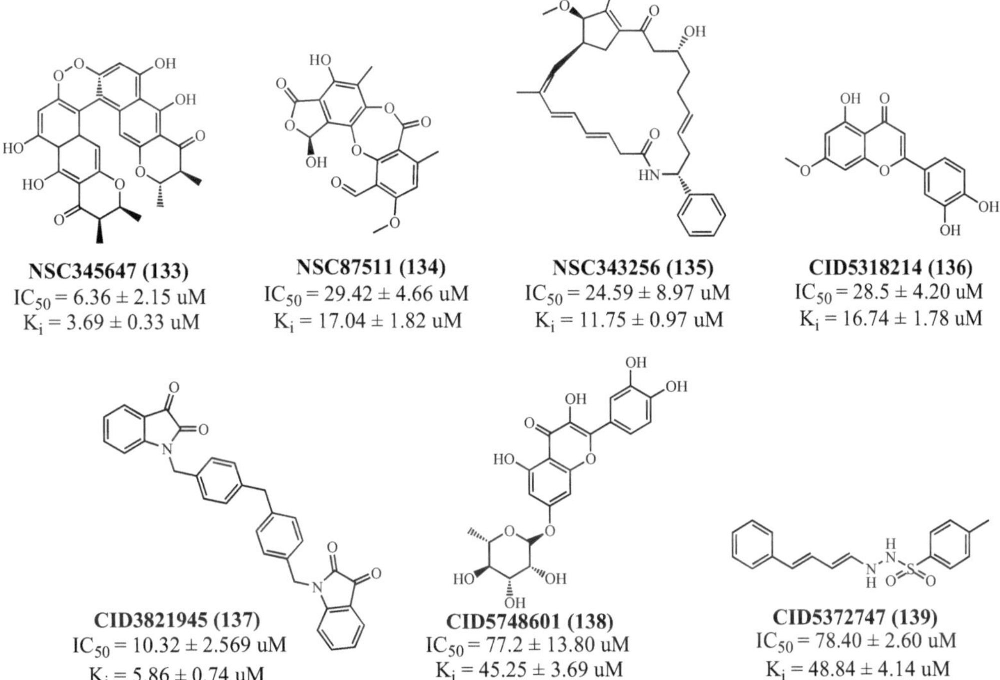

NSC345647 (133)
IC$_{50}$ = 6.36 ± 2.15 uM
K$_i$ = 3.69 ± 0.33 uM

NSC87511 (134)
IC$_{50}$ = 29.42 ± 4.66 uM
K$_i$ = 17.04 ± 1.82 uM

NSC343256 (135)
IC$_{50}$ = 24.59 ± 8.97 uM
K$_i$ = 11.75 ± 0.97 uM

CID5318214 (136)
IC$_{50}$ = 28.5 ± 4.20 uM
K$_i$ = 16.74 ± 1.78 uM

CID3821945 (137)
IC$_{50}$ = 10.32 ± 2.569 uM
K$_i$ = 5.86 ± 0.74 uM

CID5748601 (138)
IC$_{50}$ = 77.2 ± 13.80 uM
K$_i$ = 45.25 ± 3.69 uM

CID5372747 (139)
IC$_{50}$ = 78.40 ± 2.60 uM
K$_i$ = 48.84 ± 4.14 uM

Fig. (28). Compounds identified by Theerawatanasirikul *et al.* 2020.

Abdallah (2019) conducted a computational study against 28 bioactive compounds derived from imidazoles to investigate their possible activity against the CoV [107]. For each of the chosen compounds, 100 conformations were generated and analyzed, where their affinity energies were calculated and ranked. In this sense, three of these showed the best results **(140-142)** (Fig. **29**), in which the main interactions presented by the compound **(140)** were hydrogen bonding interactions (Arg[188], Leu[141], and Ser[144]) and π-π interactions, similar to interactions of compounds **(141)** and **(142)**. The authors concluded that the high-affinity energy of the compounds is due to the strong interactions with the amino acid residues.

Fig. (29). Imidazoles and benzothiazole identified as promising 3CL[pro] inhibitors.

Another computational study was carried out by Gao and coworkers (2020), based on a virtual screening in the ChEMBL database [14]. Then, 115 compounds were selected as promising molecules against SARS-CoV. Also, 4,463 molecules were selected from the PDB database. Then, the authors proposed that the 15 best compounds **(143-157)** can be promising against CoV because they have high affinity, mainly related to the greater possibility of hydrogen bonding interactions formation at the active site (Fig. **30**).

Drug Repurposing

A very interesting strategy that is gaining more attention from the scientific community is drug repurposing. This strategy is based on finding new therapeutic uses for known, commercialized, discontinued, or even drug candidates [108 - 110]. The advantage of repurposing a drug lies in the fact that they are compounds that already have proven safety and adequate pharmacokinetic, thus avoiding problems related to toxicity and stability, and being more economical viable [108, 111]. This strategy is mainly associated with bioinformatics, which performing an *In silico* screening, it is possible to propose a new activity for different previously approved drugs [109, 110]. Thus, several drugs have been reused in the search for new treatments against viral infections, such as ZIKV, EBOV, DENV, and more recently against the SARS-CoV-2 [112]. Later in this chapter, it will be shown the discovery of anti-CoV activity of various drugs on the market, such as ribavirin **(166)**, hexachlorophene **(222)**, and nitazoxanide **(187)** [113].

(143)
-10.56 kcal/mol

(144)
-9.71 kcal/mol

(145)
-9.55 kcal/mol

(146)
-9.55 kcal/mol

(147)
-9.45 kcal/mol

(148)
-9.35 kcal/mol

(149)
-9.31 kcal/mol

(150)
-8.36 kcal/mol

(151)
-8.87 kcal/mol

(152)
-8.87 kcal/mol

(153)
-8.86 kcal/mol

(154)
-8.85 kcal/mol

(155)
-8.55 kcal/mol

(156)
- 8.85 kcal/mol

(157)
-8.85 kcal/mol

Fig. (30). 3CL^{pro} inhibitors identified from the ChEMBL database.

Based on this strategy, in 2003, it was discovered that the compounds lopinavir **(158)** and ritonavir **(159)** had activity against SARS-CoV, as well as niclosamide **(160)** (anti-parasite) and promazine **(161)** (anti-psychotic) were promising as well (Fig. **31**). In this sense, Zhang and collaborators (2004) conducted an *In silico* study with these drugs, as well as two other compounds, PNU **(162)** and UC2 **(163)** (Fig. **31**), which are structurally related to niclosamide and promazine, respectively [114]. These compounds were promising as HIV-1 reverse transcriptase inhibitors. Furthermore, these compounds were found to be active upon the 3CL^{pro} SARS-CoV. Through docking studies and based on the binding modes presented by Chou and coworkers (2003), it was verified that part of the lopinavir structure does not fit into the catalytic site, as well as the side chain of benzene present in ritonavir structure, it is also difficult to fit at the active site. These results demonstrate why these compounds have low effectiveness against the SARS-CoV. However, the authors mention that when combined with ribavirin

(166) and corticosteroids, they can reduce the incubation and mortality rates of the virus. As for niclosamide **(160)**, promethazine **(161)**, and PNU **(162)**, similarly to the others, they did not fit well in the active site mainly because they have a very long side chain. Finally, UC2 **(163)** connects in a region far from the active site.

Fig. (31). Potential drugs with activity against SARS-CoV 3CL^{pro}.

A computational approach that produces effective results is pharmacophore modeling, based on the superposition of a set of molecules in which their common characteristics are observed, looking the interactions of a ligand in a binding site, resulting in a three-dimensional (3D) arrangement used to search for compounds that have both structure and similar interactions [115, 116]. This approach has been constantly used in medical chemistry laboratories, especially when it comes to virtual screenings, as well as lead optimization applied in the discovery of new drugs [116].

In this context, using the compounds from previous work and the CMK peptide (Asn-Ser-Thr-Leu-Gln), Zhang and collaborators (2005) [117] developed a 3D-pharmacophore model against SAR-CoV to provide more solid information for designing new drugs. Then, the results were evaluated and applied to the anti-HIV and anti-opportunistic infection chemical compound database, containing approximately 100,000 compounds that have anti-HIV activity and against opportunistic infections. As results, 30 drugs were selected and, only 6 of them presented experimental results against SARS-CoV, such as azauridine **(164)**, pyrazofurin **(165)**, ribavirin **(166)**, 2,3-dideoxycytidine **(167)**, dideoxyganosine **(168)**, and 5-bromo-2-deoxycytidine **(169)**, shown in Fig. **(32)**.

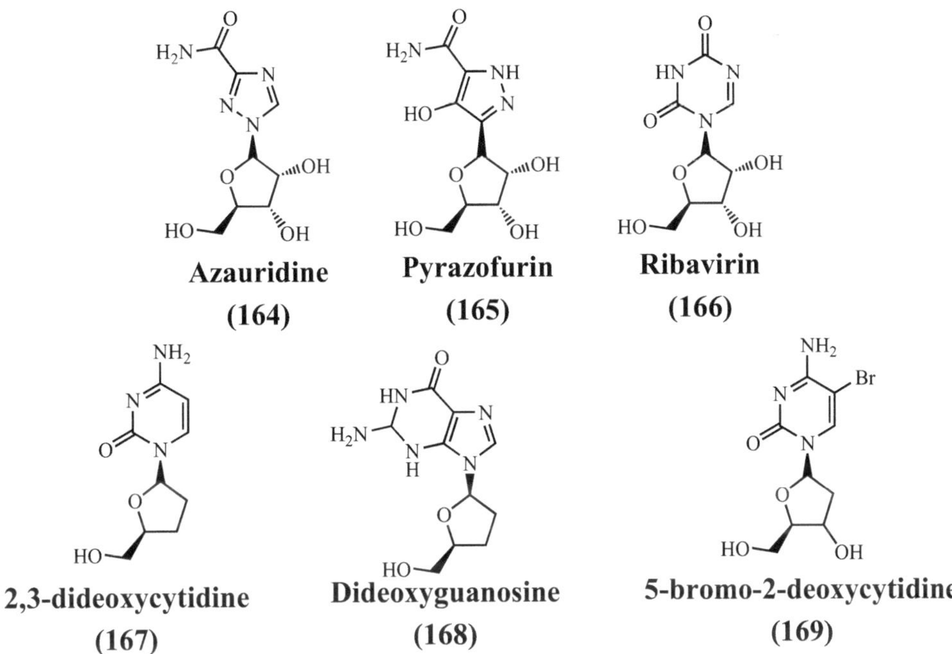

Fig. (32). Compounds identified from the anti-HIV and anti-opportunistic infection chemical compound database.

Other studies have revealed that the ribavirin **(166)** is a promising anti-CoV agent, as well as its combination with interferon-α2b. Thus, Al-Tawfiq and colleagues (2014) conducted a clinical study with the combination of these drugs in five patients infected with MERS-CoV [118]. In three cases, some adverse effects of this combination were observed, such as elevation of pancreatic enzymes and hemolysis, as well as laboratory abnormalities. Despite these effects, and due to the urgent need to find a treatment for this disease, the authors concluded that this combination can be promising if used with caution and with monitoring of adverse effects.

The promising potential of remdesivir **(170)** (Fig. **33**) was investigated by Sheahan and collaborators (2020) against MERS-CoV through *in vitro* and *in vivo* assays [119]. Thus, this drug presented an EC_{50} value of 0.09 µM, with no apparent toxicity at 10 µM, and SI >100. In mice, prophylactic and therapeutic use reduced viral load, leading to improved lung function. The results indicate that this drug may be useful in the treatment of infected patients with MERS-CoV, observing a decrease in pathogenesis, as well as a reduction of viral load, showing to be a potential drug that can be added to the therapy of the disease. Another suggestion by the authors was that the combination of lopinavir **(158)** and ritonavir **(159)** may be promising in the treatment. With this promising potential, remdesivir **(170)** was intravenously used, leading the patient recovery. Also, Li and colleagues (2020) conducted to phase III clinical trials in patients with SARS-CoV-2 and then confirmed the promising potential of these drugs [120].

Remdesivir

(170)

Fig. (33). Chemical structure of remdesivir.

As *VS* campaigns are commonly applied to drug repurposing, Xu and coworkers (2020) conducted a molecular docking study on 1,903 compounds approved as drugs obtained from the DrugBank database, as well as by homology studies [95]. All compounds were virtually screened toward SARS-CoV-2 3CL^{pro}. The authors identified that this enzyme is 96% similar to existing SARS-CoV. Thus, a homology model was carried out, as well as the screening of approved drugs. Then, only 15 drugs were selected, where four molecules were performed screened. Finally, nelfinavir **(171)** was identified as a potential drug for the treatment of SARS-CoV-2, so that pitavastatin **(172)**, perampanel **(173)** and praziquantel **(174)**, also showing moderate activity (Fig. **34**).

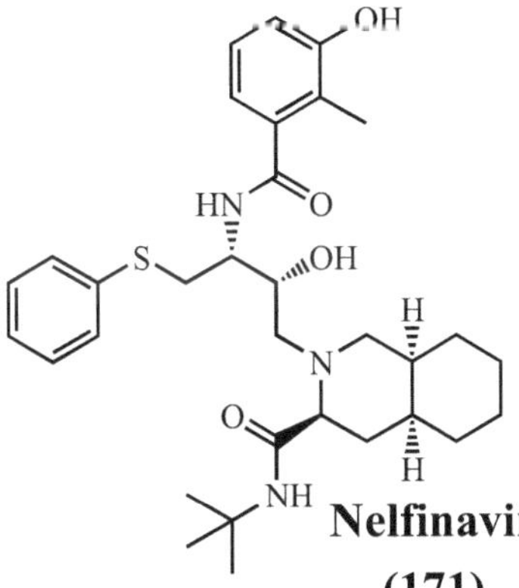

Nelfinavir

(171)

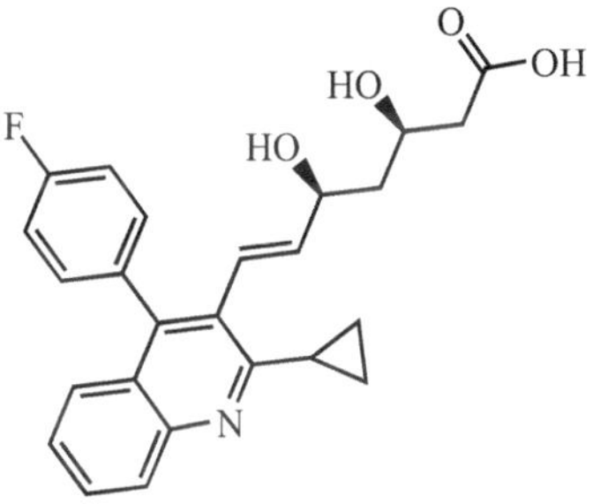

Pitavastatin

(172)

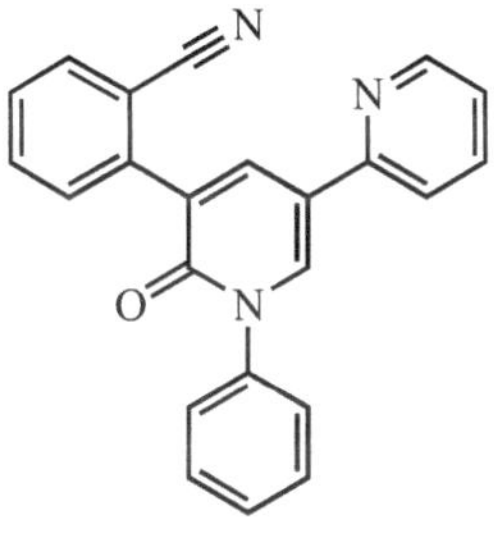

Perampanel

(173)

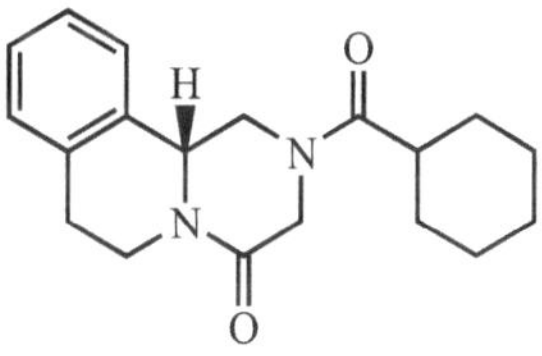

Praziquantel

(174)

Fig. (34). Chemical structures of pitavastatin, perampanel, and praziquantel drugs.

An interesting methodology developed by Zhou and colleagues (2020) was based on the systematic identification of drugs, as well as combinations of drugs that may be useful in repurposing against HCoV, integrating drug-target networks, induction of HCoV transcriptome in human cells, interactions between HCoV and host, and protein-protein interactions (PPI) [121]. Thus, the authors proposed 12 drugs **(175-186)**, as well as three combinations (Sirolimus + dactinomycin; Toremifene + emodin; Melatonin + mercaptopurine) as a potential treatment (Fig. **35**). The authors stated that although the compounds have the possibility of use in treatment, preclinical validation is necessary before being used by patients. Despite this, the study offers a powerful methodology based on a rapid drug identification network that can be repositioned for the treatment of HCoV.

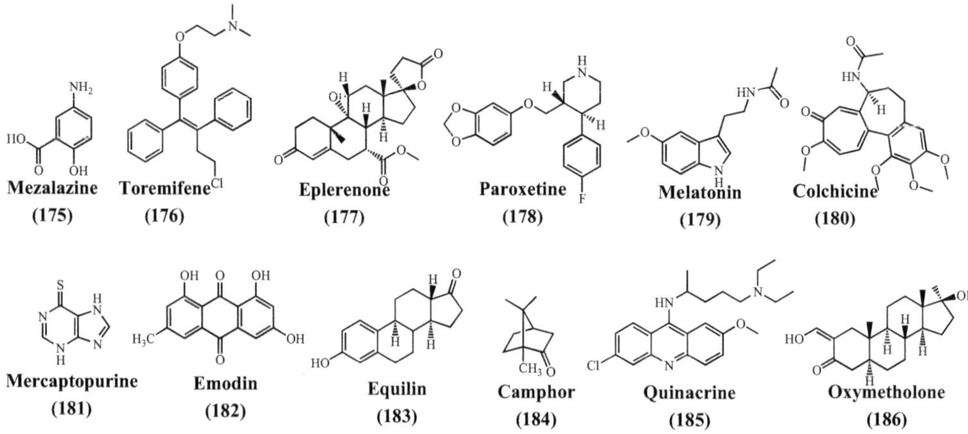

Fig. (35). Compounds identified by Zhou *et al.* 2020.

Instigated to discover new treatments more quickly against CoV, Wang and coworkers (2020) evaluated the effectiveness of seven drugs on the market (Fig. **37**), such as ribavirin **(166)**, nitazoxanide **(187)**, penciclovir **(188)**, nafamostat **(190)** and chloroquine **(191)**, as well as two others with broad-spectrum antiviral activity remdesivir **(170)** and favipiravir **(189)** against a clinical isolate of SARS-CoV-2 [122]. Thus, after evaluating their cytotoxicity in *Vero E6* cells (ATCC-1586), the cells were infected with SARS-CoV-2 for the evaluation of the drugs. The results (Fig. **36**) showed that the most effective compounds in controlling SARS-CoV-2 infection were remdesivir **(170)** and chloroquine **(191)**, suggesting that they can be promising in treatment and should be evaluated in infected patients by CoV. From this perspective, Keyaerts and colleagues (2004) also proposed chloroquine **(191)** as a promising drug against SARS-CoV, presenting an IC$_{50}$ value of 8.8 μM [123]. In addition to this study, others point to nitazoxanide **(187)** as promising in the treatment of some types of viral infections, such as the CoV. Thus, Rossignol and collaborators (2016) through a literature review, showing *in vitro* potential against MERS-CoV for nitazoxanide **(187)**, as well as its pro-inflammatory cytokine and IL-6 inhibitions, and reduction of influenza virus symptoms in humans [124]. So, the authors suggested as potent drug candidates in the treatment of this disease.

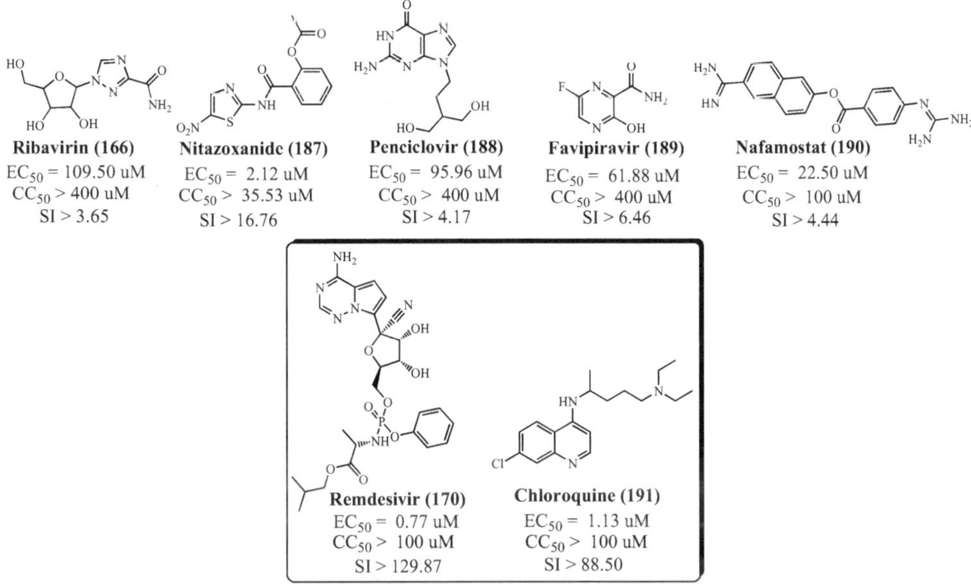

Fig. (36). Compounds identified as promisors against SARS-CoV-2 by Wang *et al.* 2020.

A molecular modeling study by Chen and collaborators (2020) proposed a 3CL^{pro} molecular model for SARS-CoV-2, followed by a virtual screening of drugs used in clinical practice [125]. The compounds used in this screening were obtained from the Drug-lib database, containing approximately 7,173 compounds. Among these 11 compounds **(192-202)** are commercially available drugs (Fig. **37**), and which can be promising in the treatment of CoV.

In the area of drug discovery, an approach that has been gaining prominence is Deep Learning (DL). This approach is a subfield of machine learning (ML), which uses various algorithms and neural networks of artificial intelligence (AI) for analyzing high levels of data [126, 127]. The implementation of methods based in AI, especially DP, can be important in drug discovery, generating a more effective identification in HTS protocols, improving lead optimization by more accurate ADMET and QSAR models, and reducing efforts to discover new compounds [93].

Fig. (37). Compounds identified from the Drug-lib database.

Zhang and coworkers (2020) used an approach based on DL for searching for new active compounds against SARS-CoV-2 [128]. The authors screened several databases of small organic molecules containing FDA-approved drugs, as well as natural compounds that have potential biological activity. From these, nine potential compounds **(203-211)** (Fig. **38**) were identified and they could be promising in the treatment of SARS-CoV-2.

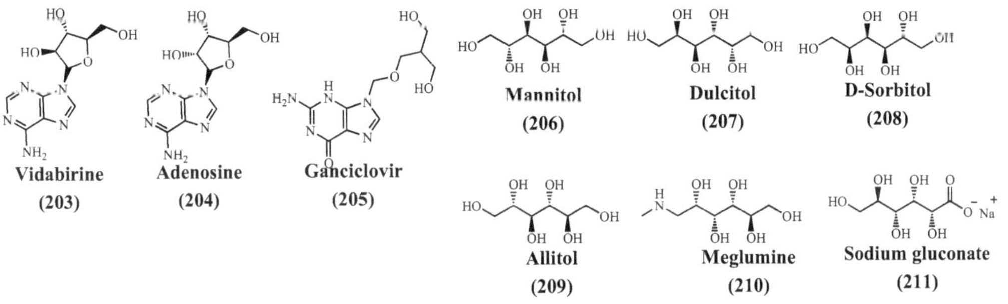

Fig. (38). Compounds identified by using an approach based on DL.

Li and collaborators (2020) carried out a high-throughput *VS* based on a library of 8,000 drugs. This study identified nelfinavir **(171)**, prulifloxacin **(212)**, tegobuvir **(213)**, and bictegravir **(214)** as potentials agents for treating CoV (Fig. **39**) [20]. Additionally, modeling studies suggested that these compounds may have the ability to stop the formation of dimers of the viral protein, as well as blocking the active sites. Finally, the authors suggested that the clinical potential of these molecules can be explored for the treatment of CoV.

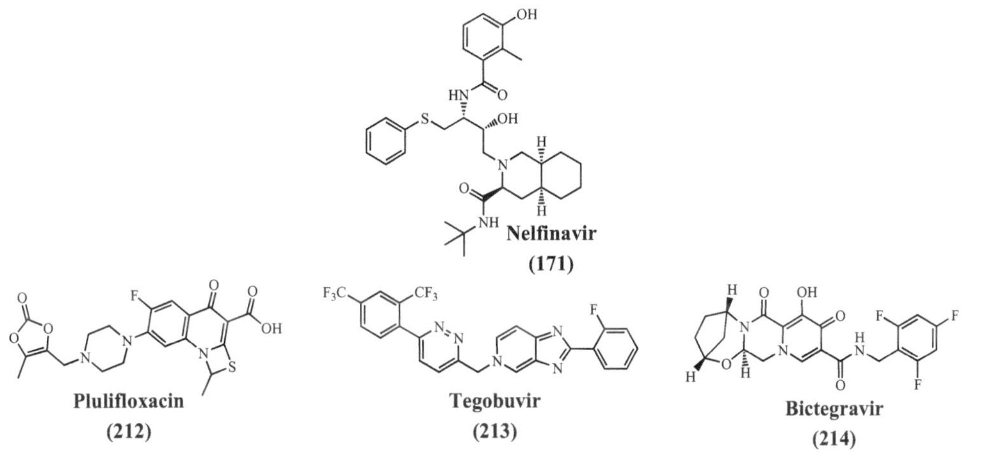

Fig. (39). Chemical structures of nelfinavir (171), prulifloxacin (212), tegobuvir (213), and bictegravir (214).

Wilde and coworkers (2017) investigated the inhibitory potential of the alisporivir **(215)** (Fig. **40**) against the replication of MERS- and SARS-CoV in cell cultures, showing that it could be a potent and broad-spectrum inhibitor, with EC_{50} values ranging from 1.5 to 8.3 µM in different cell lines, and acting in the inhibition of alpha- and beta-CoV [129]. However, the authors suggested that further studies should be carried out to elucidate this mechanism of action. Another drug that had its activity against MERS-CoV and SARS-CoV PL^{pro} enzymes is disulfiram **(216)** (Fig. **40**). In a study conducted by Lin and colleagues (2018) was demonstrated that this compound acts as a non-competitive and competitive (or mixed) inhibitor for MERS- and SARS-CoV, respectively [130]. Additionally, the authors proposed that the inhibition of SARS-CoV PL^{pro} is a covalent interaction with the Cys^{112} residue.

Alisporivir

(215)

Dissulfiram

(216)

Fig. (40). Chemical structures of alisporivir and disulfiram.

High-Throughput Screening (HTS) for Discovering New Antiviral Agents

The HTS has been evolving since the 90s, constituting a powerful tool in the identification of new hits compounds [131 - 133]. This approach is based on biochemical assays against large compound libraries, with the possibility of testing approximately 20,000 compounds *per* week against enzyme targets, providing fast and effective results [134, 135]. It has great importance for the identification of new compounds, given that the synthesis and combinatorial chemistry leads to the production of several compounds, being necessary the HTS assays for the quick evaluation of the molecules, and can also reduce costs related to the discovery of new drugs [136].

Using this approach, Blanchard and coworkers (2004) described a HTS procedure in a library of approximately 50,000 compounds [137]. Initially, 572 compounds were identified on the primary screening, being categorized into 126 groups based on their molecular similarity. The most active compound from each group was selected for a second screening. For the remaining compounds, a dose-response curve was performed at 100 μM of the substrate and 1 μM 3CL^{pro}, using 90– 00 μM of the compounds, in which 72 molecules presented good results and 54 did not present satisfactory results. From these 72 compounds, a test was carried out in the presence of BSA to eliminate non-specific inhibitors that may show "promiscuous" activity. In this sense, three molecules were discarded, resulting in 69 potential drug candidates. Thus, five compounds **(217-221)** were identified (Fig. **41**) with activity against SARS-CoV 3CL^{pro}, with IC$_{50}$ values ranging from 0.5 to 7 μM.

MAC - 5576

(217)

IC$_{50}$ = 0.5 ± 0.3 uM

MAC - 8120

(218)

IC$_{50}$ = 4.3 ± 0.5 uM

MAC - 13985

(219)

IC$_{50}$ = 7.0 ± 2.0 uM

MAC - 22272

(220)

IC$_{50}$ = 2.6 ± 0.4 uM

MAC - 30731

(221)

IC$_{50}$ = 7.0 ± 3.0 uM

Fig. (41). Thiophene, thiazolidine, and furan derivatives as promising anti-SARS-CoV 3CL^{pro} agents.

The study conducted by Liu and collaborators (2005) was an HTS campaign in a library of 1000 commercially available compounds [138]. After this procedure, it was detected that the compounds nelfinavir **(171)**, hexachlorophene **(222)**, and triclosan **(223)** (Fig. **42**) showed potential activity against 3CL^{pro}. Hexachlorophene **(222)** showed to be the most promising, with an IC$_{50}$ value of 5 μM. The other compounds had lower potency, with IC$_{50}$ values of 75 and 46 μM, respectively. Given these results, a docking study was carried out, showing that the main interactions of hexachlorophene **(222)** are hydrogen bonding interactions with Glu^{166}, His^{163}, Cys^{145}, Ser^{144}, and Asn^{142}. Additionally, the authors modified the hexachlorophene **(222)**, obtaining nine new compounds **(224-232)**, with IC$_{50}$ values ranging from 7.6 to 84.5 μM (Fig. **43**). Thus, compounds HL-5 and HL-6 were the most promising (IC$_{50}$= 9.2 and 7.6 μM, respectively), generating new scaffolding for the design of new $3CL^{pro}$ inhibitors.

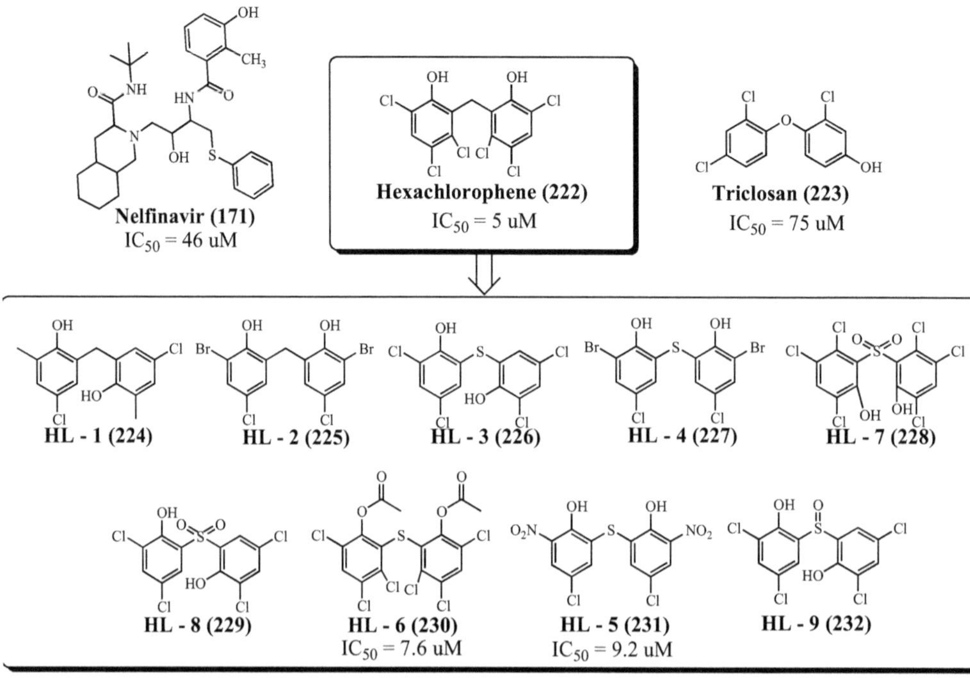

Fig. (42). Compounds identified by Liu *et al.* 2005.

Ge and coworkers (2008) used HTS assay under the replicon (BHK cell line) and SARS-CoV cell line to identify new antiviral compounds that could be promising in the treatment of CoV [139]. The assays were performed against a library of 7,035 compounds, where seven compounds **(233-239)** (Fig. **43**) were found to be promising, with IC_{50} values ranging from 1.4 to 5.8 μM against BHK, and 3.2-11.3 μM against SARS-CoV (*Vero* cells).

Replicon (BHK-233) $IC_{50} = 3.1 \pm 0.19$ uM
SARS-CoV (Vero) $IC_{50} = 7.3 \pm 2.09$ uM

Replicon (BHK-234) $IC_{50} = 5.8 \pm 0.31$ uM
SARS-CoV (Vero) $IC_{50} = 4.5 \pm 1.31$ uM

Replicon (BHK-235) $IC_{50} = 3.2 \pm 0.37$ uM
SARS-CoV (Vero) $IC_{50} = 11.3 \pm 2.56$ uM

Replicon (BHK-236) $IC_{50} = 2.0 \pm 0.45$ uM
SARS-CoV (Vero) $IC_{50} = 8.9 \pm 1.17$ uM

Replicon (BHK-237) $IC_{50} = 2.1 \pm 0.09$ uM
SARS-CoV (Vero) $IC_{50} = 7.6 \pm 1.21$ uM

Replicon (BHK-238) $IC_{50} = 1.4 \pm 0.11$ uM
SARS-CoV (Vero) $IC_{50} = 3.2 \pm 1.97$ uM

Replicon (BHK-239) $IC_{50} = 2.1 \pm 0.16$ uM
SARS-CoV (Vero) $IC_{50} = 6.8 \pm 1.87$ uM

Fig. (43). BHK compounds identified as promising anti-SARS-CoV agents.

The strategy used by Jacobs and collaborators (2012) was to carry out an HTS campaign followed by the structural optimization of the hit compound (Fig. **44**) for the discovery of new compounds against CoV [140]. The HTS assays were carried out against 3CL[pro] in a library containing approximately 293,000 compounds, where from the 44 most active molecules, the compound **(240)** was identified as the most promising candidate. Structural modifications were proposed, generating a new series of 80 compounds, where the compounds **(241-242)** were found to be the most active. Through the crystallographic analysis, it was determined that the main interactions of compound **(241)** occurs with the residues of His[163] and Gly[143] amino acid residues, being proposed a new series of

10 compounds. In contrast, they did not show satisfactory activity. Thus, it was proposed to separate the compound **(241)** enantiomers, showing that the (*R*)-enantiomer **(244)** shows activity and it is a modest non-covalent inhibitor of 3CL^{pro}.

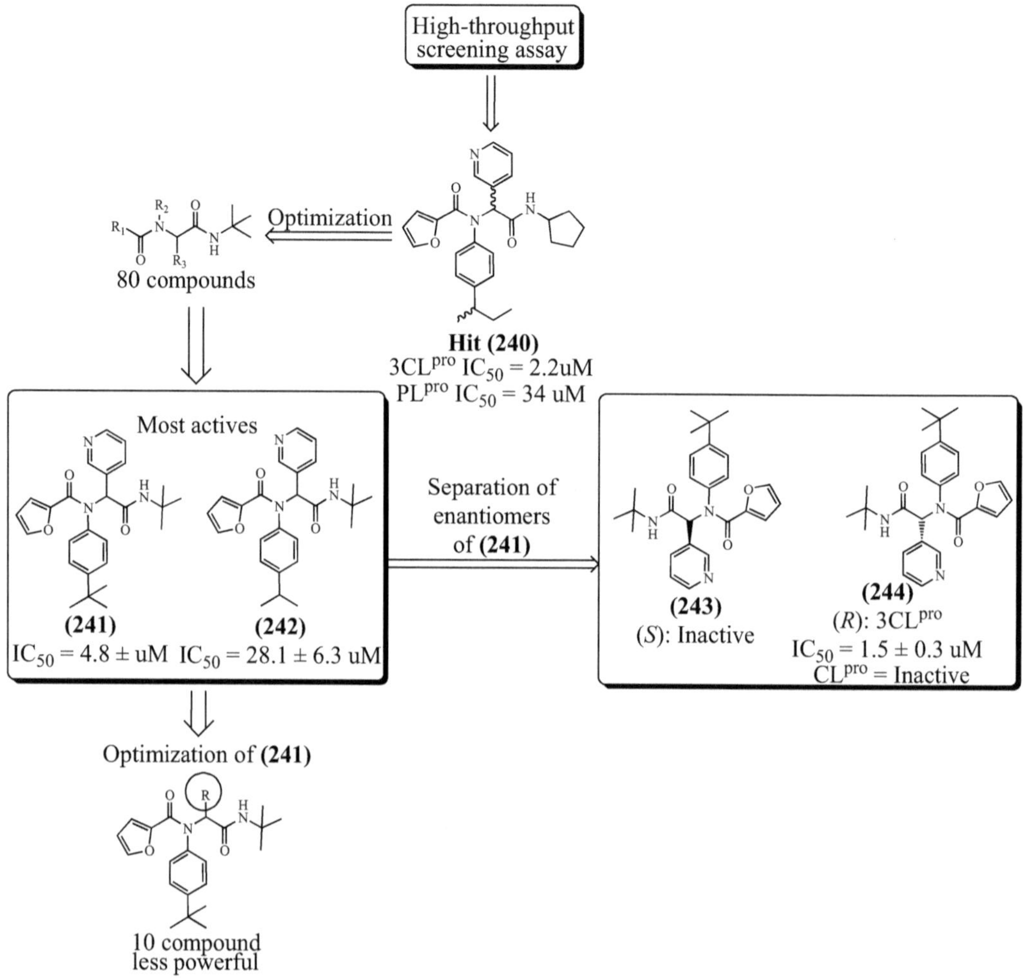

Fig. (44). Discovery of compound (244) (*R*)-enantiomer.

Based on an HTS study, Lee and collaborators (2019) applied this procedure to PL^{pro} in different databases (FDA-approved Prestwick, Maybridge, and Chembridge libraries) containing approximately 30,000 compounds, selecting only those approved by the FDA [141]. Of these compounds, 48 molecules that showed inhibitory activity against MERS-CoV PL^{pro} above 35% at 50 μM concentration were selected for the second analysis, based on the visual inspection of the compounds in which those that had reactive groups and that could generate toxicity were eliminated. Thus, 30 compounds were tested in triplicates, where 23 molecules were selected for the validation of the HTS procedure through the dose-response curve. The compounds showed IC_{50} values ranging from 20 to 125 μM (Fig. **45**). Compounds **(245)** and **(251)** were identified as the most promising analogs, with IC_{50} values of 25 and 20 μM, respectively. Instigated to improve the activity of the compound **(251)**, the authors performed screening in a library of small fragments to increase the inhibitory capacity of this compound. From the 352 fragments, 11 showed an inhibitory activity above 60%, and 5 fragments increased the activity of the compound **(251)**, being its combination with ZT626 **(255)** that improved significantly the activity through additive effect.

Fig. (45). Compounds identified by Lee *et al.* 2019.

CONCLUSION AND FUTURE OUTLOOK

Newly declared SARS-CoV-2 pandemic represents a global health emergency, which is having severe consequences for the lives of infected individuals, as well as an economic recession of worldwide proportions since China is a strategic country for the productive architecture of all continents. This worldwide problem is aggravated by the fact that currently there is no pharmacological treatment available on the market, as well as licensed antiviral vaccines. However, several studies demonstrated in this chapter, whether related to natural, synthetic or computational chemistry, present promising molecules, with low toxicity and addressed to enzymatic targets, which represent a trend in selectivity.

The emerging pandemic generates an urgent need for new treatments, and it is evident that the drug repurposing strategy is the most used by research groups worldwide, as it generates satisfactory results, at a lower financial cost, given that most studies use virtual screening among libraries containing drugs known in clinical practice that are safe for use in humans, providing faster results and immediate application.

Among the repurposed drugs, hopes for a cure against the SARS-CoV-2 are deposited in drugs of class antivirals and antimalarials, such as remdesivir, nelfinavir, hydroxychloroquine, chloroquine, favipiravir, and others, representing drugs undergoing clinical trials, in which the hopes of health agencies around the world are placed. In this way, in the medium and long term, the SARS-CoV-2 outbreak, as well as SARS and MERS demonstrate that it is necessary to reach broad-spectrum antiviral agents as soon as possible, as well as the development of vaccines for the prophylaxis of these infections. Finally, we believe that this review will be essentially important for designing and developing new antiviral molecules, especially enzyme inhibitors, that could be more effective, safe, selective, and low-costs of production.

CONSENT FOR PUBLICATION

Not applicable.

CONFLICT OF INTEREST

The authors confirm that this chapter content has no conflict of interest.

ACKNOWLEDGEMENTS

The authors thank to Coordenação de Aperfeiçoamento Pessoal de Nível Superior (CAPES), National Council for Scientific and Technological Development (CNPq), Fundação de Amparo à Pesquisa do Estado de Alagoas (FAPEAL), and

Financier of Studies and Projects (FINEP) for their support to the Post-Graduate Program in Chemistry and Biotechnology (PPGQB).

REFERENCES

[1] Azhar EI, Hui DSC, Memish ZA, Drosten C, Zumla A. The Middle East Respiratory Syndrome (MERS). Infect Dis Clin North Am 2019; 33(4): 891-905.
[http://dx.doi.org/10.1016/j.idc.2019.08.001] [PMID: 31668197]

[2] Khan G, Sheek-Hussein M. Chapter 8 - The Middle East Respiratory Syndrome Coronavirus: An Emerging Virus of Global Threat. In: Ennaji MM, Ed. Emerging and Reemerging Viral Pathogens. Cambridge: Academic Press 2020; pp 151-67

[3] Chapter 24-Coronaviridae. Fenner's Veterinary Virology Fifth Edition., MacLachlan NJ, Dubovi EJ, Eds. E Publisher: Academic Press 2017; 435-61.
[http://dx.doi.org/10.1016/B978-0-12-800946-8.00024-6]

[4] Báez-Santos YM, St John SE, Mesecar AD. The SARS-coronavirus papain-like protease: structure, function and inhibition by designed antiviral compounds. Antiviral Res 2015; 115: 21-38.
[http://dx.doi.org/10.1016/j.antiviral.2014.12.015] [PMID: 25554382]

[5] WHO Director-General's opening remarks at the media briefing on COVID-19 - 11 March 2020

[6] Chen N, Zhou M, Dong X, *et al.* Epidemiological and clinical characteristics of 99 cases of 2019 novel coronavirus pneumonia in Wuhan, China: a descriptive study. Lancet 2020; 395(10223): 507-13.
[http://dx.doi.org/10.1016/S0140-6736(20)30211-7] [PMID: 32007143]

[7] Kasmi Y, Khataby K, Souiri A, Ennaji MM. Coronaviridae: 100,000 years of emergence and reemergence. Emerg Reemerging Viral Pathog 2020; pp. 127-49.

[8] WHO. https://www.who.int/neglected_diseases/diseases/en/

[9] Li YH, Hu CY, Wu NP, Yao HP, Li LJ. Molecular characteristics, functions, and related pathogenicity of MERS-CoV proteins. Engineering (Beijing) 2019; 5(5): 940-7.
[http://dx.doi.org/10.1016/j.eng.2018.11.035] [PMID: 32288963]

[10] The coronavirus is more dangerous for the economy than SARS - Bloomberg nd 2019.

[11] China's Xi Jinping knew of coronavirus earlier than first thought | Financial Times nd 2019.

[12] Sohrabi C, Alsafi Z, O'Neill N, *et al.* World health organization declares global emergency: A review of the 2019 novel coronavirus (COVID-19). Int J Surg 2020; 76: 71-6.https://doi.org/https://doi.org/10.1016/j.ijsu.2020.02.034
[http://dx.doi.org/10.1016/j.ijsu.2020.02.034] [PMID: 32112977]

[13] Pillaiyar T, Meenakshisundaram S, Manickam M. Recent discovery and development of inhibitors targeting coronaviruses. Drug Discov Today 2020; 25(4): 668-88.
[http://dx.doi.org/10.1016/j.drudis.2020.01.015] [PMID: 32006468]

[14] Gao K, Nguyen DD, Wang R, Wei G-W. Machine intelligence design of 2019-nCoV drugs 2020; 2507: 1-9.

[15] Lu H. Drug treatment options for the 2019-new coronavirus (2019-nCoV). Biosci Trends 2020; 14(1): 69-71.
[http://dx.doi.org/10.5582/bst.2020.01020] [PMID: 31996494]

[16] RCSB PDB - 6LU7: The crystal structure of COVID-19 main protease in complex with an inhibitor N3 nd 2019.

[17] Malik YS, Sircar S, Bhat S, *et al.* Emerging novel coronavirus (2019-nCoV)-current scenario, evolutionary perspective based on genome analysis and recent developments. Vet Q 2020; 40(1): 68-76.
[http://dx.doi.org/10.1080/01652176.2020.1727993] [PMID: 32036774]

[18]   Beigel JH, Nam HH, Adams PL, *et al.* Advances in respiratory virus therapeutics - A meeting report from the 6th isirv Antiviral Group conference. Antiviral Res 2019; 167: 45-67.
[http://dx.doi.org/10.1016/j.antiviral.2019.04.006] [PMID: 30974127]

[19]   Huang C, Wang Y, Li X, *et al.* Clinical features of patients infected with 2019 novel coronavirus in Wuhan, China. Lancet 2020; 395(10223): 497-506.
[http://dx.doi.org/10.1016/S0140-6736(20)30183-5] [PMID: 31986264]

[20]   Li Y, Zhang J, Wang N, *et al.* Therapeutic drugs targeting 2019-ncov main protease by high-throughput screening. BioRxiv 2020; 922922.

[21]   Kruse RL. Therapeutic strategies in an outbreak scenario to treat the novel coronavirus originating in Wuhan, China. F1000 Res 2020; 9: 72.
[http://dx.doi.org/10.12688/f1000research.22211.2] [PMID: 32117569]

[22]   Momattin H, Al-Ali AY, Al-Tawfiq JA. A systematic review of therapeutic agents for the treatment of the middle east respiratory syndrome coronavirus (MERS-CoV). Travel Med Infect Dis 2019; 30: 9-18.
[http://dx.doi.org/10.1016/j.tmaid.2019.06.012] [PMID: 31252170]

[23]   Hu CS, Tkebuchava T. SARS and its treatment strategies. Asian Pac J Trop Med 2019; 12: 95-7.
[http://dx.doi.org/10.4103/1995-7645.254934]

[24]   Veljkovic V, Vergara-Alert J, Segalés J, Paessler S. Use of the informational spectrum methodology for rapid biological analysis of the novel coronavirus 2019-nCoV: prediction of potential receptor, natural reservoir, tropism and therapeutic/vaccine target. F1000 Res 2020; 9: 52.
[http://dx.doi.org/10.12688/f1000research.22149.3] [PMID: 32419926]

[25]   Jin Y-H, Cai L, Cheng Z-S, *et al.* A rapid advice guideline for the diagnosis and treatment of 2019 novel coronavirus (2019-nCoV) infected pneumonia (standard version). Mil Med Res 2020; 7(1): 4.
[http://dx.doi.org/10.1186/s40779-020-0233-6] [PMID: 32029004]

[26]   Chang L, Yan Y, Wang L. Coronavirus disease 2019: Coronaviruses and blood safety. Transfus Med Rev 2020; 34(2): 75-80.https://doi.org/https://doi.org/10.1016/j.tmrv.2020.02.003
[http://dx.doi.org/10.1016/j.tmrv.2020.02.003] [PMID: 32107119]

[27]   Lai CC, Liu YH, Wang CY, *et al.* Asymptomatic carrier state, acute respiratory disease, and pneumonia due to severe acute respiratory syndrome coronavirus 2 (SARS-CoV-2): Facts and myths. J Microbiol Immunol Infect 2020; 53(3): 404-12.
[http://dx.doi.org/10.1016/j.jmii.2020.02.012] [PMID: 32173241]

[28]   Rothan HA, Byrareddy SN. The epidemiology and pathogenesis of coronavirus disease (COVID-19) outbreak. J Autoimmun 2020; 109: 102433. https://doi.org/https://doi.org/10.1016/j.jaut.2020.102433
[http://dx.doi.org/10.1016/j.jaut.2020.102433] [PMID: 32113704]

[29]   Lupia T, Scabini S, Mornese Pinna S, Di Perri G, De Rosa FG, Corcione S. 2019 novel coronavirus (2019-nCoV) outbreak: A new challenge. J Glob Antimicrob Resist 2020; 21: 22-7.
[http://dx.doi.org/10.1016/j.jgar.2020.02.021] [PMID: 32156648]

[30]   Lai C-C, Shih T-P, Ko W-C, Tang H-J, Hsueh P-R. Severe acute respiratory syndrome coronavirus 2 (SARS-CoV-2) and coronavirus disease-2019 (COVID-19): The epidemic and the challenges. Int J Antimicrob Agents 2020; 55(3): 105924.
[http://dx.doi.org/10.1016/j.ijantimicag.2020.105924] [PMID: 32081636]

[31]   Farooq HZ, Davies E, Ahmad S, *et al.* Middle east respiratory syndrome coronavirus (MERS-CoV) - Surveillance and testing in North England from 2012 to 2019. Int J Infect Dis 2020; 93: 237-44.
[http://dx.doi.org/10.1016/j.ijid.2020.01.043] [PMID: 32004690]

[32]   Tang B, Bragazzi NL, Li Q, Tang S, Xiao Y, Wu J. An updated estimation of the risk of transmission of the novel coronavirus (2019-nCov). Infect Dis Model 2020; 5: 248-55.
[http://dx.doi.org/10.1016/j.idm.2020.02.001] [PMID: 32099934]

[33]   Kumar S. Drug and vaccine design against novel coronavirus (2019-nCoV) spike protein through computational approach. Preprints 2020; 2020020071.

[34]   Yang Y, Peng F, Wang R, *et al.* The deadly coronaviruses: The 2003 SARS pandemic and the 2020 novel coronavirus epidemic in China. J Autoimmun 2020; 109: 102434.
[http://dx.doi.org/10.1016/j.jaut.2020.102434] [PMID: 32143990]

[35]   Mizumoto K, Chowell G. Transmission potential of the New Corona (COVID-19) onboard the Princess Cruises Ship, 2020. MedRxiv 2020; 5: 20027649.
[http://dx.doi.org/10.1101/2020.02.24.20027649]

[36]   Li X, Geng M, Peng Y, Meng L, Lu S. Molecular immune pathogenesis and diagnosis of COVID-19. J Pharm Anal 2020; 10(2): 102-8.
[http://dx.doi.org/10.1016/j.jpha.2020.03.001] [PMID: 32282863]

[37]   Shen M, Zhou Y, Ye J, *et al.* Recent advances and perspectives of nucleic acid detection for coronavirus. J Pharm Anal 2020; 10(2): 97-101.
[http://dx.doi.org/10.1016/j.jpha.2020.02.010] [PMID: 32292623]

[38]   Xie C, Jiang L, Huang G, *et al.* Comparison of different samples for 2019 novel coronavirus detection by nucleic acid amplification tests. Int J Infect Dis 2020; 93: 264-7.
[http://dx.doi.org/10.1016/j.ijid.2020.02.050] [PMID: 32114193]

[39]   Phan T. Novel coronavirus: From discovery to clinical diagnostics. Infect Genet Evol 2020; 79: 104211.
[http://dx.doi.org/10.1016/j.meegid.2020.104211] [PMID: 32007627]

[40]   Al-Tawfiq JA, Memish ZA. Diagnosis of SARS-CoV-2 infection based on CT scan vs RT-PCR: reflecting on experience from MERS-CoV. J Hosp Infect 2020; 105(2): 154-5.
[http://dx.doi.org/10.1016/j.jhin.2020.03.001] [PMID: 32147407]

[41]   Cordes AK, Heim A. Rapid random access detection of the novel SARS-coronavirus-2 (SARS-CoV-2, previously 2019-nCoV) using an open access protocol for the Panther Fusion. J Clin Virol 2020; 125: 104305.
[http://dx.doi.org/10.1016/j.jcv.2020.104305] [PMID: 32143123]

[42]   Rebensburg S, Helfer M, Schneider M, *et al.* Potent *in vitro* antiviral activity of Cistus incanus extract against HIV and Filoviruses targets viral envelope proteins. Sci Rep 2016; 6: 20394.
[http://dx.doi.org/10.1038/srep20394] [PMID: 26833261]

[43]   Shaikh F, Zhao Y, Alvarez L, *et al.* Structure-Based *In silico* screening identifies a potent ebolavirus inhibitor from a traditional chinese medicine library. J Med Chem 2019; 62(6): 2928-37.
[http://dx.doi.org/10.1021/acs.jmedchem.8b01328] [PMID: 30785281]

[44]   Ling CQ. Traditional chinese medicine is a resource for drug discovery against 2019 novel coronavirus (SARS-CoV-2). J Integr Med 2020; 18(2): 87-8.
[http://dx.doi.org/10.1016/j.joim.2020.02.004] [PMID: 32122812]

[45]   Zhang DH, Wu KL, Zhang X, Deng SQ, Peng B. *In silico* screening of Chinese herbal medicines with the potential to directly inhibit 2019 novel coronavirus. J Integr Med 2020; 18(2): 152-8.
[http://dx.doi.org/10.1016/j.joim.2020.02.005] [PMID: 32113846]

[46]   Cinatl J, Morgenstern B, Bauer G, Chandra P, Rabenau H, Doerr HW. Glycyrrhizin, an active component of liquorice roots, and replication of SARS-associated coronavirus. Lancet 2003; 361(9374): 2045-6.
[http://dx.doi.org/10.1016/S0140-6736(03)13615-X] [PMID: 12814717]

[47]   Chen F, Chan KH, Jiang Y, *et al. In vitro* susceptibility of 10 clinical isolates of SARS coronavirus to selected antiviral compounds. J Clin Virol 2004; 31(1): 69-75.
[http://dx.doi.org/10.1016/j.jcv.2004.03.003] [PMID: 15288617]

[48]   Li SY, Chen C, Zhang HQ, *et al.* Identification of natural compounds with antiviral activities against

SARS-associated coronavirus. Antiviral Res 2005; 67(1): 18-23.
[http://dx.doi.org/10.1016/j.antiviral.2005.02.007] [PMID: 15885816]

[49]   Mishra A, Behura A, Mawatwal S, *et al.* Structure-function and application of plant lectins in disease biology and immunity. Food Chem Toxicol 2019; 134: 110827.
[http://dx.doi.org/10.1016/j.fct.2019.110827] [PMID: 31542433]

[50]   Ribeiro AC, Ferreira R, Freitas R. Chapter 1-Plant Lectins: Bioactivities and Bioapplications. Studies in Natural Products Chemistry. 1st ed. Elsevier B.V. 2018; pp. 1-42.

[51]   Mitchell CA, Ramessar K, O'Keefe BR. Antiviral lectins: Selective inhibitors of viral entry. Antiviral Res 2017; 142: 37-54.
[http://dx.doi.org/10.1016/j.antiviral.2017.03.007] [PMID: 28322922]

[52]   Kaur R, Neetu , Mudgal R, Jose J, Kumar P, Tomar S. Glycan-dependent chikungunya viral infection divulged by antiviral activity of NAG specific chi-like lectin. Virology 2019; 526: 91-8.
[http://dx.doi.org/10.1016/j.virol.2018.10.009] [PMID: 30388630]

[53]   Keyaerts E, Vijgen L, Pannecouque C, *et al.* Plant lectins are potent inhibitors of coronaviruses by interfering with two targets in the viral replication cycle. Antiviral Res 2007; 75(3): 179-87.
[http://dx.doi.org/10.1016/j.antiviral.2007.03.003] [PMID: 17428553]

[54]   Kim HY, Shin HS, Park H, *et al. In vitro* inhibition of coronavirus replications by the traditionally used medicinal herbal extracts, Cimicifuga rhizoma, Meliae cortex, Coptidis rhizoma, and Phellodendron cortex. J Clin Virol 2008; 41(2): 122-8.
[http://dx.doi.org/10.1016/j.jcv.2007.10.011] [PMID: 18036887]

[55]   Ryu YB, Jeong HJ, Kim JH, *et al.* Biflavonoids from Torreya nucifera displaying SARS-CoV 3CL(pro) inhibition. Bioorg Med Chem 2010; 18(22): 7940-7.
[http://dx.doi.org/10.1016/j.bmc.2010.09.035] [PMID: 20934345]

[56]   Galasiti Kankanamalage AC, Kim Y, Damalanka VC, *et al.* Structure-guided design of potent and permeable inhibitors of MERS coronavirus 3CL protease that utilize a piperidine moiety as a novel design element. Eur J Med Chem 2018; 150: 334-46.
[http://dx.doi.org/10.1016/j.ejmech.2018.03.004] [PMID: 29544147]

[57]   Lim L, Gupta G, Roy A, *et al.* Structurally- and dynamically-driven allostery of the chymotrypsin-like proteases of SARS, Dengue and Zika viruses. Prog Biophys Mol Biol 2019; 143: 52-66.
[http://dx.doi.org/10.1016/j.pbiomolbio.2018.08.009] [PMID: 30217495]

[58]   Park JY, Kim JH, Kim YM, *et al.* Tanshinones as selective and slow-binding inhibitors for SARS-CoV cysteine proteases. Bioorg Med Chem 2012; 20(19): 5928-35.
[http://dx.doi.org/10.1016/j.bmc.2012.07.038] [PMID: 22884354]

[59]   Park JY, Kim JH, Kwon JM, *et al.* Dieckol, a SARS-CoV 3CL(pro) inhibitor, isolated from the edible brown algae Ecklonia cava. Bioorg Med Chem 2013; 21(13): 3730-7.
[http://dx.doi.org/10.1016/j.bmc.2013.04.026] [PMID: 23647823]

[60]   Kim DE, Min JS, Jang MS, *et al.* Natural bis-benzylisoquinoline alkaloids-tetrandrine, fangchinoline, and cepharanthine, inhibit human coronavirus oc43 infection of mrc-5 human lung cells. Biomolecules 2019; 9(11): E696.
[http://dx.doi.org/10.3390/biom9110696] [PMID: 31690059]

[61]   Semwal DK, Badoni R, Semwal R, Kothiyal SK, Singh GJP, Rawat U. The genus stephania (Menispermaceae): Chemical and pharmacological perspectives. J Ethnopharmacol 2010; 132(2): 369-83.
[http://dx.doi.org/10.1016/j.jep.2010.08.047] [PMID: 20801207]

[62]   Wang ST, Qian WQ, He P, Feng MQ, Kang Y, Wang YQ, *et al.* Two new glycoalkaloids from Stephania succifera. Phytochem Lett 2019; 34: 99-102.
[http://dx.doi.org/10.1016/j.phytol.2019.10.001]

[63]   Wang R, Liu Y, Shi G, *et al.* Bioactive bisbenzylisoquinoline alkaloids from the roots of *Stephania*

tetrandra 2020; 98: 103697.
[http://dx.doi.org/10.1016/j.bioorg.2020.103697]

[64]   Keck JG, Wang PH, Lien EJ, Lai MMC. Inhibition of murine coronavirus RNA synthesis by hydroxyguanidine derivatives. Virus Res 1989; 14(1): 57-63.
[http://dx.doi.org/10.1016/0168-1702(89)90069-5] [PMID: 2554614]

[65]   Caliguiri LA, Tamm I. Guanidine. Oxford: Pergamon Press 1972; 1: pp. 181-230.

[66]   Martina E, Stiefl N, Degel B, *et al.* Screening of electrophilic compounds yields an aziridinyl peptide as new active-site directed SARS-CoV main protease inhibitor. Bioorg Med Chem Lett 2005; 15(24): 5365-9.
[http://dx.doi.org/10.1016/j.bmcl.2005.09.012] [PMID: 16216498]

[67]   Chen LR, Wang YC, Lin YW, *et al.* Synthesis and evaluation of isatin derivatives as effective SARS coronavirus 3CL protease inhibitors. Bioorg Med Chem Lett 2005; 15(12): 3058-62.
[http://dx.doi.org/10.1016/j.bmcl.2005.04.027] [PMID: 15896959]

[68]   Shie JJ, Fang JM, Kuo TH, *et al.* Inhibition of the severe acute respiratory syndrome 3CL protease by peptidomimetic α,β-unsaturated esters. Bioorg Med Chem 2005; 13(17): 5240-52.
[http://dx.doi.org/10.1016/j.bmc.2005.05.065] [PMID: 15994085]

[69]   Xu Z, Zhao SJ, Lv ZS, *et al.* Fluoroquinolone-isatin hybrids and their biological activities. Eur J Med Chem 2019; 162: 396-406.
[http://dx.doi.org/10.1016/j.ejmech.2018.11.032] [PMID: 30453247]

[70]   Chou CY, Chien CH, Han YS, *et al.* Thiopurine analogues inhibit papain-like protease of severe acute respiratory syndrome coronavirus. Biochem Pharmacol 2008; 75(8): 1601-9.
[http://dx.doi.org/10.1016/j.bcp.2008.01.005] [PMID: 18313035]

[71]   Parmet S. Childhood Leukemia. The Journal of the American Medical Association 2004; 291(4): 514.
[http://dx.doi.org/10.1001/jama.291.4.514]

[72]   Lee C, Lee JM, Lee NR, *et al.* Aryl diketoacids (ADK) selectively inhibit duplex DNA-unwinding activity of SARS coronavirus NTPase/helicase. Bioorg Med Chem Lett 2009; 19(6): 1636-8.
[http://dx.doi.org/10.1016/j.bmcl.2009.02.010] [PMID: 19233643]

[73]   Keum YS, Jeong YJ. Development of chemical inhibitors of the SARS coronavirus: viral helicase as a potential target. Biochem Pharmacol 2012; 84(10): 1351-8.
[http://dx.doi.org/10.1016/j.bcp.2012.08.012] [PMID: 22935448]

[74]   Yang CW, Lee YZ, Kang IJ, *et al.* Identification of phenanthroindolizines and phenanthroquinolizidines as novel potent anti-coronaviral agents for porcine enteropathogenic coronavirus transmissible gastroenteritis virus and human severe acute respiratory syndrome coronavirus. Antiviral Res 2010; 88(2): 160-8.
[http://dx.doi.org/10.1016/j.antiviral.2010.08.009] [PMID: 20727913]

[75]   Sen S, Chakraborty R. Revival, modernization and integration of Indian traditional herbal medicine in clinical practice: Importance, challenges and future. J Tradit Complement Med 2016; 7(2): 234-44.
[http://dx.doi.org/10.1016/j.jtcme.2016.05.006] [PMID: 28417092]

[76]   Balasubramanian G, Sarathi M, Kumar SR, Hameed ASS. Screening the antiviral activity of Indian medicinal plants against white spot syndrome virus in shrimp. Aquaculture 2007; 263: 15-9.
[http://dx.doi.org/10.1016/j.aquaculture.2006.09.037]

[77]   Zhao Z, Dai X, Li C, *et al.* Pyrazolone structural motif in medicinal chemistry: Retrospect and prospect. Eur J Med Chem 2020; 186: 111893.
[http://dx.doi.org/10.1016/j.ejmech.2019.111893] [PMID: 31761383]

[78]   Ramajayam R, Tan KP, Liu HG, Liang PH. Synthesis and evaluation of pyrazolone compounds as SARS-coronavirus 3C-like protease inhibitors. Bioorg Med Chem 2010; 18(22): 7849-54.
[http://dx.doi.org/10.1016/j.bmc.2010.09.050] [PMID: 20947359]

[79]   Kim MK, Yu MS, Park HR, *et al.* 2,6-Bis-arylmethyloxy-5-hydroxychromones with antiviral activity against both hepatitis C virus (HCV) and SARS-associated coronavirus (SCV). Eur J Med Chem 2011; 46(11): 5698-704.
[http://dx.doi.org/10.1016/j.ejmech.2011.09.005] [PMID: 21925774]

[80]   Chuck CP, Chen C, Ke Z, Wan DC, Chow HF, Wong KB. Design, synthesis and crystallographic analysis of nitrile-based broad-spectrum peptidomimetic inhibitors for coronavirus 3C-like proteases. Eur J Med Chem 2013; 59: 1-6.
[http://dx.doi.org/10.1016/j.ejmech.2012.10.053] [PMID: 23202846]

[81]   Ábrányi-Balogh P, Petri L, Imre T, *et al.* A road map for prioritizing warheads for cysteine targeting covalent inhibitors. Eur J Med Chem 2018; 160: 94-107.
[http://dx.doi.org/10.1016/j.ejmech.2018.10.010] [PMID: 30321804]

[82]   Silva DG, Ribeiro JFR, De Vita D, *et al.* A comparative study of warheads for design of cysteine protease inhibitors. Bioorg Med Chem Lett 2017; 27(22): 5031-5.
[http://dx.doi.org/10.1016/j.bmcl.2017.10.002] [PMID: 29054358]

[83]   Prior AM, Kim Y, Weerasekara S, *et al.* Design, synthesis, and bioevaluation of viral 3C and 3C-like protease inhibitors. Bioorg Med Chem Lett 2013; 23(23): 6317-20.
[http://dx.doi.org/10.1016/j.bmcl.2013.09.070] [PMID: 24125888]

[84]   Ku T, Lopresti N, Shirley M, *et al.* Synthesis of distal and proximal fleximer base analogues and evaluation in the nucleocapsid protein of HIV-1. Bioorg Med Chem 2019; 27(13): 2883-92.
[http://dx.doi.org/10.1016/j.bmc.2019.05.019] [PMID: 31126822]

[85]   Peters HL, Jochmans D, de Wilde AH, *et al.* Design, synthesis and evaluation of a series of acyclic fleximer nucleoside analogues with anti-coronavirus activity. Bioorg Med Chem Lett 2015; 25(15): 2923-6.
[http://dx.doi.org/10.1016/j.bmcl.2015.05.039] [PMID: 26048809]

[86]   Kumar V, Tan KP, Wang YM, Lin SW, Liang PH. Identification, synthesis and evaluation of SARS-CoV and MERS-CoV 3C-like protease inhibitors. Bioorg Med Chem 2016; 24(13): 3035-42.
[http://dx.doi.org/10.1016/j.bmc.2016.05.013] [PMID: 27240464]

[87]   Chan HCS, Shan H, Dahoun T, Vogel H, Yuan S. Advancing drug discovery *via* artificial intelligence. Trends Pharmacol Sci 2019; 40(8): 592-604.
[http://dx.doi.org/10.1016/j.tips.2019.06.004] [PMID: 31320117]

[88]   Cerqueira NMFSA, Gesto D, Oliveira EF, *et al.* Receptor-based virtual screening protocol for drug discovery. Arch Biochem Biophys 2015; 582: 56-67.
[http://dx.doi.org/10.1016/j.abb.2015.05.011] [PMID: 26045247]

[89]   Beck KR, Kaserer T, Schuster D, Odermatt A. Virtual screening applications in short-chain dehydrogenase/reductase research. J Steroid Biochem Mol Biol 2017; 171: 157-77.
[http://dx.doi.org/10.1016/j.jsbmb.2017.03.008] [PMID: 28286207]

[90]   Murgueitio MS, Bermudez M, Mortier J, Wolber G. *In silico* virtual screening approaches for anti-viral drug discovery. Drug Discov Today Technol 2012; 9(3): e219-25.
[http://dx.doi.org/10.1016/j.ddtec.2012.07.009] [PMID: 24990575]

[91]   Danishuddin M, Khan AU. Structure based virtual screening to discover putative drug candidates: necessary considerations and successful case studies. Methods 2015; 71: 135-45.
[http://dx.doi.org/10.1016/j.ymeth.2014.10.019] [PMID: 25448480]

[92]   Slater O, Kontoyianni M. The compromise of virtual screening and its impact on drug discovery. Expert Opin Drug Discov 2019; 14(7): 619-37.
[http://dx.doi.org/10.1080/17460441.2019.1604677] [PMID: 31025886]

[93]   Panteleev J, Gao H, Jia L. Recent applications of machine learning in medicinal chemistry. Bioorg Med Chem Lett 2018; 28(17): 2807-15.
[http://dx.doi.org/10.1016/j.bmcl.2018.06.046] [PMID: 30122222]

[94]   Ghosh AK, Xi K, Johnson ME, Baker SC, Mesecar AD. Progress in Anti-SARS Coronavirus Chemistry, Biology and Chemotherapy. Annu Rep Med Chem 2007, 41. 183-96.
[http://dx.doi.org/10.1016/S0065-7743(06)41011-3] [PMID: 19649165]

[95]   Xu Z, Peng C, Shi Y, *et al.* Nelfinavir was predicted to be a potential inhibitor of 2019 nCov main protease by an integrative approach combining homology modelling, molecular docking and binding free energy calculation. bioRxiv 2020.
[http://dx.doi.org/10.1101/2020.01.27.921627]

[96]   Stoermer M. Homology Models of the Papain-Like Protease PLpro from Coronavirus 2019. nCoV 2020.
[http://dx.doi.org/10.26434/chemrxiv.11799705.v1.]

[97]   Pruijssers AJ, Denison MR. Nucleoside analogues for the treatment of coronavirus infections. Curr Opin Virol 2019; 35: 57-62.
[http://dx.doi.org/10.1016/j.coviro.2019.04.002] [PMID: 31125806]

[98]   Chou K-C, Wei D-Q, Zhong W-Z. Binding mechanism of coronavirus main proteinase with ligands and its implication to drug design against SARS. Biochem Biophys Res Commun 2003; 308(1): 148-51.
[http://dx.doi.org/10.1016/S0006-291X(03)01342-1] [PMID: 12890493]

[99]   Niu C, Yin J, Zhang J, Vederas JC, James MNG. Molecular docking identifies the binding of 3-chloropyridine moieties specifically to the S1 pocket of SARS-CoV Mpro. Bioorg Med Chem 2008; 16(1): 293-302.
[http://dx.doi.org/10.1016/j.bmc.2007.09.034] [PMID: 17931870]

[100]   Mukherjee P, Desai P, Ross L, White EL, Avery MA. Structure-based virtual screening against SARS-3CL(pro) to identify novel non-peptidic hits. Bioorg Med Chem 2008; 16(7): 4138-49.
[http://dx.doi.org/10.1016/j.bmc.2008.01.011] [PMID: 18343121]

[101]   Nguyen TT, Ryu HJ, Lee SH, *et al.* Virtual screening identification of novel severe acute respiratory syndrome 3C-like protease inhibitors and *in vitro* confirmation. Bioorg Med Chem Lett 2011; 21(10): 3088-91.
[http://dx.doi.org/10.1016/j.bmcl.2011.03.034] [PMID: 21470860]

[102]   Zhu L, George S, Schmidt MF, Al-Gharabli SI, Rademann J, Hilgenfeld R. Peptide aldehyde inhibitors challenge the substrate specificity of the SARS-coronavirus main protease. Antiviral Res 2011; 92(2): 204-12.
[http://dx.doi.org/10.1016/j.antiviral.2011.08.001] [PMID: 21854807]

[103]   Turlington M, Chun A, Tomar S, *et al.* Discovery of N-(benzo[1,2,3]triazol-1-y-)-N-(benzyl)acetamido)phenyl) carboxamides as severe acute respiratory syndrome coronavirus (SARS-CoV) 3CLpro inhibitors: identification of ML300 and noncovalent nanomolar inhibitors with an induced-fit binding. Bioorg Med Chem Lett 2013; 23(22): 6172-7.
[http://dx.doi.org/10.1016/j.bmcl.2013.08.112] [PMID: 24080461]

[104]   Lee H, Mittal A, Patel K, *et al.* Identification of novel drug scaffolds for inhibition of SARS-CoV 3-Chymotrypsin-like protease using virtual and high-throughput screenings. Bioorg Med Chem 2014; 22(1): 167-77.
[http://dx.doi.org/10.1016/j.bmc.2013.11.041] [PMID: 24332657]

[105]   Wang L, Bao BB, Song GQ, *et al.* Discovery of unsymmetrical aromatic disulfides as novel inhibitors of SARS-CoV main protease: Chemical synthesis, biological evaluation, molecular docking and 3D-QSAR study. Eur J Med Chem 2017; 137: 450-61.
[http://dx.doi.org/10.1016/j.ejmech.2017.05.045] [PMID: 28624700]

[106]   Theerawatanasirikul S, Kuo CJ, Phetcharat N, Lekcharoensuk P. *In silico* and *in vitro* analysis of small molecules and natural compounds targeting the 3CL protease of feline infectious peritonitis virus. Antiviral Res 2020; 174: 104697.
[http://dx.doi.org/10.1016/j.antiviral.2019.104697] [PMID: 31863793]

[107]   Abdallah HH. Theoretical study for the inhibition ability of some bioactive imidazole derivatives against the Middle-East respiratory syndrome corona virus (MERS-Co). Zanco J Pure Appl Sci 2019; 31
[http://dx.doi.org/10.21271/zjpas.31.2.10]

[108]   Mercorelli B, Palù G, Loregian A. Drug Repurposing for Viral Infectious Diseases: How Far Are We? Trends Microbiol 2018; 26(10): 865-76.
[http://dx.doi.org/10.1016/j.tim.2018.04.004] [PMID: 29759926]

[109]   Bellera CL, Balcazar DE, Vanrell MC, *et al.* Computer-guided drug repurposing: identification of trypanocidal activity of clofazimine, benidipine and saquinavir. Eur J Med Chem 2015; 93: 338-48.
[http://dx.doi.org/10.1016/j.ejmech.2015.01.065] [PMID: 25707014]

[110]   Bellera CL, Balcazar DE, Alberca L, Labriola CA, Talevi A, Carrillo C. Application of computer-aided drug repurposing in the search of new cruzipain inhibitors: discovery of amiodarone and bromocriptine inhibitory effects. J Chem Inf Model 2013; 53(9): 2402-8.
[http://dx.doi.org/10.1021/ci400284v] [PMID: 23906322]

[111]   Kumar R, Harilal S, Gupta SV, *et al.* Exploring the new horizons of drug repurposing: A vital tool for turning hard work into smart work. Eur J Med Chem 2019; 182: 111602.
[http://dx.doi.org/10.1016/j.ejmech.2019.111602] [PMID: 31421629]

[112]   Zhavoronkov A, Aladinskiy V, Zhebrak A, Zagribelnyy B, Terentiev V, Bezrukov DS, *et al.* Potential 2019-nCoV 3C-like Protease Inhibitors Designed Using Generative Deep Learning Approaches 2019.
[http://dx.doi.org/10.26434/CHEMRXIV.11829102.V1]

[113]   Mustafa S, Balkhy H, Gabere MN. Current treatment options and the role of peptides as potential therapeutic components for Middle East Respiratory Syndrome (MERS): A review. J Infect Public Health 2018; 11(1): 9-17.
[http://dx.doi.org/10.1016/j.jiph.2017.08.009] [PMID: 28864360]

[114]   Zhang XW, Yap YL. Old drugs as lead compounds for a new disease? Binding analysis of SARS coronavirus main proteinase with HIV, psychotic and parasite drugs. Bioorg Med Chem 2004; 12(10): 2517-21.
[http://dx.doi.org/10.1016/j.bmc.2004.03.035] [PMID: 15110833]

[115]   Wolber G, Seidel T, Bendix F, Langer T. Molecule-pharmacophore superpositioning and pattern matching in computational drug design. Drug Discov Today 2008; 13(1-2): 23-9.
[http://dx.doi.org/10.1016/j.drudis.2007.09.007] [PMID: 18190860]

[116]   Yang SY. Pharmacophore modeling and applications in drug discovery: challenges and recent advances. Drug Discov Today 2010; 15(11-12): 444-50.
[http://dx.doi.org/10.1016/j.drudis.2010.03.013] [PMID: 20362693]

[117]   Zhang XW, Yap YL, Altmeyer RM. Generation of predictive pharmacophore model for SARS-coronavirus main proteinase. Eur J Med Chem 2005; 40(1): 57-62.
[http://dx.doi.org/10.1016/j.ejmech.2004.09.013] [PMID: 15642409]

[118]   Al-Tawfiq JA, Momattin H, Dib J, Memish ZA. Ribavirin and interferon therapy in patients infected with the Middle East respiratory syndrome coronavirus: an observational study. Int J Infect Dis 2014; 20: 42-6.
[http://dx.doi.org/10.1016/j.ijid.2013.12.003] [PMID: 24406736]

[119]   Sheahan TP, Sims AC, Leist SR, *et al.* Comparative therapeutic efficacy of remdesivir and combination lopinavir, ritonavir, and interferon beta against MERS-CoV. Nat Commun 2020; 11(1): 222.
[http://dx.doi.org/10.1038/s41467-019-13940-6] [PMID: 31924756]

[120]   Li G, De Clercq E. Therapeutic options for the 2019 novel coronavirus (2019-nCoV). Nat Rev Drug Discov 2020; 19(3): 149-50.
[http://dx.doi.org/10.1038/d41573-020-00016-0] [PMID: 32127666]

[121] Zhou Y, Hou Y, Shen J, Huang Y, Martin W, Cheng F. Network-based Drug Repurposing for Human Coronavirus 2020.
[http://dx.doi.org/10.1101/2020.02.03.20020263]

[122] Wang M, Cao R, Zhang L, *et al.* Remdesivir and chloroquine effectively inhibit the recently emerged novel coronavirus (2019-nCoV) *in vitro.* Cell Res 2020; 30(3): 269-71.
[http://dx.doi.org/10.1038/s41422-020-0282-0] [PMID: 32020029]

[123] Keyaerts E, Vijgen L, Maes P, Neyts J, Van Ranst M. *In vitro* inhibition of severe acute respiratory syndrome coronavirus by chloroquine. Biochem Biophys Res Commun 2004; 323(1): 264-8.
[http://dx.doi.org/10.1016/j.bbrc.2004.08.085] [PMID: 15351731]

[124] Rossignol JF. Nitazoxanide, a new drug candidate for the treatment of Middle East respiratory syndrome coronavirus. J Infect Public Health 2016; 9(3): 227-30.
[http://dx.doi.org/10.1016/j.jiph.2016.04.001] [PMID: 27095301]

[125] Chen YW, Yiu CB, Wong K. Prediction of the 2019-nCoV 3C-like protease (3CL pro) structure : virtual screening reveals velpatasvir , ledipasvir , and other drug repurposing candidates 2019; 1-15.

[126] Chen H, Engkvist O, Wang Y, Olivecrona M, Blaschke T. The rise of deep learning in drug discovery. Drug Discov Today 2018; 23(6): 1241-50.
[http://dx.doi.org/10.1016/j.drudis.2018.01.039] [PMID: 29366762]

[127] Lavecchia A. Deep learning in drug discovery: opportunities, challenges and future prospects. Drug Discov Today 2019; 24(10): 2017-32.
[http://dx.doi.org/10.1016/j.drudis.2019.07.006] [PMID: 31377227]

[128] Zhang H, Saravanan KM, Yang Y, Hossain T. Deep learning based drug screening for novel coronavirus 2019-nCov 2020; 19: 1-17.

[129] de Wilde AH, Falzarano D, Zevenhoven-Dobbe JC, *et al.* Alisporivir inhibits MERS- and SARS-coronavirus replication in cell culture, but not SARS-coronavirus infection in a mouse model. Virus Res 2017; 228: 7-13.
[http://dx.doi.org/10.1016/j.virusres.2016.11.011] [PMID: 27840112]

[130] Lin MH, Moses DC, Hsieh CH, *et al.* Disulfiram can inhibit MERS and SARS coronavirus papain-like proteases *via* different modes. Antiviral Res 2018; 150: 155-63.
[http://dx.doi.org/10.1016/j.antiviral.2017.12.015] [PMID: 29289665]

[131] Yang ZY, He JH, Lu AP, Hou TJ, Cao DS. Frequent hitters: nuisance artifacts in high-throughput screening. Drug Discov Today 2020; 25(4): 657-67.
[http://dx.doi.org/10.1016/j.drudis.2020.01.014] [PMID: 31987936]

[132] Volochnyuk DM, Ryabukhin SV, Moroz YS, *et al.* Evolution of commercially available compounds for HTS. Drug Discov Today 2019; 24(2): 390-402.
[http://dx.doi.org/10.1016/j.drudis.2018.10.016] [PMID: 30399443]

[133] Cronk D. High-throughput screening. Drug Discov Dev Technol Transit 2013; pp. 95-117.

[134] Rizk MA, El-Sayed SAE, Nassif M, Mosqueda J, Xuan X, Igarashi I. Assay methods for *in vitro* and *in vivo* anti-Babesia drug efficacy testing: Current progress, outlook, and challenges. Vet Parasitol 2020; 279: 109013.
[http://dx.doi.org/10.1016/j.vetpar.2019.109013] [PMID: 32070899]

[135] Deng H, Lei Q, Wu Y, He Y, Li W. Activity-based protein profiling: Recent advances in medicinal chemistry. Eur J Med Chem 2020; 191: 112151.
[http://dx.doi.org/10.1016/j.ejmech.2020.112151] [PMID: 32109778]

[136] Szymański P, Markowicz M, Mikiciuk-Olasik E. Adaptation of high-throughput screening in drug discovery-toxicological screening tests. Int J Mol Sci 2012; 13(1): 427-52.
[http://dx.doi.org/10.3390/ijms13010427] [PMID: 22312262]

[137] Blanchard JE, Elowe NH, Huitema C, *et al.* High-throughput screening identifies inhibitors of the

SARS coronavirus main proteinase. Chem Biol 2004; 11(10): 1445-53.
[http://dx.doi.org/10.1016/j.chembiol.2004.08.011] [PMID: 15489171]

[138]   Liu Y-C, Huang V, Chao T-C, *et al.* Screening of drugs by FRET analysis identifies inhibitors of SARS-CoV 3CL protease. Biochem Biophys Res Commun 2005; 333(1): 194-9.
[http://dx.doi.org/10.1016/j.bbrc.2005.05.095] [PMID: 15950190]

[139]   Ge F, Xiong S, Lin FS, Zhang ZP, Zhang XE. High-throughput assay using a GFP-expressing replicon for SARS-CoV drug discovery. Antiviral Res 2008; 80(2): 107-13.
[http://dx.doi.org/10.1016/j.antiviral.2008.05.005] [PMID: 18584889]

[140]   Jacobs J, Grum-Tokars V, Zhou Y, *et al.* Discovery, synthesis, and structure-based optimization of a series of N-(tert-butyl)-2-(N-arylamido)-2-(pyridin-3-yl) acetamides (ML188) as potent noncovalent small molecule inhibitors of the severe acute respiratory syndrome coronavirus (SARS-CoV) 3CL protease. J Med Chem 2013; 56(2): 534-46.
[http://dx.doi.org/10.1021/jm301580n] [PMID: 23231439]

[141]   Lee H, Ren J, Pesavento RP, *et al.* Identification and design of novel small molecule inhibitors against MERS-CoV papain-like protease *via* high-throughput screening and molecular modeling. Bioorg Med Chem 2019; 27(10): 1981-9.
[http://dx.doi.org/10.1016/j.bmc.2019.03.050] [PMID: 30940566]

CHAPTER 3

Opportunities Offered by Fragment-Based Drug Design in Antibiotic Development

Sanjay Yapabandara[1], Lorna Wilkinson-White[2], Sandro Ataide[1] and Ann H. Kwan[1,*]

[1] *School of Life and Environmental Sciences, University of Sydney, NSW 2006, Australia*

[2] *Sydney Analytical Core Research Facility, University of Sydney, NSW 2006, Australia*

Abstract: In recent years, the discovery of new and effective antibiotics has slowed dramatically due to the rapid and widespread development of bacterial drug resistance and many pharmaceutical companies exiting the field. Reliance on conventional drug discovery methods, while effective in the past, has led to significant present-day challenges that are becoming increasingly difficult to overcome. A fundamental challenge to the development of new antibiotics against multi-drug resistant bacteria is the high cost of development relative to expected revenues. Fragment-based drug design (FBDD), which involves screening low molecular weight ligands, can help to drastically reduce the cost of finding initial hits compared with traditional high-throughput screening (HTS). In addition, a knowledge-driven and multi-pronged approach to the subsequent expansion of amenable fragments into high-affinity inhibitors may assist with overcoming hurdles in the hit-to-lead (H2L) optimisation process. Favourable pharmacological and physicochemical properties, as well as strategies against the development of resistance, can be incorporated as part of the fragment expansion process. This chapter discusses the features of the FBDD approach that are relevant and beneficial for antibiotic development. Successful examples and barriers to progress from hit discovery to H2L development, as well as patents, are presented. Finally, the outlook for FBDD in the field of antibiotic development, including the latest FBDD advances and challenges, is discussed.

Keywords: Antibiotic, Antibacterial, Antimicrobial, Drug design, Drug discovery, Drug lead, FBDD, FBLD, Fragment, Hit-to-lead, H2L, Resistance.

INTRODUCTION

The discovery of antibiotics was one of the most significant medical achievements of the 20th century and has revolutionised modern medicine. However, their widespread overuse and misuse have resulted in the rise of antibacterial resistance

* **Corresponding author Ann H. Kwan:** School of Life and Environmental Sciences, University of Sydney, NSW 2006, Australia; Tel: +612 93513911; Email: ann.kwan@sydney.edu.au

Atta-ur-Rahman and M. Iqbal Choudhary (Eds.)
All rights reserved-© 2020 Bentham Science Publishers

across all drug classes. The emergence of multi-drug resistance in bacterial pathogens is of particular concern, specifically in Gram-negative bacteria which already have limited treatment options. International agencies such as the World Health Organization (WHO) have warned that unless urgent action is taken, the world may be about to enter a 'post-antibiotic' era, where once easily treatable infections will cause significant mortality or morbidity. It has been estimated that as many as 5–20 novel drugs would need to enter clinical development to keep pace with the high attrition rates of our current drug discovery model [1].

Despite these dire predictions, the last three decades have seen a distinct lack of discoveries of novel antibiotics. This can be partly attributed to the abandonment of antibiotic discovery methods by major pharmaceutical companies, for reasons that include the lack of revenue generated from competitive pricing, short-term use, the rapid rise of drug resistance and very high development costs. However, scientific challenges remain a fundamental cause of stagnation in the field [1].

High throughput screening (HTS) is a well-established and commonly used small-molecule drug discovery method employed by pharmaceutical companies. It has yielded the majority of the drugs in clinical use or undergoing clinical trials to date [2]. The fundamental requirement of HTS is the successful identification from the screening library of at least one compound with high potency (sub μM affinity; a "hit") that can progress through the hit-to-lead (H2L) development phase. HTS libraries typically need to contain $> 10^5$ drug-like compounds (~300–500 Da) to cover enough structural scaffolds and functional chemical space to provide a reasonable chance of finding hits. As such, HTS is often a very expensive process and rarely affordable for academic researchers and smaller biotechnology companies. Despite the cost, a number of large pharmaceutical companies have attempted HTS for antibacterials but it has not been effective in bringing new antibiotics into the drug discovery pipeline. For example, between 1995 and 2001, GlaxoSmithKline (GSK) led a concerted HTS campaign during which 300 bacterial target genes were independently screened against over half a million compounds. However, only five potential leads were identified with all failing to progress to clinical trials due to a lack of broad-spectrum activity and drug-like properties [3]. This is by no means an exception and similar experiences have resulted in only a handful of large companies remaining engaged with antibiotic development today [4].

The successful revitalisation of the development of new antibiotics requires a concerted effort. To drive scientific breakthroughs, new research strategies must be explored, innovative government policies to change funding schemes implemented, and market subsidies to promote investment in the sector provided. An increasing number of policy statements and publications (such as reviewed by

Shlaes and Bradford [5]) have supported "fixing the broken antibiotic market" and some progress has been made. For example, there have been discussions in the United States about the possibility of funding antibiotic innovations with vouchers [6], as well as significant buy-ins from non-government charitable agencies. With this backdrop, it is ever more important that researchers, both from industry and academia, re-join the research and development effort to produce new antibiotics while utilising more time- and cost-efficient methodologies and tools to overcome the problems that have plagued the field. In this chapter, we first outline the potential merits of the fragment-based drug design (FBDD) approach for antibiotic development. Four case studies, including relevant patents, are then presented to showcase how FBDD has assisted to resolve some of the key scientific challenges in the antibiotic discovery pipeline. Finally, we discuss recent technical advances that can be incorporated into a FBDD research workflow to assist future antibiotic development efforts.

POTENTIAL ADVANTAGES OF FBDD FOR DEVELOPMENT OF ANTIBIOTICS

Over the last two decades, FBDD has been established as a mainstream approach and a success story for developing new small molecule drugs for treating a range of conditions [7]. Despite this relatively short timeframe, FBDD has already led to 40+ lead molecules in clinical trials and four drugs on the market (Table **1**, see https://practicalfragments.blogspot.com/2020/3/fragments-in-clinic-2020- edition. html for the latest update) [8]. In some cases, FBDD has yielded lead molecules where HTS has failed. This has given hope that FBDD may provide a system for the development of drugs against otherwise "impossible" targets and establish pathways for finding new antibiotics in the face of rising drug resistance.

A number of excellent reviews have recently described FBDD methodology and its advantages and caveats [9 - 11], from library design [12] to new and integrated screening methodologies [13], including a focus on specific protein classes such as kinases [14, 15]. Therefore, herein only a very brief summary of the technique is provided in order to introduce terms and abbreviations frequently used in the literature and in this chapter. Very briefly, an FBDD campaign begins with screening a library of low molecular weight compounds (termed fragments) which are only a fraction of the size of more typical drug-like molecules utilised in HTS. The small size of FBDD library compounds means only a few thousand fragments can effectively sample the chemical and structural space required to yield hits against a target. Compared to HTS, this makes FBDD more cost-effective and accessible to researchers. However, because of the small size of library fragments, the affinity of binding fragments for the target is typically very weak (hundreds of μM or even low mM). As such, FBDD relies on a plethora of techniques (*e.g.* surface plasmon resonance, SPR; Nuclear magnetic resonance spectroscopy, NMR; X-ray crystallography; microscale thermophoresis, MST) that can accurately measure these molecular interactions and/or provide detailed molecular information about the binding site. This allows the evolution and expansion of the fragment hits into high-affinity binders, in a similar fashion to the H2L process used in HTS.

Table 1. A brief history of the development of the first four drugs identified by FBDD and taken to market.

Drug	Target (s); Indications	Original Fragment (Target: IC_{50})	Final IC_{50}	Project Started; Drug Approved
Vemurafenib	Pim-1/B-Raf; Metastatic melanoma	(Pim-1: >200 µM)	B-Raf: 0.031 µM	2005; 2011
Venclexta™	Bcl-xL/Bcl-2; Chronic lymphocytic leukemia	(Bcl-xL: 300 µM) (Bcl-xL: 6 mM)	Bcl-xL: 0.048 µM Bcl-2: < 0.0001 µM	1996; 2016
Pexidartinib	CSF1R/KIT; Symptomatic tenosynovial giant cell tumor	(CSF1R: >100 µM)	CSF1R: 0.013 µM KIT: 0.027 µM	2013; 2019
Erdafitinib	FGFR3/VEGRF2; Urothelial carcinomas	(FGFR3: 120 µM) (VEGRF2: 140 µM)	FGFR3: 0.003 µM VEGRF2: 0.037 µM	2006; 2019

As shown in Fig. (**1**), following library screening and validation, the development of fragments typically utilises the approach of linking, merging or growing the initial hits into larger more drug-like molecules [16]. To guide this process, structural information at the atomic level is often invaluable. For example, if two fragments are found to have bound in adjacent binding sites, a linking approach may be employed to chemically join these fragments, with the aim of creating a single molecule that can fulfil interactions at both sites simultaneously (Fig. **1A**). One challenge in this approach is the identification of linkers that can maintain the desired spacing and relative orientations of the initial fragments in their respective bound states. Similarly, fragment merging can be employed when fragments are found to have bound in overlapping regions within a binding pocket (Fig. **1B**). In this case, a new series of larger compounds can be designed with the aim of better complementing the overall shape of the binding pocket by incorporating desirable structural and chemical features from contributing fragments. Lastly, if only single fragments are identified at the targeted region, or little structural information is available, then a growing approach is the most likely path forward (Fig. **1C**). A series of "growing" compounds with the addition of a broad array of functional groups based on the original fragment is generated. As for linking and merging fragments, structural information can inform on the type and position of functional groups to be added to the parent fragment and fast track the pathway to better binders.

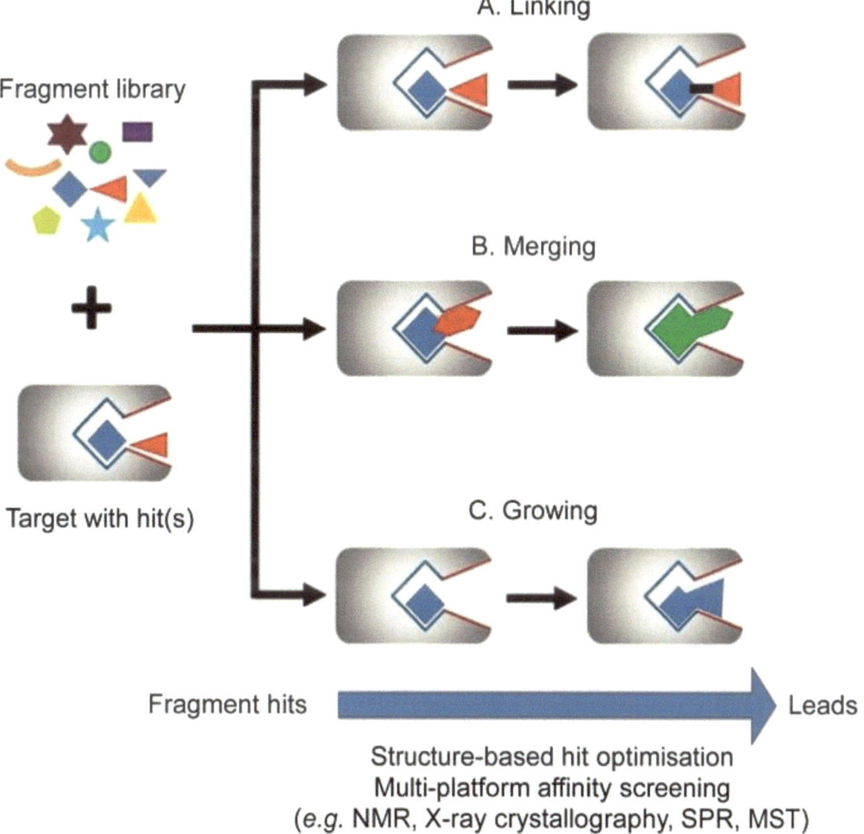

Fig. (1). Schematic diagram showing the key steps of the FBDD pathway and common methodologies used in the H2L development process. Figure based on http://luckprepopp.com/pharma-biotech/fbdd/attachment/190222_fbdd_fragment-development/.

In all cases, the new molecules that are generated will have their binding and/or activity assessed using a combination of *in vitro* and *in vivo* assay techniques and this data, along with new structural information, will be used to inform further cycles of fragment development. Typically, the dissociation constant (K_D) is used as the primary measure to rank the binding affinity of evolving compounds, while ligand efficiency (LE) is used as a secondary measure. LE is defined as the ratio between the ligand's total binding energy relative to the number of heavy atoms and can, therefore, provide a good indication of increasing favourable interactions as fragments increase in size.

During the lead development phase, desirable drug-like properties are also considered and introduced where appropriate, along with information from functional screens, such as toxicity and efficacy screens, ADME (absorption, distribution, metabolism, and excretion) profiling and optimisation. In short, FBDD is a multi-pronged approach with the aim of accurately determining structure-activity relationships (SARs) that ultimately result in the development of drugs from initial fragment hits to drug leads.

One key advantage of FBDD is that smaller fragments better complement their target of interest. Hann's framework of molecular complexity suggests that as a molecule increases in size and structural complexity, it has more interactions with the target that can be favourable or unfavourable. In the case of a perfectly complementary interaction between a small molecule and protein, a single misplaced functional group can disrupt strong binding [17]. Thus, the screening of more complex, structurally diverse molecules in HTS will inevitably lead to lower hit rates. While there has been moderate success in designing target-biased HTS libraries to favour known interactions, this strategy cannot be applied to antibiotics, generally due to a lack of consensus on the specific chemical properties that define antibacterial activity [18]. In addition, typical selection criteria such as Lipinski's 'rule of five' are not readily applicable to antibacterial drugs, as other criteria such as bacterial membrane permeability and efflux rate may be far more important. Therefore, smaller fragments are advantageous as they can more easily fulfil perfect complementary interactions while their progressive expansion offers the opportunity to combine favourable interactions as well as accommodate other selection criteria such as aqueous solubility and other desirable pharmacokinetic properties. Overall, fragment-derived drugs can be smaller and more efficient than HTS-derived molecules in their mechanism of action, without compromising drug safety and efficacy which are particularly strict requirements for antibiotics.

Another significant FBDD advantage is that the use of fragments greatly reduces the complexity of complementing the targeted protein surface, requiring at most one to two bonding interactions for binding due to the small size of the fragments. This enables a relatively unconstrained exploration of the protein surface and aids in the identification of specific 'hot spots' or novel pockets that can be eventually targeted simultaneously to produce antibiotic drugs with high affinity, selectivity, and, most importantly, a low propensity for development of bacterial resistance [19]. In some cases, it may also be possible to divide the protein's molecular architecture into simpler binding motifs during the screening process to enable targeting of secondary binding sites. Such strategies are highly advantageous, as resistance to compounds that bind to multiple targets is unlikely to develop rapidly due to a low probability of simultaneous mutagenesis in distinct binding pockets [20].

Given these advantages, it is perhaps not surprising that over the last decade FBDD has been increasingly applied in antibiotic development projects and this has generated several promising H2L examples as discussed below. It is worth noting that in many cases the targets have been unsuccessfully pursued at length with alternative drug discovery methods (*e.g.* HTS). Indeed, several targets are enzymes involved in key cellular processes or antibiotic resistance mechanisms which have been deemed to possess "non-druggable" binding pockets due to their depth, narrowness and hydrophobic nature [21]. The following sections outline four case studies to illustrate how FBDD has enabled significant breakthroughs in the antibiotic development arena and has produced molecules against "non-druggable" pockets, as well as incorporated features that can counteract resistance development. The first two case studies focus on the bacterial DNA gyrase and biotin carboxylase which also feature in a recent review by Lamoree and Hubbard [22]. The last two case studies showcase how FBDD can be used to target multiple enzymes in one pathway (Fatty Acid Synthesis) and against a multidrug resistant organism (*Mycobacterium tuberculosis*). In all cases, the capacity of FBDD to translate complex molecular architecture into simpler motifs provides a distinct benefit.

CASE STUDIES OF NEW ANTIBIOTIC DEVELOPMENT UTILISING FBDD

The following sections explore the success of applying FBDD approaches to four selected targets, with relevant scientific publications and patents presented.

Case Study 1: β-Lactamase

β-Lactams are an extensively used class of antibiotics that target bacterial cell wall synthesis *via* inhibition of penicillin-binding proteins. Resistance to these antibiotics has been primarily mediated *via* a family of hydrolases known as β-lactamases, which catalyse β-lactam inactivation. β-Lactamases can be classified into two subgroups: serine β-lactamases which include Classes A, C and D hydrolases and utilise a serine to catalyse hydrolysis, and Class B lactamases which are metallo enzymes [23]. Novel β-lactam drugs, such as cephalosporins and carbapenems, have been designed to either evade or inhibit β-lactamase activity, yet their efficacy is short-lived due to an invariable occurrence of mutations in the bacteria or generation of enzymes that enable the recognition and subsequent inactivation of these late generation antibiotics [24].

The combined use of a β-lactam inhibitor and additional antibiotic has been the primary strategy utilised to tackle resistance. Classical β-lactamase inhibitors are largely ineffective in modern multi-drug resistant (MDR) environments due to both their lack of broad-spectrum activity against β-lactamases and their readily targetable β-lactam ring structure for which resistance already exists. This has necessitated the search for novel β-lactamase inhibitor chemotypes with unique mechanisms of action. HTS campaigns against serine and metallo β-lactamases have produced mixed results. There has been relative success in targeting the metalloenzymes largely due to their shallow and easily accessible active sites, which lower the probability of steric clashes for tested inhibitors [25]. In contrast, serine-β-lactamases lack one significant binding feature within their active sites and that inhibits matching of the binding affinities of metal-ligand interactions observed for Class B enzymes. Given that multiple binding interactions need to be satisfied, the probability of identifying HTS hits of adequate affinity is considered very low.

Fortunately, the presence of numerous binding sub-sites makes these enzyme classes well suited to FBDD. Indeed, FBDD has proven to be a promising platform for targeting both serine and metallo β-lactamases, specifically in the context of serine hydrolases, as reviewed in [26]. The so-called CTX-M β-lactamases, which can be further divided into five subgroups, are the most commonly encountered β-lactamases and they effectively hydrolyse third generation cephalosporins such as cefotaxime and ceftazidime. The CTX-M family has been the primary focus of FBDD efforts to date with a series of fragment screens and optimisation conducted for subgroup CTX-M-9. This work incorporated high-resolution X-ray crystallography of protein:fragment complexes to drive molecule development by providing suitable templates for computational modelling and the rapid identification of notable features within binding sites. This has resulted in new compounds with sub micromolar affinities, including an 89-nM inhibitor that potentiated the effects of cefotaxime by reducing its MIC between 32-64-fold in *E. coli* isolates expressing CTX-M-9 [27]. More recently, mechanistic considerations taking into account the reaction coordinate and time spent in different chemical states have also been used to complement high-resolution X-ray structures of the β-lactamase:inhibitor complexes and a "fragmented" approach to improve inhibitor binding. This approach has contributed to five new inhibitors entering the market [28].

Case Study 2: Bacterial DNA Gyrase/Topoisomerase IV

Bacterial topoisomerases are essential modulators of DNA topology and are well established antibacterial drug targets due to their vital roles in DNA replication and repair. Two classes of antibiotics, quinolones and aminocoumarins, have been devised [29]. However, only quinolone-based drugs are still in use, albeit with decreasing efficacy due to emerging resistant strains. To prevent promotion of cross-resistance, non-quinolone-based compounds which act *via* novel binding sites found within two particular enzymes, DNA gyrase and its paralogue topoisomerase IV, have been suggested [29]. DNA gyrase is comprised of two GyrA subunits and two GyrB subunits (A_2B_2), while topoisomerase IV contains two ParC subunits and two ParE subunits (C_2E_2), which are homologous to GyrA and GyrB, respectively [29]. Fragment-based targeting of these enzymes has been conducted due to the potential for dual target inhibition, which would drastically reduce the chance of resistance development [30].

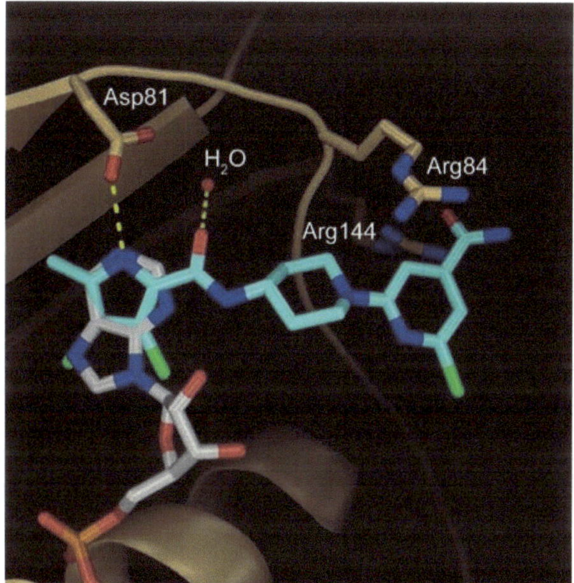

Fig. (2). Crystal structure of the 24-kDa N-terminal ATP-binding domain of *Staphylococcus aureus* GyrB in complex with a pyrrole fragment derivative overlaid with native substrate ATP. The carbon atoms of the pyrrole derivative are coloured cyan while those from ATP are coloured grey. Other heavy atoms are shown in standard colouring. The GyrB protein is presented as a gold ribbon with key residues shown as sticks. Hydrogen bonds are indicated as yellow dotted lines between the adenine component of ATP, amino acid residue, Asp81, and a water molecule (red sphere). Figure is based on [30] and prepared using PDB code 3U2K.

Virtual screening and fragment-based methods have been utilised to identify several classes of either independent or dual GyrB/ParE inhibitors. A pertinent example was the development of DNA gyrase pyrrolamide inhibitors which targeted the ATP binding site of GyrB to prevent functional coupling of DNA supercoiling to ATP hydrolysis [30]. Approximately 1000 chemically diverse compounds, including fragments deconstructed from known GyrB inhibitors, were screened against GyrB ATPase domain using NMR methods. Of the fragment hits identified, a low-affinity pyrrole carboxylate demonstrated a binding mode amenable to further expansion within the adenine pocket (Fig. **2**).

Despite the pyrrole carboxylate (termed Fragment 7) only displaying initial affinities in the millimolar range, the conserved engagement with aspartate and water motifs upon expansion of the fragment (Fig. **3**) indicated the formation of a high-quality interaction that was thermodynamically advantageous, and was favourable enough to offset the loss of rotational and translational freedom associated with the rigid bonding. This points to another advantage of FBDD, as fragments that register as hits have already accounted for this entropic debt and it was postulated that additions made to the fragments would directly strengthen binding affinity to the targets.

In the same screen, another fragment (Fragment 8), while considered a weak binder and an inefficient ligand, bound to a distinct distal aminocoumarin-binding site, providing motivation for further expansion. Subsequent design of a novel fragment library by elaboration of the quinoline structure led to pyrrole-containing compounds being screened for inhibition of ATPase activity in a specific *E. coli* DNA gyrase assay. This eventuated in the identification of pyrrolamides (Fragments 9 and 10), a chemotype that displayed broad-spectrum potency against Gram-positive pathogens, including resistant strains. A follow-up study focused on optimising Fragment 10, which displayed both bacteriostatic and bactericidal activity against *Staphylococcus aureus* and efflux pump deficient *E. coli*. Stereochemical adjustments were made to the piperidine ring, a key contributor to the binding orientations of the pyrrole and thiazole rings which subsequently influence ligand binding affinity. The final product with optimised physicochemical properties was compound 11 (AZD5099). AZD5099 also showed notable efficacy in a mouse neutropenic *S. aureus* infection model. Development of resistance was low and there were few reports of clinical resistance due to alteration of the target.

AZD5099 progressed through a Phase I, single-centre, double-blind, randomized, placebo-controlled, parallel-group trial but did not progress further. However, two new DNA gyrase inhibitors from AstraZeneca developed from whole cell screening assays are currently undergoing clinical trials. One such drug,

Zoliflodacin (AZD0914), completed Phase II against gonorrhoea in 2017, with Phase III recruiting as of December 2019.

Fragment 7

K_D 1 mM

LE 0.37

Fragment 8

K_D 2 mM

LE 0.22

Fragment 9

IC50 3 μM

LE 0.3

Fragment 11 (AZD5099)

S. aureus MIC$_{90}$ 0.06 μg/mL

Fragment 10

IC$_{50}$ 0.025 μM

LE 0.41

S. aureus MIC 8 μg/mL

Fig. (3). Optimisation of GyrB inhibitors, with progression of pyrrole hit **7** into clinical candidate AZD5099 **11**. IC$_{50}$ = Half maximal inhibitory concentration. MIC$_{90}$ = Minimum inhibitory concentration required to inhibit 90% of tested strains. LE= Ligand efficiency. Figure adapted from [22].

While AZD5099 has not progressed to Phase II trials to date, FBDD development of compounds that target similar processes is ongoing. For example, 2016 saw provisional patenting (US20190248836A1) of compounds involved in targeting of both bacterial primase and gyrase enzymes. This patent, for which a combined NMR-based FBDD and virtual screen was used to identify scaffolds that initially bind T7 DNA primase, remained under examination in 2019. The scaffolds were then used as a filter to select larger drug-like compounds from the ZINC database before virtual screening. Afterwards, selected compounds were assessed for their ability to inhibit T7 DNA replication as well as *Mycobacterium tuberculosis* DnaG primase, with some compounds demonstrating complete primase inhibition. Because DNA primase shares active site motifs with GyrB, it was proposed that some of the designed molecules could potentially target bacterial gyrase and lead to GyrB antibiotics; indeed, effective inhibition of DNA Gyrase was then confirmed. Furthermore, in a more recent patent (CN108504647A filed in 2018), a thermal shift assay-based FBDD approach was used to target DNA gyrase – specifically GyrB. Follow up work from the initial screen identified compounds that were also able to show inhibitory activity in an enzyme assay. It therefore seems promising for more FBDD-derived inhibitors of DNA Gyrase to proceed to clinical trials in the near future.

Case Study 3: Fatty Acid Synthesis (FAS) Pathways

Fatty acids are integral structural components of bacterial cell walls that contribute to membrane permeability and transport processes; as a result, their biosynthesis has been targeted extensively for generation of novel antibiotics [31]. Biosynthetic pathways differ significantly between humans and bacteria: mammalian cells utilise a Type I system which involves the action of a single, multifunctional fatty acid synthase; in contrast, bacterial cells utilise a Type II system which incorporates a separate enzyme for each reaction. *In vitro* and *in vivo* data from organisms and natural whole-cell screened inhibitors validated this system's suitability for drug targeting [32]. The production of malonyl-CoA from acetyl-CoA (Ac-CoA) is the initial step in the fatty acid synthesis (FAS) pathway. In bacteria this reaction is primarily driven by the acetyl-CoA carboxylase complex (ACC). Bacterial ACCs are multi-unit biotin-dependent complexes, composed of three separate proteins: a homodimeric biotin carboxylase (BC) subunit, BC carrier protein (BCCP), and carboxyltransferase (CT). Two half reactions ensue: the first involves an ATP-dependent carboxyl group transfer from bicarbonate to BCCP; the second involves transfer of the carboxyl group from carboxy-biotinylated BCCP to Ac-CoA, producing malonyl-CoA. The resulting malonyl-CoA is then utilised as a template substrate in which the developing fatty acid is elongated *via* an iterative series of reduction, dehydration, reduction, and condensation reactions catalysed by fatty acid biosynthesis enzymes [31].

Biotin Carboxylase

BC was selected for a FBDD-centric campaign by Mochalkin and co-workers [33] due to its principal role in the first step of fatty acid synthesis, its structural tractability for X-ray crystallography and its amenability to sensitive high-throughput enzymatic assays. This campaign was carried out *via* two complementary fragment-based approaches conducted in parallel. The first consisted of a virtual, 3D-shape similarity-based screening of ligands followed by a validation of hits *via* a high-concentration acetyl-CoA carboxylase assay. This approach selectively sampled the chemical space for a novel chemotype by utilising an HTS-based pyridopyrimidine BC inhibitor as the starting point for screening of structural modifications. The second approach involved the use of the same assay against an established fragment library, coupled with an NMR approach to further characterise the binding epitope of fragment hits in complex with BC. This parallel approach eventuated in the identification of several fragment hits with distinct BC inhibitor chemotypes. Similar binding modes were confirmed through co-crystallisation and subsequent fragment optimisation to generate several leads, with some demonstrating bactericidal activity.

Despite sharing similar pharmacophoric features to the HTS-identified hit, fragment-derived leads demonstrated substantially reduced efflux pump susceptibility and markedly enhanced cell penetration and antibacterial activity, possibly because of their higher LE. Despite the ATP binding site in BC being homologous to that in many human kinases, the lead inhibitors in this study, the amino-oxazoles, selectively inhibited BC when screened against 40 human protein kinases [33].

Ketoacyl Synthase

Ketoacyl synthase (KAS) enzymes in the FAS-II pathway, have also been targeted in drug discovery projects. Patents US9056851B2 and US20140113941 (published in 2014 and 2015) and WO2012135027A2/WO2012135027 (published 2012 and 2013) all describe targeting of this pathway with a focus on utilising FBDD to develop new analogues based on an existing molecule – thiolactomycin (TLM). TLM is a natural product known to be a selective and reversible inhibitor of KAS. Kinetic and structural data indicated TLM acted specifically as a competitive inhibitor of malonyl-ACP. It binds preferentially with slow onset kinetics to the covalently modified reaction intermediate, preventing the catalysed reaction of malonyl-ACP to 3-ketoacyl-ACP and thus blocking a key step in the FAS pathway.

An NMR-based FBDD approach was used to initially identify small molecules that bound adjacent to the TLM binding site. To guide further development, NMR spectroscopy was then used to specifically determine the interactions between the fragments and the protein. This was coupled with X-ray crystallographic analysis of the protein complexed to both TLM and binding fragments at adjacent sites. This led to production of a series of analogues containing a pantetheine fragment coupled with the TLM molecule, from which further expansions to the TLM moiety were undertaken to improve contacts between the ligand and the enzyme. This approach has resulted in new high affinity molecules as drug leads.

Case Study 4: *Mycobacterium Tuberculosis (Mtb)*

Tuberculosis (TB) is the leading cause of death from a single infectious disease agent and is caused by the bacterial pathogen, *M. tuberculosis* (*Mtb*), a species that has evolved several strains which are either MDR, extensively drug resistant (XDR), or totally drug resistant (TDR). Current therapies rely on dated drug combinations that are no longer able to treat these new strains; as a result, there has been a decade-long search for effective TB drugs that might circumvent the resistance mechanisms that have developed [34]. Despite the identification of highly potent anti-TB compounds *in vitro* from HTS and phenotypic screening campaigns conducted during this period, these substances were ineffective *in vivo*. This has been attributed to poorly constructed chemical libraries [35] and the prioritisation of larger drug-like molecules over those that were smaller and more efficacious. High attrition rates during clinical trials due to the complex nature of TB also affected successful outcomes. More specifically, within a patient there may be multiple replication states of *Mtb* and a variety of lesions with diverse local environments that prevent sufficient penetration and accumulation of adequate drug concentrations [36, 37]. Consequently, there is a need to utilise novel drug discovery approaches to find effective TB drugs, and the recent application of FBDD, which enables a greater sampling of chemical space, has shown promise across several *Mtb* targets which are discussed below.

Pantothenate Synthetase (PanC)

Coenzyme A is a ubiquitous cofactor required for an array of metabolic pathways including fatty acid biosynthesis and metabolism. It is generated *via* two separate pathways, the first of which is involved in producing pantothenic acid (Vitamin B_5), a critical intermediate [34]. Enzymes involved in this pathway are essential for *Mtb* survival and display low sequence identity to those in humans, making them ideal targets for the development of broad-spectrum antibacterial agents [37]. In recent years several of these enzymes have been investigated with the most prominent being pantothenate synthetase (PanC), an enzyme that synthesises the CoA precursor molecule, Vitamin B5. In addition to the host of genetic studies that have validated its status as an *Mtb* target [38], the vast array of X-ray crystal structures, whether in apo form or in complex with substrates, have provided sufficient structural information to facilitate structure-guided drug design following the identification of fragment hits [39]. As a result, PanC has proven to be a suitable FBDD target. A screen of a 1250 compound fragment library was carried out using thermal shift assays, with validation of hits carried out using ligand-based NMR techniques. Dissociation constants (K_D) of binding fragments in the low millimolar range were subsequently obtained from isothermal titration calorimetry (ITC) [13] (Fig. **4**).

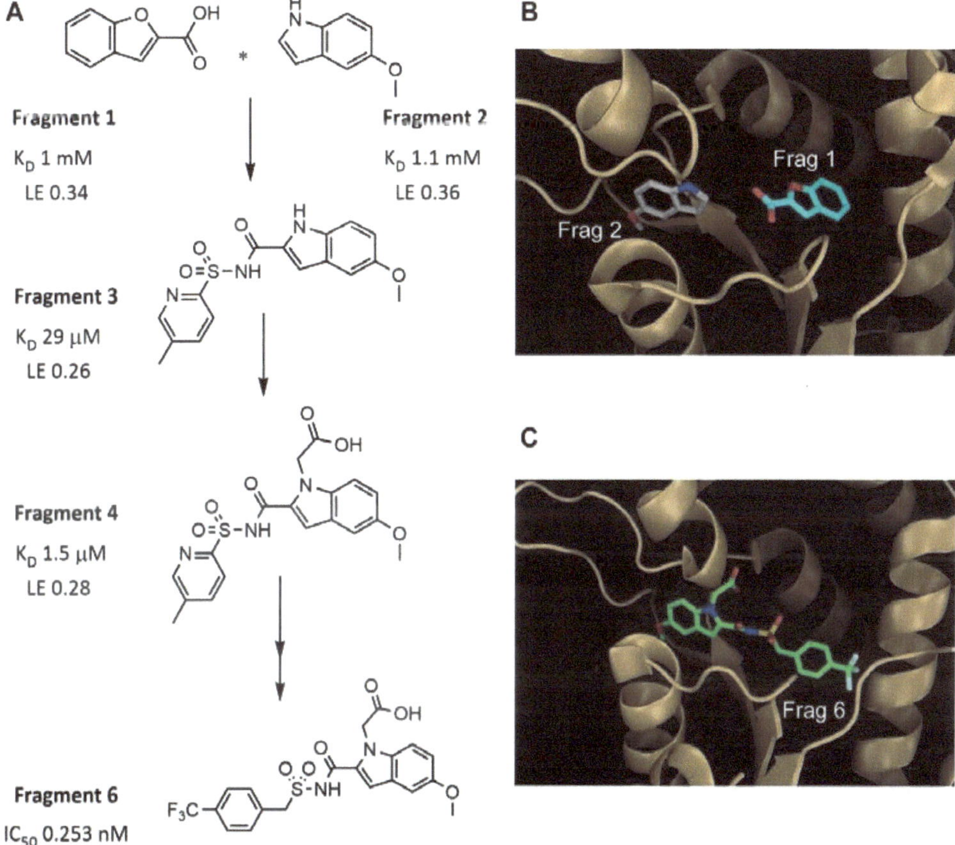

Fig. (4). **(A)** Optimisation of PanC inihibitors, with progression of a benzofuran-based and methoxyindole fragments (1 and 2) through growing and linking to become drug lead 6. IC_{50} = Half maximal inhibitory concentration. LE = Ligand efficiency. K_D = dissociation constant. **(B)** and **(C)** Crystal structures of PanC in complex with fragments 1 and 2, as well as 6, respectively. The carbon atoms of fragments 1, 2 and 6 are coloured cyan, grey and green, respectively. Other heavy atoms are shown in standard colouring. PanC is presented as a gold ribbon. Figure is based on [34] and prepared using PDB codes 3IMG and 4MUK.

Furthermore, X-ray crystallography enabled identification of three binding pockets within PanC's active site, one of which was targeted using a fragment-growing approach. Subsequent optimisation yielded products that retained the binding mode of the initial fragment hits and eventuated in a compound with nanomolar affinity [30].

Mtb Transcriptional Repressor (EthR)

A defining aspect of *Mtb* is that their cell wall incorporates a variety of lipid-rich elements to form a covalently bound peptidoglycan-arabinogalactan-mycolic complex. The formation of this complex is well characterised, and many essential steps have been countered by drugs such as ethionamide, which inhibits the synthesis of mycolic acid, a component that heavily contributes to *Mtb* pathogenicity [40]. Ethionamide is a second-line anti-TB prodrug that requires activation by mycobacterial mono-oxygenase EthA. However, the drug's efficacy is hindered by the activity of a TetR-type transcriptional repressor, EthR, which lowers EthA expression levels [41]. Current treatment of MDR-TB with ethionamide necessitates a high dosage that is frequently associated with liver toxicity. Fragment-based inhibition of EthR has been investigated as a means of elevating EthA expression levels to potentiate ethionamide's efficacy and prevent administration of toxic dosages [22].

Given the assumed lack of possible H-bonding interactions to potential ligands, developing drugs that target the long and hydrophobic binding pocket of EthR, which routinely accommodates fatty acids, had proven to be a considerable challenge [42]. However, a fragment-based screen identified novel H-bonding opportunities within the hydrophobic cavity that were previously unexplored by natural ligands [43]. A follow-up study employed an optimisation process to fragment hits but merged and linked fragments generally demonstrated lower potencies [44]. This was attributed to either lowered solubility as molecular complexity increased, or that the focus to maintain ideal interactions when merging/linking fragment scaffolds led to limited functionality of connecting groups [44]. Fortunately, several research efforts have generated lead inhibitors which penetrated the mycobacterial cell wall and subsequently produced an ethionamide-boosting effect *in vitro* and within macrophage infection models [43].

Mycocyclosin Synthase (CYP121)

The disproportionately large number of cytochrome P450 enzymes encoded within the 4.4-Mb mycobacterial genome when compared to the substantially larger 3-Gb human genome (*i.e.* 20 *vs* 57 respectively), underlines the centrality of these enzymes to the organism's virulence and survival. These cytosolic mono-oxygenase enzymes utilise a heme cofactor and separate electron donor system to oxidise substrates; as a result, they represent robust targets for selective inhibitors [34]. CYP121, an enzyme exclusive to *Mtb*, has been established as a promising target for fragment-based drug development. This susceptibility is due to its unique yet highly constrained binding site that has been ascertained from a high resolution apo X-ray crystal structure [45]. A fragment-based screening campaign utilising differential scanning fluorimetry (DSF), NMR and ITC identified several hits that bound to the active site *via* two distinct binding modes, with the higher affinity mode involving heme coordination. Subsequent fragment merging strategies were employed and resulted in the generation of compounds with low micromolar affinity that retained parent fragment binding modes but displayed low ligand efficiency (LE) [46]. This LE deficiency highlights a limitation of fragment development methods, as certain expansions may provide greater potency overall but at the expense of other essential drug parameters such as LE or solubility. Novel retro-fragmentation strategies were employed to circumvent this issue by analysing and sequentially rebuilding component fragments to achieve a higher overall LE [47]. This culminated in the design of a highly potent and selective inhibitor with low nanomolar affinity. However, this lead failed to demonstrate antimycobacterial activity which was hypothesised to be associated with an inability to combat drug-efflux mechanisms and achieve sufficient permeability [47]. This highlights the importance of screening of antimy-cobacterial activity in the early stages of the drug development process.

Fructose 1,6-bisphosphate Aldolase (FBA)

The targeting of *Mtb*, specifically the Class II enzyme fructose 1,6-bisphosphate aldolase (FBA) is part of patents WO2014182954A1/US9394254B2. As of 2015, the WO patent had entered national phase and the US patent had been fully granted. The patents focus on the targeting of antibiotics and anti-parasitic agents to inhibit Class II fructose 1,6-bisphosphate aldolase (FBA). They aim to produce minimal off-target effects in humans by targeting Class II FBA and not Class I FBAs. To identify new antibiotics targeting *Mtb* FBA (mtFBA), an FBDD approach was used with chemical fragments screened for their ability to block the enzymatic reaction – specifically targeting MtFBA's active site Zn(II), while lacking groups that might interfere with pharmaceutical development. 8-Hydroxyquinoline-2-carboxylic acid (HCA) and several derivatives were identified as having inhibitory activity. These were of particular interest as they bind through an induced fit, with the drug essentially creating its own binding pocket.

RECENT ADVANCES IN FBDD

There is no doubt that FBDD has become a powerful method for identification of new biologically active fragments and can aid in the development of new antibiotics and pharmacophores. Due to its modular nature, many new advances in screening, structure determination, chemical synthesis and other methodologies are readily applicable to FBDD. Advances in FBDD methodologies range from development of new heterocyclic spirocycles [48] and multimeric fragments (US20150087043), the use of membrane associated scaffolds [49], *in situ* click chemistry (WO2016210239A1), combined with *in silico* screening [50], differential scanning fluorimetry (DSF) screening [51], to cryogenic electron microscopy (cyro-EM) structural characterisation [52]. Some of these are briefly discussed below.

Library selection is a crucial starting point in the success of FBDD since compounds in the H2L pipeline are built on fragment scaffolds. In a search for new scaffolds targeting membranes, Li and colleagues [49] used a xanthone-based scaffold to develop new fragments and search for membrane-active microbials. By exploring the hydrophobic chemical environment of membranes, FBDD can now be used to target the cell membrane of Gram-negative bacteria to overcome drug resistance. Libraries containing scaffolds with structural constraints are important for a successful FBDD approach and the expansion of the scaffold chemical space will improve the identification of new binding sites and fragments that could not be identified previously due to a lack of structural constraints. Using structurally divergent heterocycles such as spirocyclic scaffolds, King *et al.* describe a new chemical approach to generating spirocyclic fragments [48]. These fragments contain synthetic handles that can be modified to cover more chemical space. Another new FBDD library development (patent US20150087043) is the use of fragments that can oligomerize in solution, transitioning from monomers to dimers, dimers to tetramers, *etc.* This technique uses a ligand moiety known to bind to a macromolecule fused to a connector followed by a linker. The linker can oligomerize and present one or more types of ligand that represent a combination of known binders with new fragments. This approach helps to identify new binding sites and can lead to a re-evaluation of weaker binders to increase their potency, potentially providing a new avenue for developing antibiotics after re-evaluation of lead compounds that previously failed to progress in the development pipeline.

Another idea to better fuse fragments that target nearby binding sites to improve potency is utilisation of click chemistry [53]. As described in a recent patent (WO2016210239A1), this method uses a library of fragments capable of undergoing click chemistry *in situ* when in proximity, such as to nearby binding sites of macromolecules. The product is then identified using chromatography and mass spectrometry. The use of a library ready for click chemistry is a promising new avenue to speed up the chemical synthesis of biologically active antibiotics.

In terms of *in silico* screening methodology, the small size of fragments combined with low binding affinities and possible multiple binding sites impose tough constraints for accurate scoring during FBDD. Bian [50] describes a combination of multiple *in silico* approaches to identify new binders against the targeted macromolecule. Casu [51] describes the use of DSF to efficiently identify fragments that bind to TraE protein in a high-throughput manner by using RT-PCR equipment readily available in most biochemistry and molecular biology laboratories. On the other hand, Saur [52] describes the use of cryo-EM to identify the interactions of fragments with large macromolecules. Recent advances in quality, resolution and reproducibility of cryo-EM structures have opened the door to the possibility of obtaining structural information of large and even relatively dynamic macromolecules bound to fragments and analogues that cannot be studied with NMR spectroscopy and X-ray crystallography. In particular, by facilitating *in silico* screens and using more cost-effective techniques such as DSF, FBDD will become more accessible which should in turn help advance the development of new antibiotics. Lastly, FBDD and HTS are not mutually exclusive techniques and there has been a suggestion that for difficult targets their integration would increase the chance of success (https://www.ddw-online.com/screening/p92852-integrating-hts-and-fragment-base--drug-discovery.html).

CONCLUSION

In summary, FBDD is a multi-pronged approach towards accurate determination of SARs to culminate in the rapid development of drug leads from initial fragment hits with weak affinities for their targets. As such and as discussed in this chapter, FBDD has overcome many of the specific challenges in new antibiotic development to combat rising antibiotic resistance. Depending on the target or system of interest, the exact FBDD pathway may be quite different and the exact technique or protocols chosen from library design, selection, screening to SAR development may differ. Ultimately, it is this adaptability that underlies the success of the technique and allows the development of new inhibitors of targets that were previously considered undruggable.

However, despite the capacity of FBDD to resolve key aspects of drug potency and selectivity, there are significant issues that have hampered the progression of several promising drug leads. The primary concern is that there is no consistent correlation between drug potency and antibacterial activity. This can be attributed to the lack of sufficient drug accumulation within bacterial cells, due to either a deficiency in drug permeation across bacterial membranes or substantial efflux of these molecules *via* drug-resistant pumps. A secondary concern is that the efficacy of single molecular target inhibitors may be affected by point mutations in the drug binding site. New developments in FBDD have been aimed at overcoming these hurdles, for example by coupling biophysical screens with whole-cell assays earlier in the process, as well as expanding the range of targets by utilising new methodologies that can provide structural and mechanistic information on multiple states while screening in more native-like environments such as inside membranes. In addition, there have been advances in FBDD detection methods as well as new strategies to help the fragment H2L process, from fragment expansion that samples larger chemical space to re-evaluation of drugs that previously failed to reach the market. All these efforts towards facilitating new drug discovery will hopefully improve success rates in antibiotic development and may finally lead to breaking of the new antibiotic drought.

CONSENT FOR PUBLICATION

Not applicable.

CONFLICT OF INTEREST

The authors confirm that this chapter content has no conflict of interest.

ACKNOWLEDGEMENTS

We thank the SPARK Oceania program and its mentors for helpful advice and discussions about the antibiotic development process and possible commercialisation pathways. We thank Bill Bubb for careful proofreading of the chapter.

REFERENCES

[1]   Jackson N, Czaplewski L, Piddock LJV. Discovery and development of new antibacterial drugs: learning from experience? J Antimicrob Chemother 2018; 73(6): 1452-9.
[http://dx.doi.org/10.1093/jac/dky019] [PMID: 29438542]

[2]   Macarron R, Banks MN, Bojanic D, *et al.* Impact of high-throughput screening in biomedical research. Nat Rev Drug Discov 2011; 10(3): 188-95.
[http://dx.doi.org/10.1038/nrd3368] [PMID: 21358738]

[3]   Payne DJ, Gwynn MN, Holmes DJ, Pompliano DL. Drugs for bad bugs: confronting the challenges of antibacterial discovery. Nat Rev Drug Discov 2007; 6(1): 29-40.
[http://dx.doi.org/10.1038/nrd2201] [PMID: 17159923]

[4]   Nass SJ, Madhavan G, Augustine NR, Madhavan G, Nass SJ, Eds. National Academies of Sciences, Engineering, and Medicine Making Medicines Affordable: A National Imperative. Washington, DC: National Academies Press 2017.
[http://dx.doi.org/10.17226/24946]

[5]   Shlaes DM, Bradford PA. Antibiotics-From There to Where?: How the antibiotic miracle is threatened by resistance and a broken market and what we can do about it. Pathog Immun 2018; 3(1): 19-43.
[http://dx.doi.org/10.20411/pai.v3i1.231] [PMID: 30993248]

[6]   Rome BN, Kesselheim AS. Transferrable Market Exclusivity Extensions to Promote Antibiotic Development: An Economic Analysis. Clin Infect Dis 2019; ciz1039.
[http://dx.doi.org/10.1093/cid/ciz1039] [PMID: 31630159]

[7]   Erlanson DA, Fesik SW, Hubbard RE, Jahnke W, Jhoti H. Twenty years on: the impact of fragments on drug discovery. Nat Rev Drug Discov 2016; 15(9): 605-19.
[http://dx.doi.org/10.1038/nrd.2016.109] [PMID: 27417849]

[8]   Jacquemard C, Kellenberger E. A bright future for fragment-based drug discovery: what does it hold? Expert Opin Drug Discov 2019; 14(5): 413-6.
[http://dx.doi.org/10.1080/17460441.2019.1583643] [PMID: 30793989]

[9]   Kashyap A, Singh PK, Silakari O. Counting on Fragment Based Drug Design Approach for Drug Discovery. Curr Top Med Chem 2018; 18(27): 2284-93.
[http://dx.doi.org/10.2174/1568026619666181130134250] [PMID: 30499406]

[10] Kirsch P, Hartman AM, Hirsch AKH, Empting M. Concepts and Core Principles of Fragment-Based Drug Design. Molecules 2019; 24(23): E4309.
[http://dx.doi.org/10.3390/molecules24234309] [PMID: 31779114]

[11] Osborne J, Panova S, Rapti M, Urushima T, Jhoti H. Fragments: where are we now? Biochem Soc Trans 2020; 48(1): 271-80.
[http://dx.doi.org/10.1042/BST20190694] [PMID: 31985743]

[12] Taylor A, Doak BC, Scanlon MJ. Design of a Fragment-Screening Library. Methods Enzymol 2018; 610: 97-115.
[http://dx.doi.org/10.1016/bs.mie.2018.09.018] [PMID: 30390807]

[13] Silvestre HL, Blundell TL, Abell C, Ciulli A. Integrated biophysical approach to fragment screening and validation for fragment-based lead discovery. Proc Natl Acad Sci USA 2013; 110(32): 12984-9.
[http://dx.doi.org/10.1073/pnas.1304045110] [PMID: 23872845]

[14] Panicker RC, Chattopadhaya S, Coyne AG, Srinivasan R. Allosteric Small-Molecule Serine/Threonine Kinase Inhibitors. Adv Exp Med Biol 2019; 1163: 253-78.
[http://dx.doi.org/10.1007/978-981-13-8719-7_11] [PMID: 31707707]

[15] Wang PF, Qiu HY, Zhu HL. A patent review of BRAF inhibitors: 2013-2018. Expert Opin Ther Pat 29; 1163(8): 595-603.

[16] de Souza Neto LR, Moreira-Filho JT, Neves BJ, *et al. In silico* Strategies to Support Fragment-to-Lead Optimization in Drug Discovery. Front Chem 2020; 8: 93.
[http://dx.doi.org/10.3389/fchem.2020.00093] [PMID: 32133344]

[17] Hann MM, Leach AR, Harper G. Molecular complexity and its impact on the probability of finding leads for drug discovery. J Chem Inf Comput Sci 2001; 41(3): 856-64.
[http://dx.doi.org/10.1021/ci000403i] [PMID: 11410068]

[18] McDowell LL, Quinn CL, Leeds JA, Silverman JA, Silver LL. Perspective on Antibacterial Lead Identification Challenges and the Role of Hypothesis-Driven Strategies. SLAS Discov 2019; 24(4): 440-56.
[http://dx.doi.org/10.1177/2472555218818786] [PMID: 30890054]

[19] Konaklieva MI. Addressing Antimicrobial Resistance through New Medicinal and Synthetic Chemistry Strategies. SLAS Discov 2019; 24(4): 419-39.
[http://dx.doi.org/10.1177/2472555218812657] [PMID: 30523713]

[20] Chilingaryan Z, Headey SJ, Lo ATY, *et al.* Fragment-Based Discovery of Inhibitors of the Bacterial DnaG-SSB Interaction. Antibiotics (Basel) 2018; 7(1): E14.
[http://dx.doi.org/10.3390/antibiotics7010014] [PMID: 29470422]

[21] Thangavelu B, Bhansali P, Viola RE. Elaboration of a fragment library hit produces potent and selective aspartate semialdehyde dehydrogenase inhibitors. Bioorg Med Chem 2015; 23(20): 6622-31.
[http://dx.doi.org/10.1016/j.bmc.2015.09.017] [PMID: 26404410]

[22] Lamoree B, Hubbard RE. Using Fragment-Based Approaches to Discover New Antibiotics. SLAS Discov 2018; 23(6): 495-510.
[http://dx.doi.org/10.1177/2472555218773034] [PMID: 29923463]

[23] Bush K, Jacoby GA, Medeiros AA. A functional classification scheme for beta-lactamases and its correlation with molecular structure. Antimicrob Agents Chemother 1995; 39(6): 1211-33.
[http://dx.doi.org/10.1128/AAC.39.6.1211] [PMID: 7574506]

[24] Fisher JF, Meroueh SO, Mobashery S. Bacterial resistance to beta-lactam antibiotics: compelling opportunism, compelling opportunity. Chem Rev 2005; 105(2): 395-424.
[http://dx.doi.org/10.1021/cr030102i] [PMID: 15700950]

[25] King DT, Worrall LJ, Gruninger R, Strynadka NC. New Delhi metallo-β-lactamase: structural insights into β-lactam recognition and inhibition. J Am Chem Soc 2012; 134(28): 11362-5.

[http://dx.doi.org/10.1021/ja303579d] [PMID: 22713171]

[26]　Nichols DA, Renslo AR, Chen Y. Fragment-based inhibitor discovery against β-lactamase. Future Med Chem 2014; 6(4): 413-27.
[http://dx.doi.org/10.4155/fmc.14.10] [PMID: 24635522]

[27]　Nichols DA, Jaishankar P, Larson W, *et al.* Structure-based design of potent and ligand-efficient inhibitors of CTX-M class A β-lactamase. J Med Chem 2012; 55(5): 2163-72.
[http://dx.doi.org/10.1021/jm2014138] [PMID: 22296601]

[28]　van den Akker F, Bonomo RA. Exploring Additional Dimensions of Complexity in Inhibitor Design for Serine β-Lactamases: Mechanistic and Intra- and Inter-molecular Chemistry Approaches. Front Microbiol 2018; 9: 622.
[http://dx.doi.org/10.3389/fmicb.2018.00622] [PMID: 29675000]

[29]　Tomašić T, Mašič LP. Prospects for developing new antibacterials targeting bacterial type IIA topoisomerases. Curr Top Med Chem 2014; 14(1): 130-51.
[http://dx.doi.org/10.2174/1568026613666131113153251] [PMID: 24236722]

[30]　Eakin AE, Green O, Hales N, *et al.* Pyrrolamide DNA gyrase inhibitors: fragment-based nuclear magnetic resonance screening to identify antibacterial agents. Antimicrob Agents Chemother 2012; 56(3): 1240-6.
[http://dx.doi.org/10.1128/AAC.05485-11] [PMID: 22183167]

[31]　Parsons JB, Rock CO. Is bacterial fatty acid synthesis a valid target for antibacterial drug discovery? Curr Opin Microbiol 2011; 14(5): 544-9.
[http://dx.doi.org/10.1016/j.mib.2011.07.029] [PMID: 21862391]

[32]　Miller JR, Dunham S, Mochalkin I, *et al.* A class of selective antibacterials derived from a protein kinase inhibitor pharmacophore. Proc Natl Acad Sci USA 2009; 106(6): 1737-42.
[http://dx.doi.org/10.1073/pnas.0811275106] [PMID: 19164768]

[33]　Mochalkin I, Miller JR, Narasimhan L, *et al.* Discovery of antibacterial biotin carboxylase inhibitors by virtual screening and fragment-based approaches. ACS Chem Biol 2009; 4(6): 473-83.
[http://dx.doi.org/10.1021/cb9000102] [PMID: 19413326]

[34]　Marchetti C, Chan DSH, Coyne AG, Abell C. Fragment-based approaches to TB drugs. Parasitology 2018; 145(2): 184-95.
[http://dx.doi.org/10.1017/S0031182016001876] [PMID: 27804891]

[35]　Koul A, Arnoult E, Lounis N, Guillemont J, Andries K. The challenge of new drug discovery for tuberculosis. Nature 2011; 469(7331): 483-90.
[http://dx.doi.org/10.1038/nature09657] [PMID: 21270886]

[36]　Prideaux B, Via LE, Zimmerman MD, *et al.* The association between sterilizing activity and drug distribution into tuberculosis lesions. Nat Med 2015; 21(10): 1223-7.
[http://dx.doi.org/10.1038/nm.3937] [PMID: 26343800]

[37]　Zumla A, Nahid P, Cole ST. Advances in the development of new tuberculosis drugs and treatment regimens. Nat Rev Drug Discov 2013; 12(5): 388-404.
[http://dx.doi.org/10.1038/nrd4001] [PMID: 23629506]

[38]　Sambandamurthy VK, Wang X, Chen B, *et al.* A pantothenate auxotroph of *Mycobacterium tuberculosis* is highly attenuated and protects mice against tuberculosis. Nat Med 2002; 8(10): 1171-4.
[http://dx.doi.org/10.1038/nm765] [PMID: 12219086]

[39]　Wang S, Eisenberg D. Crystal structures of a pantothenate synthetase from M. tuberculosis and its complexes with substrates and a reaction intermediate. Protein Sci 2003; 12(5): 1097-108.
[http://dx.doi.org/10.1110/ps.0241803] [PMID: 12717031]

[40]　Mendes V, Blundell TL. Targeting tuberculosis using structure-guided fragment-based drug design. Drug Discov Today 2017; 22(3): 546-54.
[http://dx.doi.org/10.1016/j.drudis.2016.10.003] [PMID: 27742535]

[41]   Engohang-Ndong J, Baillat D, Aumercier M, *et al.* EthR, a repressor of the TetR/CamR family implicated in ethionamide resistance in mycobacteria, octamerizes cooperatively on its operator. Mol Microbiol 2004; 51(1): 175-88.
[http://dx.doi.org/10.1046/j.1365-2958.2003.03809.x] [PMID: 14651620]

[42]   Frénois F, Engohang-Ndong J, Locht C, Baulard AR, Villeret V. Structure of EthR in a ligand bound conformation reveals therapeutic perspectives against tuberculosis. Mol Cell 2004; 16(2): 301-7.
[http://dx.doi.org/10.1016/j.molcel.2004.09.020] [PMID: 15494316]

[43]   Surade S, Ty N, Hengrung N, *et al.* A structure-guided fragment-based approach for the discovery of allosteric inhibitors targeting the lipophilic binding site of transcription factor EthR. Biochem J 2014; 458(2): 387-94.
[http://dx.doi.org/10.1042/BJ20131127] [PMID: 24313835]

[44]   Villemagne B, Flipo M, Blondiaux N, *et al.* Ligand efficiency driven design of new inhibitors of *Mycobacterium tuberculosis* transcriptional repressor EthR using fragment growing, merging, and linking approaches. J Med Chem 2014; 57(11): 4876-88.
[http://dx.doi.org/10.1021/jm500422b] [PMID: 24818704]

[45]   McLean KJ, Carroll P, Lewis DG, *et al.* Characterization of active site structure in CYP121. A cytochrome P450 essential for viability of *Mycobacterium tuberculosis* H37Rv. J Biol Chem 2008; 283(48): 33406-16.
[http://dx.doi.org/10.1074/jbc.M802115200] [PMID: 18818197]

[46]   Hudson SA, McLean KJ, Surade S, *et al.* Application of fragment screening and merging to the discovery of inhibitors of the *Mycobacterium tuberculosis* cytochrome P450 CYP121. Angew Chem Int Ed Engl 2012; 51(37): 9311-6.
[http://dx.doi.org/10.1002/anie.201202544] [PMID: 22890978]

[47]   Kavanagh ME, Coyne AG, McLean KJ, *et al.* Fragment-Based Approaches to the Development of *Mycobacterium tuberculosis* CYP121 Inhibitors. J Med Chem 2016; 59(7): 3272-302.
[http://dx.doi.org/10.1021/acs.jmedchem.6b00007] [PMID: 27002486]

[48]   King TA, Stewart HL, Mortensen KT, North AJP, Sore HF, Spring DR. Cycloaddition Strategies for the Synthesis of Diverse Heterocyclic Spirocycles for Fragment-Based Drug Discovery. Eur J Org Chem 2019; 2019(31-32): 5219-29.
[http://dx.doi.org/10.1002/ejoc.201900847] [PMID: 31598091]

[49]   Li J, Liu S, Koh JJ, *et al.* A novel fragment based strategy for membrane active antimicrobials against MRSA. Biochim Biophys Acta 2015; 1848(4): 1023-31.
[http://dx.doi.org/10.1016/j.bbamem.2015.01.001] [PMID: 25582665]

[50]   Bian Y, Xie XS. Computational Fragment-Based Drug Design: Current Trends, Strategies, and Applications. AAPS J 2018; 20(3): 59.
[http://dx.doi.org/10.1208/s12248-018-0216-7] [PMID: 29633051]

[51]   Casu B, Arya T, Bessette B, Baron C. Fragment-based screening identifies novel targets for inhibitors of conjugative transfer of antimicrobial resistance by plasmid pKM101. Sci Rep 2017; 7(1): 14907.
[http://dx.doi.org/10.1038/s41598-017-14953-1] [PMID: 29097752]

[52]   Saur M, Hartshorn MJ, Dong J, *et al.* Fragment-based drug discovery using cryo-EM. Drug Discov Today 2020; 25(3): 485-90.
[PMID: 31877353]

[53]   Kolb HC, Finn MG, Sharpless KB. Click Chemistry: Diverse Chemical Function from a Few Good Reactions. Angew Chem Int Ed Engl 2001; 40(11): 2004-21.
[http://dx.doi.org/10.1002/1521-3773(20010601)40:11<2004::AID-ANIE2004>3.0.CO;2-5] [PMID: 11433435]

CHAPTER 4

Phage Therapy as a Tool for Control of Foodborne Diseases: Advantages and Limitations

S. Pacios-Michelena[1,2], R. Rodríguez-Herrera[1], A. C. Flores-Gallegos[1], M.L Chávez González[2], E.P. Segura-Ceniceros[2], R. Ramos-González[3] and A. Ilyina[2,*]

[1] *Research Group in Molecular Biology. Postgraduate Program in Food Science and Technology. Faculty of Chemical Sciences of the Autonomous University of Coahuila. Blvd. V. Carranza e Ing. José Cárdenas V., Col. República, Saltillo, CP 25280, Coahuila, Mexico*

[2] *Nanobioscience Research Group. Postgraduate Program in Food Science and Technology. Faculty of Chemical Sciences of the Autonomous University of Coahuila. Blvd. V. Carranza e Ing. José Cárdenas V., Col. República, Saltillo, CP 25280, Coahuila, Mexico*

[3] *CONACYT- Autonomous University of Coahuila. Postgraduate Program in Food Science and Technology. Faculty of Chemical Sciences of the Autonomous University of Coahuila. Blvd. V. Carranza e Ing. José Cárdenas V., Col. República, Saltillo, CP 25280, Coahuila, Mexico*

Abstract: It is estimated that only in USA, foodborne pathogens cause 48 million illnesses, with 128,000 hospitalizations and 3,000 deaths each year. The growing global emergence of multi-drug-resistant infections raises the need to find alternative methods for the effective treatment of infectious illnesses. Phages possess properties that make them interesting but challenging candidates for different applications, including phage therapy against foodborne bacteria. The results of different clinical studies confirm the safety and efficiency of the use of bacteriophages for this purpose. Bacteriophage applications include water and food safety, agriculture and animal health. There are already several products available in the market. Studies indicate that phages have potent immunomodulatory and anti-inflammatory properties, and are recognized as an important part of the immune system. The use of bacteriophages for the control of foodborne infections should lead to promising alternative therapy. This review focuses on the application of bacteriophages as an antimicrobial alternative for therapies against antibiotic-resistant bacterial infections.

Keywords: Antibiotic-resistant bacteria, Antimicrobial, Bacteria, Bacteriophage, Biological control, Food, Foodborne pathogens, Foodborne diseases, Phage therapy, Safety food.

---

* **Corresponding author A. Ilyina:** Nanobioscience Research Group. Postgraduate Program in Food Science and Technology. Faculty of Chemical Sciences of the Autonomous University of Coahuila. Blvd. V. Carranza e Ing. José Cárdenas V., Col. República, Saltillo, CP 25280, Coahuila, Mexico; Tel: +528444159534; E-mail: anna_ilina@hotmail.com

Atta-ur-Rahman and M. Iqbal Choudhary (Eds.)
All rights reserved-© 2020 Bentham Science Publishers

INTRODUCTION

Foodborne pathogens cause 48 million illnesses with 128,000 hospitalizations and 3000 deaths each year in the USA; 9.4 million of them are caused by 31 known pathogens of bacterial, viral, and parasitic origin. Around 800 annual outbreaks are reported, and the most frequent bacterial pathogens include *Campylobacter* sp., *Salmonella enterica* non-typhoid, *Clostridium botulinum*, *Escherichia coli*, and *Listeria monocytogenes* [1, 2].

Recently, some strategies have been explored to reduce foodborne bacterial disease incidence. The uncontrolled use of antibiotics in antimicrobial therapies brings a negative impact on human health. Improper use of antibiotics has promoted bacterial resistance that reduces the effectiveness of antibiotic treatments [3, 4]. The worldwide increase in multi-drug resistant bacteria is alarming. Bacteria that form biofilms are particularly resistant to antibiotics [5]. Thus, substantial efforts are made to produce antibiotics and non-antibiotic derivatives, such as vaccines, immunostimulants, adjuvants, and probiotics. However, the production of drugs is not enough to cover their global demand [6]. Finding alternative ways to treat infectious diseases is necessary. These factors have aroused interest in phage therapy around the world with clinical studies confirming the safe use of bacteriophages. This review focuses on the application of bacteriophages as an antimicrobial alternative for therapies against antibiotic-resistant bacterial infections.

BACTERIOPHAGE

History

The term bacteriophage was coined by the Canadian bacteriologist Felix d'Herelle in 1917, to describe both: the phenomenon of a spontaneous decrease in bacterial culture's turbidity and the presence of a hypothetical agent behind this process. d'Herelle believed in the presence of a virus or a small microbe that could pass through the best bacteriological filters [7]. The English bacteriologist Frederick Twort had described a similar phenomenon in 1915, observing the bactericidal effect of these viruses [8].

Moreover, in the 1920s, d'Herelle published extensive work on phage biology after performing numerous studies on the isolation, characterization, and clinical evaluation of them. d'Herelle proposed the existence of viruses capable of infecting bacteria. This work allowed him to start as an assistant at the International Institute of Bacteriophages in Georgia. During his studies, he made filtrates without bacteria from fecal specimens from patients suffering dysentery and mixed them and incubated with *Shigella* strains isolated from patients. In an agar culture, d'Herelle observed the appearance of small and precise areas that contained no bacteria, which were later called plaques [7].

Shortly after the discovery, d'Herelle used phages to treat dysentery. Probably it was the first description of using bacteriophage as a therapeutic agent. The studies were performed in the *Hôpital des enfants-malades* in Paris in 1919 under the clinical supervision of Professor Victor-Henri Hutinel, pediatrics head of the hospital. d'Herelle, Hutinel and several hospital workers ingested the phage preparation to confirm its safety before administering it the next day to a 12-yea--old child with severe dysentery. The symptoms of the patient ceased after a single administration of the phage, and the child recovered entirely in a few days [9]. The laboratory of d'Herelle in Paris produced at least five phage preparations against various bacterial infections that were marketed. Later it became the well-known French company L'Oréal [10].

Therapeutic phages were also produced in the United States. In 1940, Eli Lilly Company (Indianapolis, Indiana) produced seven phage products for human use, including targeted preparations against *Staphylococcus*, *Streptococcus*, *Escherichia coli*, and other bacterial pathogens. Initially, the bacteriophages seemed to offer great potential as first-line therapies against infectious diseases in the pre-antibiotic era. Until World War II, many countries used phage therapy [11]. In almost the entire western world, the production of phages as therapies ceased due to the arrival of antibiotics. However, in Eastern Europe and the former Soviet Union, phages continued to be therapeutically used altogether with or instead of other therapeutic medicines [11].

General Phage Characteristics

Phages are the most abundant biological entities on Earth, estimated to be a total of 10^{30} to 10^{32} viral particles throughout the planet and play a decisive role in the balance of bacterial ecosystems [12]. It is thought that phages play a key ecological role in the modulation of ecological equilibria, in preventing bacterial population overgrowth in nature, and helps in the recycling of nutrients *via* lysis of bacterial cells in these environmental niches [13]. Additionally, prokaryotic evolution is mediated by phages through gene transfer processes, such as transduction and lysogenic conversion. Phages are present in soil, oceans and sediments, river, underground water, pants, animal biomass, waste streams from agricultural and food industries, households, human waste, hospitals, schools, airports and municipal sewage [14].

Bacteriophages are viruses that lack genomic attributes to generate ATP. Hence, they are obligate intracellular parasites, do not have a cytoplasmic membrane and are quite complex macromolecules of nucleic acids and proteins. They are inert in their extracellular form, replicating only after being recognized and infecting a suitable bacterial host cell [14].

The International Committee on Taxonomy of Viruses (ICTV) reported that almost 90% of the studied phages possess a tail and an icosahedral head that surrounds a double-stranded DNA molecule (Table **1**). The order *Caudovirales* contain most phages [15]. Three families form this order: *Myoviridae, Siphoviridae,* and *Podoviridae* [16]. The other families are not grouped in higher taxonomic categories, and they are *Microviridae, Corticoviridae, Tectiviridae, Leviviridae, Cystoviridae, Inoviridae, Lipothrixiviridae, Rudiviridae, Plasmavirus, Fuselloviridae,* and *Guttaviridae* [4].

Table 1. Molecular and morphological characteristics of phages.

Family	Nucleic Acid	Morphology Characteristics	Phage	Host	Reference
Myoviridae	Double-stranded DNA	Rigid, long and contractile tail, no envelope, icosahedral capsid.	T4- like	Enteric bacteria	[17]
Siphoviridae	Double-stranded DNA	Non-contractile, long and flexible tail	phage ΦCD6356	*Clostridium difficile*	[17]
Podoviridae	Double-stranded DNA	Non-contractile and short tail	Phage φ KMV	*Salmonella* sp.	[17]
Corticoviridae	Double-stranded circular DNA	Icosahedral, internal-membran--containing virions, single capsid protein P2, and a single spike protein P1	Phage PM2	*Pseudomonas* sp.	[18]
Microviridae,	Single-stranded circular DNA	Icosahedral capsid, size ~27 nm.	Phage φ X174	*Escherichia coli*	[17]
Tectiviridae	Double-stranded DNA	Icosahedral capsid, inner lipid vesicle, pseudo- tail, size ~60 nm.	Phage PRD1	*E. coli* *S. enteric* *P. aeruginosa*	[17]
Guttaviridae	Double-Stranded RNA	Ovoid, enveloped viruses, a diameter of 55–80 nm and a length of 75–130 nm	Phage APOV1	*Aeropyrum pernix*	[19]
Fuselloviridae	Double-Stranded RNA	Pleomorphic	Phage SSV1	*Sulfolobus shibatae*	[17]
Leviviridae	Single-Stranded RNA	Icosahedral symmetric protein layers, size ~23 nm.	Phage MS2	*E. coli*	[17]
Cystoviridae	Double-Stranded RNA	Icosahedral symmetric protein layers. Enveloped virions. Spikes protrude from the virion surface. Size between 70-80 nm.	Phage φ6	*Pseudomonas* sp.	[20]
Plasmavirus	Double-Stranded RNA	Pleomorphic, lipidic envelope, no capsid, 80 nm	Phage MVL2	*Acholeplasma laidlawii*	[21]

Replication Cycle

Adsorption to the Bacterial Cell Wall

A main characteristic of phages is the presence of receptor-binding proteins (RBP) in the tail. This protein determines the phage's specificity in recognizing the host bacterial cell. The structural differences of RBP between phages are due to their morphology and guarantee a specific binding mechanism of the viral particle to the bacterium. In some cases, these proteins act with Ca^{2+} for a necessary conformational change to perform their function. In other cases, the presence of Ca^{2+} is not essential for their activation [22, 23]. Their nature and localization also vary between genera: *Myovirus* contain the RBP in their long or short tails or are associated with the viral baseplate (Fig. **1A**) [24, 25]. For the *Siphovirus* family such as *Lactococcus lactis* phage TP901-1, they were found on the surface of the tails base. In contrast, *Bacillus subtilis* phage SPP1 has its RBP associated with its tail fibers (Fig. **1B**) [25]. Phages belonging to the *Podoviridae* family such as P22 phage specific to *Salmonella enterica* serotype Typhimurium, bind to the cellular receptors *via* homotrimeric tail fibers (Fig. **1C**). For infectivity, at least three to six tail fibers are required [26].

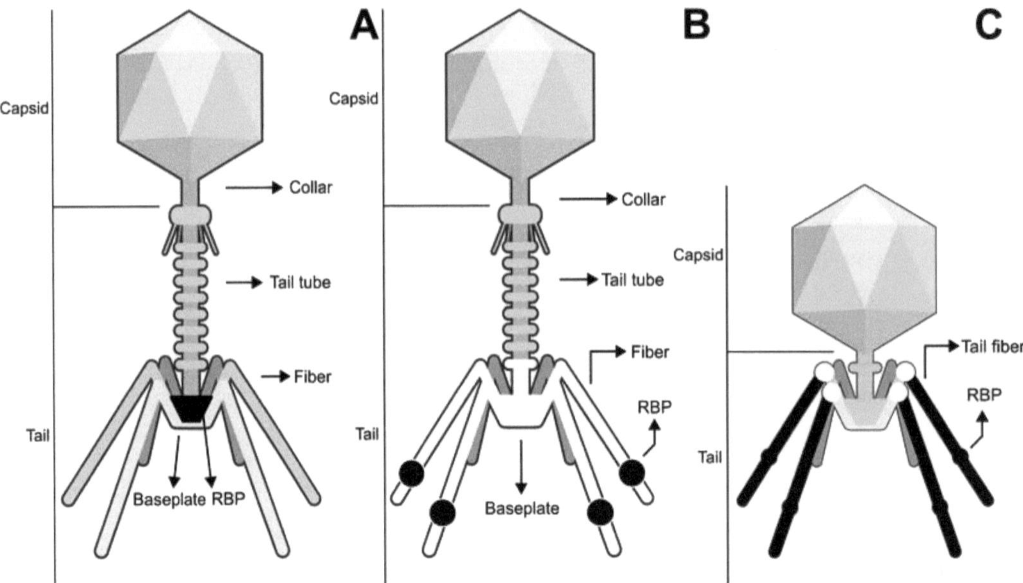

Fig. (1). Schematic representation of phage structures of the different families: *Myoviridae* (A), *Syphoviridae* (B), and *Podoviridae* (C). (The RBP are marked with black circles).

The nature and localization of the phage-like host bacteria receptor also vary. Bacteriophage bind to molecules located on the walls of Gram-positive [27] or

Gram-negative [28] bacteria and to various appendages (*e.g.*, pili [29] and flagella [30]). This diversity of receptors and associated structures is evidence of the presence of mechanisms developed by phage and host bacteria as evolutionary strategies of adoption to changes [31]. In some cases, the phage may have RBP for reversible and irreversible junctions in the bacterial cell wall. The phage proteins and host receptors involved in reversible adsorption are not always the same as those involved in irreversible binding. For example, in the case of the absorption of phage T5 to the Gram-negative bacterium *E. coli*, reversible adsorption occurs through the union of the L-shaped fibers to the polymannose portion of the host cell's lipopolysaccharide (LPS) O antigen. The irreversible binding is achieved by the connection of the pb5 protein of the phage tail with the outer membrane protein receptor FhuA [32]. In the case of phage SPP1 that infects the Gram-positive bacterium *Bacillus subtilis*, the host's glucosylated cell wall teichoic acid (WTA) residues are targeted for reversible binding. In contrast, the interaction between the phage's gp21 protein and the cell membrane protein YueB leads to the irreversible adsorption [33].

If the receptors become inaccessible or non-complementary to the phage receptor-binding protein (RBP), a phage loses the ability to infect its host effectively. Consequently, receptors play a crucial role in the emergence of bacterial resistance to phage attack. Bacteria have developed strategies to avoid phage attacks. For example, they can block phage receptors with the production of capsule or exopolysaccharides that obstruct phage access to the surface of the host cell or with the presence of competitive inhibitors like ferrichrome compounds [31]. But modifications of the receptor structure or even complete loss of the phage receptor leads to adsorption resistance [34].

Some studies of the phage genome of the *Siphoviridae* family show that these phages infect Gram-positive bacteria and encode for certain endolysins. These genes are among the *tmp* genes encoding for Tmp proteins that determine the tail length [35]. *dit* is a highly conserved gene within the family. This gene encodes for the distal tail protein (Dit) responsible for the viral particle basal plaque formation. The *tal* gene, which encodes for an endolysin (lysin) associated with the tail (*tal*), is usually located after *dit*. Tal has murolithical activity associated with the virion and facilitates the phage penetration of the cell by the degradation of the cell wall's peptidoglycan [23, 35, 36]. Structural differences between phage have been found in the same family [25]. These genes are essential for phage adsorption and virulence for certain bacterial infections [37].

The diversity of cell wall components between Gram-positive and Gram-negative bacteria causes structural differences between phages and leads to their diversity. In the case of Gram-positive bacteria, the peptidoglycan, or murein and teichoic acid moieties, are essential components of the bacterial cell wall and are often involved in bacteriophage adsorption. However, in the case of Gram-negative bacteria, it was challenging to identify phage receptors in their complex cell walls, because the cell wall is composed of several different moieties that can contribute to or interfere with phage adsorption [38]. A lipid bilayer with proteins, polysaccharides, comprise the outer membrane (cell wall) of Gram-negative bacteria. The last two molecules form the lipopolysaccharides (LPS) layer. LPS consists of three parts: lipid A, the central polysaccharide domain, and a repetitive glycosylated polymer referred to as the O antigen or O polysaccharide. Some studies showed that coliphage and *Salmonella* phage used proteins, sugar moieties, or both types of receptors. On the other hand, some *Pseudomonas* phages surveyed adsorb onto polysaccharide receptors [39].

Other bacterial structures that serve as a phage receptor are flagella and Fimbriae. Flagella are long thin helical structures that confer motility to cells. Flagellar filaments are composed of many subunits of a single protein called flagellin. The adhesion of phage to the filament structure is generally reversible. The helical movement of the flagellum favors the approach of the phage to the cell surface until reaching the receptors located on the bacterial surface near the base of the flagellum [29].

Fimbriae or pili are filamentous appendages used for bacterial conjugation (sex pilus) and colonization onto surfaces (adherence factors). The sex pili or type IV secretion systems extend from the donor cell to receptors in the wall of the recipient cell. Binding proteins on their surfaces achieved the depolymerization of the pilus, which then causes its retraction, bringing both cells closer for transference of the genetic material on a plasmid. Phage adsorption through pili is not well understood, and most phages that use this system belong to the families *Cystoviridae* and *Inoviridae* [32]. Adsorption of phages to capsules or slime layers is mediated by enzymatic cleavage of the exopolysaccharides that compose these structures [31].

Replication

After phage adsorption takes place through reversible or irreversible interactions, enzymatic degradation of the bacterial cell wall occurs before the insertion of its genome in the host cell [15]. Once internalized, the genome is methylated by an adenine-methylase where the methylase enzyme introduces clumps into the carbon 5 of the DNA pyrimidine ring to protect it from the restriction endonucleases of the host cell cytoplasm [40, 41].

The second step is replication. The bacterial cell provides the molecules and enzymes needed to replicate the genetic material of the phage to produce progeny.

Four different infection cycles have been observed, depending on the phage type. The first is the lysogenic cycle (or temperate). It is favored when the bacteriophage is higher concentration that host cell numbers. It is known as the multiplicity of infection (MOI) [4]. In the lysogenic cyclc, the viral genome integrates into the bacterial genome, where it is replicated during each cell cycle for a specified period. The virus remains latent. When the host cell is under some stressful growth situation, induced by bacterial SOS responses like antibiotic treatment, oxidative stress, or DNA damage, the integrated phage induces its lytic cycle. In this cycle, replication of the viral genome is initiated through the synthesis of its proteins, maturation of progeny occurs, and virion genomes are passed down to all daughter cells. The viral genome uses part or all of the biosynthetic machinery of the host cell for its replication. Recently, the mechanism by which bacteriophage elect when to perform each step of the cycle was described. Molecular communication between phage particles was found. This communication involves small molecules that are released into the medium by the bacteriophage after entering a lysogenic cycle. These molecules inform other viral particles to perform a lysogenic cycle instead of a lytic cycle. This communication system was termed "arbitrary" by Erez *et al.* [42]. It allows communication between virions from one generation to another, estimates the number of recent infections, and decides whether to use the lytic or lysogenic cycle [42, 43].

Lytic phages (virulent) infect bacterial cells causing inhibition of the host's metabolism and directing it exclusively to produce progeny. The result is the lysis of the bacterium accompanied by the release of multiple phage particles. New phage can then infect and propagate in other host cells. The time for the whole cycle to take is usually 1 to 2 h, and the number of phages produced depends on the type of phage [44].

In the continuous development cycle, phages are formed uninterruptedly within the host cell without causing lysis and are released when the maturation of the virion is completed [4].

The pseudolysogenic replication cycle has been studied to a lesser extent. Therefore, its molecular and physiological basis is not well understood. The constant production of phages in the presence of a great abundance of host cells allows the co-existence of both. Miller and Day [45] proposed that the pseudolysogenic process occurs when host cells are in limited nutrient conditions. Consequently, there is no energy available for the phage to produce a lysogenic or lytic cycle response. With the right conditions of nutrients for the cell and optimal levels of metabolic energy, the phage can use this energy for its gene expression and produce lysogenic or lytic phage. In many hostile environments, virions inactivate the cycle, resulting in pseudo-lysogenicity, which ultimately serves to protect and extend the useful life of the viral genome under stressful host growth conditions [45].

Release of Viral Progeny and Cell Lysis

The first step in the release of viral particles is caused by smoothing of the host cell wall due to the activity of holins, enzymes encoded by phages which produce pores in the host cell membranes, and by lysins, which digest the bacterial peptidoglycan. The function of the holins is to pierce the cytoplasmic membrane of the host cell, thus allowing the endolysins to access the peptidoglycan layer of the cell wall [46]. The holins determine the time of bacterial lysis and control the access of phage endolysins to the cell wall murein. Therefore, they synchronize the activity of the holin-lysin system with late-phase events of the phage replication cycle [47]. The primary structure of the holins is not well preserved in evolution. However, differences in amino acid sequences between holins do not have a significant impact on their function [46]. S105 is the product of the expression of λ phage S gene and causes lethal lesions in lipid bilayer [47].

Phage endolysins are the enzymes responsible for the degradation of the cell wall. These enzymes are amidase, glycosidases, transglycosidases, and can hydrolyze cell wall peptidoglycans [48]. There are structural differences between lysins that act against Gram-positive and Gram-negative bacteria. Differences were observed between substrates and degradation sites of the enzymes. The cell wall structure of Gram-negative bacteria limits accesses to the cell wall. Endolysins targeted to Gram-negative bacteria are small globular proteins composed of a single domain, called the Enzymatically Active Domain (EAD) [49]. Endolysins directed against Gram-positive organisms have a cell wall binding domain (CBD) and therefore remain immobilized on the surface of peptidoglycan [50, 51]. CBD participates in the hydrolytic effects of endolysin by synergy with EAD that performs a catalytic function of the enzyme protein. During this process, the endolysin remains tightly bound to a site associated with the peptidoglycan. The time of bacterial lysis depends on the ratio between holin and its antagonist, antiholins. The holin-antiholins rate is strictly regulated by controlling its expression at the translation level. The loss of the plasma membrane integrity, followed by the elevation of the holin-antiholins rate, allows the endolysin to reach the periplasm and begin to degrade the peptidoglycan of the host [52]. The progeny is then released, ready to infect other cells and start the cycle again [4, 25].

Other Components in the Replication Cycle

During the synthesis of the viral enzymes within the replication cycle, encoded endolysins and phage accumulate within the bacterial cytoplasm until the assembly of the viral particles is complete. Bacteria secrete endolysins, which remain inactive, anchored to the membrane until the membrane potential collapses [53]. This process is triggered by holins, a small membrane protein that controls endolysin function. Holin molecules accumulate in the host cytoplasmic and form small pores that dissipate the potential of the membrane [54]. Even though the natural mode of action of endolysins is internal, the endolysins can degrade the peptidoglycan layer of Gram-positive bacteria when applied exogenously. This mechanism has sparked interest in its use as an alternative to antimicrobials [55].

Three enzyme groups exist which are implicated in the viral replication cycle:

1. The glycosidase group of enzymes includes N-acetyl-β-D-glucosaminidases, which hydrolyzed the β-1,4 linkage between GlcNAc and MurNAc subunits of the bacterial peptidoglycan. N-acetyl-β-D-muramidase hydrolyzes the β-1,4 link between MurNAc and GlcNAc; and transglycosylases that are very similar to muramidase. The difference in their mechanism of action is that they break the β-1,4 bond between the MurNAc and GlcNAc, and they form a 1,6-anhydrous residue of MurNAc [56].
2. Amidases: The N-acetylmuramic-L-alanine amidase activity catalyzes the hydrolysis of the amide bond between MurNAc and the first amino acid of the stem peptide [57].
3. Endopeptidases: The endopeptidases hydrolyze the bond between two amino acids, thus cleaving the peptides within the peptidoglycan [57].

BACTERIOPHAGE USE FOR PHAGE THERAPY

Phages possess properties that make them interesting but challenging candidates for different applications. The medical and veterinary fields and the hygiene, sanitation, food, agriculture, and environment sectors could potentially apply phages. Advances in the field of phage biology have found multiple applications in different science areas, especially in biotechnology, including vaccine development, bacterial detection systems, nanotechnology, antimicrobials production, and foodborne pathogens control [58 - 60].

Health Applications

The use of antimicrobials is the most affordable alternative for controlling and eliminating pathogenic bacteria. These can act by inhibiting the biosynthesis of the nucleic acids or molecules linked to the cell wall structure, causing damage to the integrity of the membranes or interfering with the wide variety of essential metabolic processes [61]. The rapid increase in multi-drug-resistant bacteria has led to an interest in phage therapy as a possible alternative to antibiotics or, at least, a complementary approach for the treatment of some bacterial infections [62 - 64]. The ease of administration is one of the essential reasons for using phage as an antimicrobial agent. They can be administered in multiple ways: topically, orally, by inhalation, directly into body tissues or intravenously. Besides, patients that are allergic to antibiotics can be treated with phages, usually without adverse effects [65]. However, the most significant concern during therapy is the development of resistance by bacteria. If phage-resistant bacteria develop during treatment, a round of detection of new phages, active against the resistant strain, can be easily and quickly configured [66].

The incorporation of phages in the combined therapy against infectious complications gave improved positive results in 81.5% of the cases, while the antibiotics alone were effective in 60.6% of the cases [67]. These authors suggest that treatment of mono-bacterial infections is efficient only with bacteriophages, but its efficiency decreases when it comes to mixed infections. However, the use of both phages and antibiotics is recommended for complicated cases [67]. In cases of patients with burns, phage therapy has shown to provide faster healing, temperature normalization, wound purification, and less mortality [68]. In the case of the treatment of suppurative foot wounds in diabetic individuals with antibiotics and phage therapy, the depuration time is shorter, and granulation and epithelization of lesions compared with the traditional treatment were also observed [69].

Studies were performed with patients with suppurative wounds to investigate the effect of phage therapy on serum levels of tumor necrosis factor-alpha (TNF-alpha) and interleukin-6 (IL-6), as well as the ability of blood cells to produce these cytokines. The release of TNF was modified according to the initial capacity to produce this cytokine: the production of TNF was reduced in high-response patients and was increased in low-response patients. These results correspond to the first study that demonstrated that phage therapy could normalize serum TNF-alpha levels and the production of IL-6 [70].

Perepanova *et al.* [71] studied the clinical and bacteriological efficacy of treatment with bacteriophage preparations in urinary tract infections. This study described the sensitivity of infectious agents to phage. The phage preparations were adapted to increase the sensitivity of the infectious agents isolated from patients with urinary tract infections. The effectiveness of the therapy amounted to 84%. So, the authors infer that phage therapy is an effective and safe therapeutic modality in the treatment of urinary tract infection in monotherapy and combination with antibiotics [71].

Moreover, studies were performed in mice to control localized and systemic infections caused by methicillin-resistant *Staphylococcus aureus*. Phages were administered in three schemes: monotherapy, multiple-dose phage cocktails, and single-dose phage cocktail. The phage cocktail and therapy with varying doses were effective in preventing and controlling localized infections. However, the single-dose phage cocktail did not control infection, and phage therapy was not effective in systemic infections [72].

Different studies have been carried out to treat health problems as dangerous as obesity, which is correlated to the composition of the intestinal microbiota. Some studies demonstrated the relationship between *Enterobacter cloacae* B29 and the intestinal microbiota in obese patients. In this sense, Gongze and Bridgewater [73] studied the lytic activity of some phages against this bacterium, suggesting phage therapy as a possible control treatment for this disease.

Currently, countries like France, Belgium, Switzerland (Phagoburn project) and the United States have included phage therapy in their health programs [74]. The Center for Phage Therapy of the Hirszfeld Institute of Immunology and Experimental Therapy in Wroclaw offers its patients phage therapies as an alternate treatment for bacterial diseases caused by *Acinetobacter, Burkholderia, Citrobacter, Enterobacter, Enterococcus, Escherichia, Klebsiella, Morganella, Proteus, Pseudomonas, Shigella, Salmonella, Serratia, Staphylococcus*, and *Stenotrophomonas* [46]. Eliava Phage Therapy Center in Tbilisi used phage for the treatment of infections caused by *Enterococcus faecalis, E. coli* (O11, O18, O20, O25, O26, O44, O55, O113, O125, O128), *Proteus vulgaris, P. mirabilis, Pseudomonas aeruginosa, Salmonella, Shigella flexneri* (serovars 1, 2, 3, 4), *Sh. Sonnei* (serovar 6), *Sh. newcastle, S. aureus, S. epidermidis, S. saprophyticus*, and *Streptococcus pyogenes, St. sanguis,* and *St. salivarius.*

Many studies have been carried out in the last decade to apply phage lysins to control pathogens topically and systemically on mucosal surfaces and biofilms [75]. Lytic phage enzymes were first tested in 2001 to prevent and treat colonization of the upper airways in mice infected with group Streptococci [76]. After two hours of administration of 500 U of PlyC lysin to colonized animals, the remaining bacteria were not detected.

Applications in the Food Industry

Many authors discussed the control of foodborne pathogens using phages at all of the stages of the food industry production chain. Examples of the use of phage in food production are shown in Table **2**.

Table 2. Some cases of phage therapy against foodborne bacteria used in the food industry.

Phage	Bacteria	Food Product	Reference
Salmonella phage SJ2	*Salmonella*	Cheddar cheese	[77]
Salmonella phage cocktails	*Salmonella*	Fruits	[78]
Salmonella phage Felix-O1	*Salmonella enterica* serotype Typhimurium	Chicken	[79]
Lytic bacteriophages	*Salmonella enterica* serotype Enteritidis	Chicken skin	[80]
Lytic bacteriophages	*Campylobacter jejuni*	Chicken skin	[80]
Phage cocktail	*Listeria monocytogenes* LCDC 81-861	Honeydew Melon Tissue	[81]
Phage cocktail	*E. coli* O157:H7	Drinking water	[82]
Phage KHI Phage SH1	*E. coli* O157:H7	Meat	[83]
S. aureus phage K	*Staphylococcus aureus*	Milk	[84]
Lytic phages	*Staphylococcus aureus*	Curd	[85]
E. sakazakii phages	*Enterobacter sakazakii*	Infant formula Milk	[86]
Listeria bacteriophages LMP1 LMP7	*L. monocytogenes* ATCC 7644, 15313, 19114, and 19115	Milk	[87]

Phages were applied as biosanitizers to decontaminate fruit and vegetables as well as surfaces of food contact equipment (Table **2**). Moreover, they were useful as biopreservatives to extend the shelf life of manufactured foods [59, 88 - 91].

The Food and Drug Administration (FDA) approved the use of phages as a preservative in food, and the interest in these bioproducts has increased in the food safety field to allow proper starter culture performance in fermented products and to keep the natural microbiota undisturbed [54, 92].

Due to their specificity, bacteriophages do not affect food's properties, do not infect other bacterial cultures used in its manufacture, as the case of probiotics or dairy, and are harmless for eukaryotic cells. These characteristics make them potentially natural food additives for biocontrol of foodborne pathogenic bacteria. There are already studies of the application of phages used to control *L. monocytogenes* [88, 93], *E. coli* [89], and *S. enterica* subspecies *enterica* serotype *Enteritidis* [91].

According to the WHO in 2015 [3], the most frequent causes of foodborne diseases are diarrheal agents, mainly *Campylobacter* spp., which causes about

230000 deaths per year, and non-typhoidal *Salmonella enterica,* which causes diarrhea, gastroenteritis, and invasive infections.

Some authors have focused on the search and application of phage therapy for the control of these bacteria in farm animals before and after being processed for human consumption [79, 94 - 98]. Atterbury *et al.* [95] showed that bacteriophages could be used to significantly reduce colonization of *Salmonella enterica* serotype *Enteritidis* and *Typhimurium* in chicken destined for human consumption. A considerable reduction of Colony Forming Units (CFU) was observed after 24 h for both bacteria compared with controls. However, in the case of *S. enterica* serotype *Hadar* treatment with phages was ineffective. They concluded that the selection of the appropriate bacteriophages and optimization of time and phage administration method are critical factors in the successful control of pathogens mediated by phages.

Wagenaar *et al.* [94] controlled disease-causing agents in chicken with bacteriophages specific for *Campylobacter jejuni* using CFU and plaque formation units (PFU). As the CFU decreased, the PFU increased, indicating productive phage replication and host cell lysis. They concluded that treatment with phages is a promising alternative to reduce colonization by *C. jejuni* in chicken. In other studies, the activity of phage proteins with endoglycosidase or hydrolase activity has been evaluated with promising results. Waseh *et al.* [99] tested Tsps P22. Tsps is a well-characterized phage protein of the *Podoviridae* family that recognizes the lipopolysaccharides of *Salmonella enterica* serotype Typhimurium. These authors demonstrated the decrease in bacterial motility, significantly reducing the colonization of these bacteria after use.

E. coli O157:H7 is one of the critical pathogens foodborne and a focus on human health because its ingestion at concentrations as low as 10-100 cells can result in potent toxin exposure. The principal reservoir for this organism is ruminants. The contamination of animal products occurs during the slaughtering process. To reduce pathogen contamination phage CEV1 was orally delivered to sheep, and in two days, a decrease of 2 logs in the intestine of *E. coli* O157:H7 was observed [100]. Some authors tested other combinations of phages in other food such as beef [47] and could not find viable cells in most cases after storage at 37 ° C.

BACTERIOPHAGE PREPARATIONS

Several products have been developed and approved to control foodborne pathogens in water and food safety, agriculture, and animal health. EBI Food Safety commercializes Listex P100 to control *Listeria* sp. in meat and cheese products [88]. In August 2006, the U.S. Food and Drug Administration (FDA) approved the use of LMP 102 phage preparation (Intralytix, Inc.) targeted to

Listeria spp in ready-to-eat meat and poultry products [101]. Ecoshield is a product marketed by the company Intralytix. It is a mixture of three phages that act against *E. coli* O157:H7, which was tested in foods with a risk of contamination by this pathogen, such as beef. The same company made ListShield™, which is a preparation that includes six phages against *L. monocytogenes*, and can be applied to foods and on surfaces that may have contact with contaminated foods. SalmFresh is a concentrated combination of six phages with positive results against *S. enterica* in red meat, chicken meat, fish, fruits, and vegetables. FDA approved all these cocktails [62].

An important aspect of phage therapy is the highest effectiveness when developing a product and its application, whether through the usage of a specific bacteriophage or the use of a phage cocktail. The application of highly particular bacteriophages, adapted to bacterial strains isolated from individual patients by a previous culture, was more effective than the treatment with a specific poly-phages cocktail [102]. The significant efficiency of this type of personalized phage therapy can be explained by phage specificity and virulence against the host strains. However, the preparation of adapted phages requires detailed characterization because they may also contain temperate phages [34].

Other ongoing experimental developments are the construction of recombinant therapeutic phages that are highly lytic and engineered for different bacterial cell receptor specificities, or that have extra genes coding for host lethal toxin proteins to enhance their killing effects [103].

Indications and Limitations

Liquid preparations were initially proposed for phage therapy and have been widely used in local situations. Still, the route of administration in patients has been extended to include other forms such as oral, subcutaneous, parental, and peritoneal preparations. It is necessary to consider the bacteriophage sensitivity to several chemical and physical conditions such as gastric acids and presence of antiseptics. Preparation of bacteriophages may also contain bacterial parts that cause some undesirable reactions such as fever and headache. So, elimination of host factors is significant in production of phage preparations for clinical use. The tolerance of these preparations to the chemical and physical conditions during its administration is difficult to predict. Still, it is an indicator that should be considered when designing quality therapy [104].

Oral administration of bacteriophages is easy and should not have side effects. It should consider, however, some antagonistic factors that, in some cases, are difficult to control. Gastric acids are a hostile barrier in oral bacteriophage intake, and the intestinal microbiota constitutes an interactive, competitive and complex environment that makes phage treatment to be uncertain. For this reason, phage therapy is personalized and a particular treatment should be used for each specific infectious event. This avoids effects on the intestinal microbiota [104].

The interaction between bacterial and viral particles increases *in vitro* by agitation conditions, while *in vivo,* it is less common. However, Loc Carrillo *et al.* demonstrated the dose-dependent decrease of more than 90% of the bacteria that colonize the intestine [105], which suggests that these bacteria were infected, but the dose was not enough for the complete elimination of host bacteria [106]. Occasionally, cells may also localize in inaccessible sites for the bacteriophage infection such as intestinal crypts or villi, which hinders the recognition of target cells by viral particles [106] and results in a physical means of protection of the host bacterial cell.

Phage DNA used for therapeutic purposes should be sequenced to ensure that it does not include genes for toxins, pathogenicity, or unwanted bacterial host genes [107]. Azeredo and Sutherland [108] report that phage is sensitive to acidic environments. Oral administration in case of phage therapy works better with an antacid since it increases the number of phages that survive through the stomach. However, the effectiveness of the treatment depends on the environment to which the virus is exposed, the concentration of pathogenic bacteria at the site of the infection and the composition of the dose applied [108].

Bacterial Resistance

Before testing bacteriophage preparations, a study should be carried out to evaluate host susceptibility to the phages before beginning treatment, which carries additional costs [34]. Bacteriophages do not always recognize all strains within the same bacterial species; by this reasoning, the spectrum of phage activity is another critical point for the development and application of phage therapies. As more phages are included in a cocktail, the possibility is greater than this formulation will cover future medical and commercial demands. However, this could have an impact on other bacteria of probiotic importance. The fact that some phage within the cocktail use bacteria with probiotic characteristics as host inside the intestine and causes its lysis, could result in an imbalance in the intestinal microbiota [109]. The characterization of the phages that are applied for this purpose is of vital importance.

In most cases, this impact is even lower than expected with typical commercial antibiotics [34]. Besides, it can promote bacterial resistance against specific phages inside the cocktail. It is important to evaluate that phages within the preparation have a strictly lytic replication cycle to avoid the emergence of bacterial resistance [106]. Modifying receptor structure through mutation and hiding receptors with additional physical barriers are some of the strategies used by the host cell to prevent phage adsorption [107]. Some bacteria can develop resistance mechanisms to phage. The phage receptor can be blocked by either the presence of inhibitors or the synthesis of a protective biofilm. However, some studies indicate that phages can overcome this hurdle by expressing lytic enzymes that can penetrate through the bacterial exopolysaccharide matrix [108]. The K1 capsule expressed by *E. coli* has shown to directly interfere with phage T7 attachment to its LPS receptor [110]. The bacterial endonucleases recognize and can destroy the injected foreign phage nucleic acid, although some phages can evade this mechanism [111]. Phage resistance mechanisms may cause phage-infected bacterial cells to die off before completing the lytic cycle [112]. In the genome of most bacteria is a genetic locus with the function as a prokaryotic immune system in conferring acquired immunity (CRISPR-Cas interference) towards exogenous genetic elements like plasmids and phages [113]. Some competing phages modulate the expression of receptors on the bacterial surface. The availability of the *P. aeruginosa* type IV pilus, which is essential in pathogenesis and biofilm formation, can be modulated by lysogenic conversion. Phage D3112 encodes a protein called Tip that binds to an ATPase from *P. aeruginosa* type IV pilus and prevents its localization, resulting in a loss of surface piliation and protection from other phages that depend on the *P. aeruginosa* type IV pilus for infection. The presence of outer membrane vesicles (OMVs) reduced Phage T4 levels, leading to the suggestion that shedding of OMVs into the environment may act as a decoy to prevent phage adsorption that would otherwise lead to a productive infection [114].

If the phage can recognize the surface receptor, bacteria have a superinfection exclusion (Sie) system that can act to block the phage DNA injection into host cells. The Sie systems are membrane-anchored or membrane-associated proteins. The TP-J34 thermophilic phage of *Streptococcus* produces the lipoprotein located in the membrane LtpTP-J34, which is thought to interact with the tape measure protein of other phages [115]. Some proteins in *Siphoviridae* are involved in the channel formation for DNA passage, LtpTP-J34 blocks the injection process and the incoming phage replication. The *E. coli* phage HK97 produces gp15, a predicted transmembrane protein that inhibits DNA entry of HK97 and the closely related phage HK75 [116]. The Sie system protects the specific cell that faces phage superinfection and the surrounding population since the phage will not be able to infect the cell [107].

There are other innate intracellular defenses to prevent the replication and release of the phage in case it manages to adsorb and inject its DNA successfully. The restriction-modification (R-M) systems are composed of a restriction endonuclease (REase) and a cognate methyltransferase (MTase). This system can destroy invading DNA [117]. REases recognize unmodified DNA and cleave it into harmless fragments, and the MTase normally methylates self-DNA at specific recognition sites, while foreign DNA is not modified [107].

Abortive infection (Abi) systems lead to death of the infected cell as a sacrifice to protect the surrounding population from viral infection. These systems can act at any stage of phage development to decrease or eliminate the production of progeny viruses [107, 118]. Chopin *et al.* [118] reported that the majority of Abis are on plasmids of Gram-positive lactococcal strains. Still, some Abi systems are in Gram-negative species, including *E. coli*, *V. cholerae*, and *Sh. dysenteriae*. From AbiA to AbiZ systems are located on *L. lactis* [118]. Fineran *et al.* [119] describe a highly effective 2-gene Abi system from the phytopathogen *Erwinia carotovora* subspecies *atroseptica*, designated ToxIN. The ToxIN Abi system also functions as a pair of toxin-antitoxin (TA). The ToxI RNA antitoxin repeated in tandem counteracts toxicity, and ToxN inhibits bacterial growth [119]. AbiA interferes with the DNA replication of small isometric phages [120]. AbiB is a constitutive protein, and its expression does not increase following phage infection. Overexpression of AbiB is toxic for both *L. lactis* and *E. coli*. It appears that a new phage product induces the synthesis or stimulates the activity of an RNase [118, 121]. AbiC reduces the synthesis of structural phage proteins [122]. AbiD1 expression is induced by the presence of the phage bIL66 infection. AbiD1 protein interacts with an isometric phage gene product (ORF1) to prevent the translation of the phage ORF3 RNA and interferes with a phage RuvC-like endonuclease [118, 123, 125]. AbiP is a membrane-anchored protein able to bind single-stranded RNA or DNA in a sequence-independent manner and acts early in the phage replication cycle to disrupt the phage DNA replication and the temporal switch from early to late gene expression [118, 124]. AbiU delays phage transcription, and AbiZ induces premature lysis of infected cells, aborting the cycle, ensuring that the viral assembly is incomplete and that infectious virions are not released [125].

SYNERGY BETWEEN BACTERIOPHAGES AND THE IMMUNE SYSTEM

Many studies demonstrated the antimicrobial activity of bacteriophages and their application in patients with bacterial infections. However, its relationship with the immune system has not been explored. Studies indicate that phage have potent immunomodulatory properties like probiotics and is recognized as an important part of the mammalian immune system by maintaining their homeostasis [126]. The immune response against bacteriophages depends on the localization of bacterial infection and the injection site of therapeutic phages. During phage therapy, an immune response is raised in which neutralizing antibodies produced against them can inhibit the effectiveness of phages from lysing the targeted bacteria *in vivo* [127, 128]. This is due to the fact that the neutralizing antibodies bind to epitopes in the virion structure that are essential for infecting the host cell [129]. Anti-phage neutralizing antibodies are probably one of the most critical factors responsible for the efficacy limitation of phage therapy. However, some studies suggest that the development of neutralizing antibodies does not represent a real problem since the kinetics of the action of the phage are much faster than the production of neutralizing antibodies from the host [130].

Phage causes anti-inflammatory effects by reducing the levels of inflammation indicators such as C-reactive protein [131]. Van Belleghem *et al.* [132] studied the immune response of human peripheral blood mononuclear cells against purified phages. They evidenced that phage blocks the expression of proinflammatory cytokines and inhibits T1 cells, NK cells, and macrophages activity; while induces a reduction of type 4 Toll-like receptor (TLR4) proinflammatory markers. Sun and Feng [133] obtained similar data. They showed that phage reduced the inflammatory response and induced high expression of interleukin (IL). Międzybrodzki *et al.* [134] showed that T4 phage acts by inhibiting the production of reactive oxygen species through endotoxins and living bacteria, by inhibiting the NF-κB activity in epithelial cells stimulated by the herpes virus type 1, as well as decreasing the cellular infiltration of allograft skin allogeneic [134, 135].

Besides, T4 phage does not only act directly on the immune system response; microorganisms, such as coliforms or *S. aureus,* caused some allergies or asthma illnesses. The application of phages could selectively eliminate these bacterial pathogens and thus alleviate or even prevent allergy symptoms [135]. In the treatment with several preparations of anti-staphylococcal bacteriophage directed to patients with Netherton Syndrome (NS) with the recurrence of bacterial infections, Zhvania *et al.* [136] reported significant improvement after seven days and very substantial changes in their symptoms and life quality after treatment for six months. One of the mechanisms recently studied showed that the activity of phage and the immune system focused on the GP12 protein, an adhesin from the tail of phage T4 that mediates binding of the phage with the lipopolysaccharide (LPS) layer of the bacterial cell wall. LPSs are also known as endotoxins and can exert a significant impact on the immune response in animals and humans. The LPS represents a Pathogen-associated Molecular Patterns (PAMP), which causes rapid activation of intracellular signaling pathways in a live system that is very similar to the signaling systems of IL-1 and IL-18 [137]. At the systemic level, this reaction means an acute inflammatory response and is a critical factor in sepsis and septic shock [138]. GP12 protein can be considered as a potential tool for modular and specifically to counteract the physiological effects related to LPS *in vivo.*

Phages contain PAMPs as genetic material, either RNA or DNA, so understanding the immune response against phage administration is necessary [139]. In addition to PAMPs, some phages may express proteins that mediate interaction with host cells and promote immune responses [140], along with possible differences in levels of endotoxin contamination that would explain the differences between levels of cytokine induction [139].

The adjuvant properties of phages are being exploited for phage-based approaches to vaccination and therapy of cancer but may also influence other types of phage therapy. For example, the recruitment of tumor-associated macrophages and tumor regression was absent in MyD88-deficient mice treated with genetically engineered phages that target tumor cells *in vivo* [139]. The absence of MyD88 or TLR9 affected the phage-mediated recognition of Ag for dendritic cells and the subsequent activation of T cells. The lack of MyD88 abolished vaccine responses to phages displaying peptides and altered in the absence of TLR9. Neutrophils were essential for successful treatment of pneumonia with anti–*P. aeruginosa* phages [139]. It showed that interactions between phage-derived ligands and host contribute to the efficacy of phage therapies.

Phages show an adaptive response to the immune system. Studies carried out with phage ΦX174 showed a specific reaction of IgM and IgG in patients with intact B cell activity [141]. In patients with absent or altered B cell activity, this response is not present [142]. For the adaptive response to take place, the viral particles must undergo a degradation process for the presentation of the Ag to occur. Some studies conducted in mice revealed that immunization using T4 phage induced high titers of anti-Hoc neutralizing antibodies, and immunomodulation of viral capsid glycoprotein expression [143]. This effect correlated with loss of protection mediated by T4 against *E. coli* [142]. The anti-phage antibodies mediated elimination of phages from the intestine and circulation, with an increase in the levels of phage-specific IgA in the feces, which correlated with the gradual absence of phages ingested orally [142].

The improvement of phage therapy could include the selection of phages with natural resistance to phagocytosis degradation, with the rational design of recombinant phages to achieve this. In this case, the induction of phage-specific adaptive immune responses would be avoided or delayed, and possibly the persistence of phages in immunocompetent individuals would be prolonged [139].

CONCLUDING REMARKS

The global increase in antibiotic-resistant pathogenic bacteria makes a priority to explore new strategies for solving this problem. The use of bacteriophages for control of these infections shows a promising alternative therapy. A combination of antibiotics can increase the efficiency of this therapy. Safe use of bacteriophages in clinical treatments will require a detailed study of the biological characteristics of phage and the properties of the product, as well as a study of the behavior of phages with target cells *in vivo* systems fundamentally.

CONSENT FOR PUBLICATION

Not applicable.

CONFLICT OF INTEREST

The authors confirm that this chapter content has no conflict of interest.

ACKNOWLEDGEMENTS

Declared none.

REFERENCES

[1]   Dewey-Mattia D, Manikonda D, Hall K, *et al.* Surveillance for Foodborne Disease Outbreaks - United States, 2009-2015 Morbidity and mortality weekly report Surveil summ 2018; 67: 1-11.

[2]   González T, Rojas R. Foodborne diseases and PCR: prevention and diagnosis. Mex Public Health 2005; 47(5): 388-90.

[3]   World Health Organization. WHO estimates of the global burden of foodborne diseases WHO 2015; 13: 13-6.

[4]   Prada-Peñaranda C, Holguín-Moreno AV, González-Barrios AF, Vives-Flórez MJ. Fagoterapia, alternativa para el control de las infecciones bacterianas. Perspectivas en Colombia. Univ Sci 2015; 20(1): 43-59.
        [http://dx.doi.org/10.11144/Javeriana.SC20-1.faci]

[5]   Balcázar JL, Subirats J, Borrego CM. The role of biofilms as environmental reservoirs of antibiotic resistance. Front Microbiol 2015; 6(1216): 1216.
        [http://dx.doi.org/10.3389/fmicb.2015.01216] [PMID: 26583011]

[6]   Tawil N. Immobilisation de plasma de bactériophages et ses applications WO Patent WO/2018/198051 2018.

[7]   Sulakvelidze A, Alavidze Z, Glenn Morris JJr. Bacteriophage therapy. Antimicrob Agents Chemother 2001; 45(3): 649-59.
        [http://dx.doi.org/10.1128/AAC.45.3.649-659.2001]

[8]   Twort FW, Long LRCP. An investigation on the nature of ultra-microscopic viruses. Lancet 1915; 186(4814): 1241-3.
        [http://dx.doi.org/10.1016/S0140-6736(01)20383-3]

[9]   Stout BF. Bacteriophage therapy. Tex State J Med 1933; 29: 205-9.

[10]   d'Herelle F, Summers WC. Felix d'Herelle and the origins of molecular biology. London: Yale University Press 1999; p. 230.

[11]   Fruciano DE, Bourne S. Phage as an antimicrobial agent: d'Herelle's heretical theories and their role

in the decline of phage prophylaxis in the West. Can J Infect Dis Med Microbiol 2007; 18(1): 19-26.
[http://dx.doi.org/10.1155/2007/976850] [PMID: 18923687]

[12]   Goyal SM. Viruses in foods. New York: Springer 2006; p. 345.
[http://dx.doi.org/10.1007/0-387-29251-9]

[13]   Appelt S, Fancello L, Le Bailly M, Raoult D, Drancourt M, Desnues C. Viruses in a 14th-century coprolite. Appl Environ Microbiol 2014; 80(9): 2648-55.
[http://dx.doi.org/10.1128/AEM.03242-13] [PMID: 24509925]

[14]   Ackermann HW. Bacteriophage observations and evolution. Res Microbiol 2003; 154(4): 245-51.
[http://dx.doi.org/10.1016/S0923-2508(03)00067-6] [PMID: 12798228]

[15]   Kutter E, Sulakvelidze A. Bacteriophages: Biology and Applications. United States of America: CRC Press 2005; p. 527.

[16]   Monk AB, Rees CD, Barrow P, Hagens S, Harper DR. Bacteriophage applications: where are we now? Lett Appl Microbiol 2010; 51(4): 363-9.
[http://dx.doi.org/10.1111/j.1472-765X.2010.02916.x] [PMID: 20796209]

[17]   Ackermann HW. Bacteriophage taxonomy. Microbiol Aust 2011; 146: 90-4.

[18]   Hanna M. Oksanen and ICTV Report Consortium. J Gen Virol 2017; 98(5): 888-9.
[http://dx.doi.org/10.1099/jgv.0.000795] [PMID: 28581380]

[19]   Prangishvili D, Mochizuki T, Krupovic M. Ictv Report Consortium. ICTV Virus Taxonomy Profile: Guttaviridae. J Gen Virol 2018; 99(3): 290-1.
[http://dx.doi.org/10.1099/jgv.0.001027] [PMID: 29458561]

[20]   Poranen MM, Mäntynen S. Ictv Report Consortium. ICTV Virus Taxonomy Profile: Cystoviridae. J Gen Virol 2017; 98(10): 2423-4.
[http://dx.doi.org/10.1099/jgv.0.001027] [PMID: 29458561]

[21]   Mart Krupovic, Ictv Report Consortium. ICTV Virus Taxonomy Profile: Plasmaviridae. J Gen Virol. Microbiol Sci 2018; 99(5): 617-8.

[22]   Veesler D, Spinelli S, Mahony J, *et al.* Structure of the phage TP901-1 1.8 MDa baseplate suggests an alternative host adhesion mechanism. Proc Natl Acad Sci USA 2012; 109(23): 8954-8.
[http://dx.doi.org/10.1073/pnas.1200966109] [PMID: 22611190]

[23]   Spinelli S, Veesler D, Bebeacua C, Cambillau C. Structures and host-adhesion mechanisms of lactococcal siphophages. Front Microbiol 2014; 5(3): 3.
[http://dx.doi.org/10.3389/fmicb.2014.00003] [PMID: 24474948]

[24]   Habann M, Leiman PG, Vandersteegen K, *et al.* Listeria phage A511, a model for the contractile tail machineries of SPO1-related bacteriophages. Mol Microbiol 2014; 92(1): 84-99.
[http://dx.doi.org/10.1111/mmi.12539] [PMID: 24673724]

[25]   Dowah ASA, Clokie MRJ. Review of the nature, diversity and structure of bacteriophage receptor binding proteins that target Gram-positive bacteria. Biophys Rev 2018; 10(2): 535-42.
[http://dx.doi.org/10.1007/s12551-017-0382-3] [PMID: 29299830]

[26]   Cvirkaite-Krupovic V. Entry of the membrane-containing bacteriophages into their hosts. PhD dissertation, 2010.

[27]   Xia G, Corrigan RM, Winstel V, Goerke C, Gründling A, Peschel A. Wall teichoic Acid-dependent adsorption of staphylococcal siphovirus and myovirus. J Bacteriol 2011; 193(15): 4006-9.
[http://dx.doi.org/10.1128/JB.01412-10] [PMID: 21642458]

[28]   Marti R, Zurfluh K, Hagens S, Pianezzi J, Klumpp J, Loessner MJ. Long tail fibres of the novel broad-host-range T-even bacteriophage S16 specifically recognize *Salmonella* OmpC. Mol Microbiol 2013; 87(4): 818-34.
[http://dx.doi.org/10.1111/mmi.12134] [PMID: 23289425]

[29]   Guerrero-Ferreira RC, Viollier PH, Ely B, *et al.* Alternative mechanism for bacteriophage adsorption to the motile bacterium Caulobacter crescentus. Proc Natl Acad Sci USA 2011; 108(24): 9963-8.
[http://dx.doi.org/10.1073/pnas.1012388108] [PMID: 21613567]

[30]   Shin H, Lee J-H, Kim H, Choi Y, Heu S, Ryu S. Receptor diversity and host interaction of bacteriophages infecting *Salmonella enterica* serovar *Typhimurium*. PLoS One 2012; 7(8): e43392.
[http://dx.doi.org/10.1371/journal.pone.0043392] [PMID: 22927964]

[31]   Bertozzi Silva J, Storms Z, Sauvageau D. Host receptors for bacteriophage adsorption. FEMS Microbiol Lett 2016; 363(4): 1-11.
[http://dx.doi.org/10.1093/femsle/fnw002] [PMID: 26755501]

[32]   Frost L. Conjugative pili and pilus-specific phages. In: Clewell DB, Ed. Bacterial Conjugation. New York: Plenum Press 1993; pp. 189-222.
[http://dx.doi.org/10.1007/978-1-4757-9357-4_7]

[33]   Rakhuba DV, Kolomiets EI, Dey ES, Novik GI. Bacteriophage receptors, mechanisms of phage adsorption and penetration into host cell. Pol J Microbiol 2010; 59(3): 145-55.
[http://dx.doi.org/10.33073/pjm-2010-023] [PMID: 21033576]

[34]   Heller KJ. Identification of the phage gene for host receptor specificity by analyzing hybrid phages of T5 and BF23. Virology 1984; 139(1): 11-21.
[http://dx.doi.org/10.1016/0042-6822(84)90325-8] [PMID: 6093378]

[35]   Vinga I, Baptista C, Auzat I, *et al.* Role of bacteriophage SPP1 tail spike protein gp21 on host cell receptor binding and trigger of phage DNA ejection. Mol Microbiol 2012; 83(2): 289-303.
[http://dx.doi.org/10.1111/j.1365-2958.2011.07931.x] [PMID: 22171743]

[36]   Hyman P, Abedon ST. Bacteriophage host range and bacterial resistance.Adv Appl Microbiol. San Diego: Elsevier Inc. 2010; Vol. 70: pp. 217-48.
[http://dx.doi.org/10.1016/S0065-2164(10)70007-1]

[37]   Li X, Koç C, Kühner P, *et al.* An essential role for the baseplate protein Gp45 in phage adsorption to *Staphylococcus aureus*. Sci Rep 2016; 6(26455): 26455.
[http://dx.doi.org/10.1038/srep26455] [PMID: 27212064]

[38]   Bielmann R, Habann M, Eugster MR, *et al.* Receptor binding proteins of *Listeria monocytogenes* bacteriophages A118 and P35 recognize serovar-specific teichoic acids. Virology 2015; 477: 110-8.
[http://dx.doi.org/10.1016/j.virol.2014.12.035] [PMID: 25708539]

[39]   Drulis-Kawa Z, Majkowska-Skrobek G, Maciejewska B. Bacteriophages and phage-derived proteins--application approaches. Curr Med Chem 2015; 22(14): 1757-73.
[http://dx.doi.org/10.2174/0929867322666150209152851] [PMID: 25666799]

[40]   Maura D, Debarbieux L. Bacteriophages as twenty-first century antibacterial tools for food and medicine. Appl Microbiol Biotechnol 2011; 90(3): 851-9.
[http://dx.doi.org/10.1007/s00253-011-3227-1] [PMID: 21491205]

[41]   Wittebole X, de Roock S, Opal SM. A historical overview of bacteriophage therapy as an alternative to antibiotics for the treatment of bacterial pathogens. Virulence 2013; 4(8): 1-10.
[PMID: 23973944]

[42]   Erez Z, Steinberger-Levy I, Shamir M, *et al.* Communication between viruses guides lysis-lysogeny decisions. Nature 2017; 541(7638): 488-93.
[http://dx.doi.org/10.1038/nature21049] [PMID: 28099413]

[43]   Gerritsen VB. Between you and me. Protein Spotlight 2017; 190: 1-2.

[44]   Guttman B, Raya R, Kutter E. Basic phage biology.Bacteriophages: Biology and applications. CRC Press 2005; pp. 28-36.

[45]   Miller R, Day M. Contribution of lysogeny, pseudolysogeny, and starvation to phage ecology. In: Stephen T Abedon, Ed. Bacteriophage ecology: population growth, evolution, and impact of bacterial

viruses. Cambridge: Cambridge University Press 2008; pp. 114-44.
[http://dx.doi.org/10.1017/CBO9780511541483.008]

[46]   Cisek AA, Dąbrowska I, Gregorczyk KP, Wyżewski Z. Phage therapy in bacterial infections treatment: One hundred years after the discovery of bacteriophages. Curr Microbiol 2017; 74(2): 277-83.
[http://dx.doi.org/10.1007/s00284-016-1166-x] [PMID: 27896482]

[47]   Dewey JS, Savva CG, White RL, Vitha S, Holzenburg A, Young R. Micron-scale holes terminate the phage infection cycle. Proc Natl Acad Sci USA 2010; 107(5): 2219-23.
[http://dx.doi.org/10.1073/pnas.0914030107] [PMID: 20080651]

[48]   Linden SB, Zhang H, Heselpoth RD, *et al.* Biochemical and biophysical characterization of PlyGRCS, a bacteriophage endolysin active against methicillin-resistant *Staphylococcus aureus*. Appl Microbiol Biotechnol 2015; 99(2): 741-52.
[http://dx.doi.org/10.1007/s00253-014-5930-1] [PMID: 25038926]

[49]   Schmelcher M, Donovan DM, Loessner MJ. Bacteriophage endolysins as novel antimicrobials. Future Microbiol 2012; 7(10): 1147-71.
[http://dx.doi.org/10.2217/fmb.12.97] [PMID: 23030422]

[50]   Borysowski J, Weber-Dabrowska B, Górski A. Bacteriophage endolysins as a novel class of antibacterial agents. Exp Biol Med (Maywood) 2006; 231(4): 366-77.
[http://dx.doi.org/10.1177/153537020623100402] [PMID: 16565432]

[51]   Loessner MJ. Bacteriophage endolysins--current state of research and applications. Curr Opin Microbiol 2005; 8(4): 480-7.
[http://dx.doi.org/10.1016/j.mib.2005.06.002] [PMID: 15979390]

[52]   Shi Y, Yan Y, Ji W, *et al.* Characterization and determination of holin protein of *Streptococcus suis* bacteriophage SMP in heterologous host. Virol J 2012; 9: 70.
[http://dx.doi.org/10.1186/1743-422X-9-70] [PMID: 22436471]

[53]   Wang IN, Smith DL, Young R. Holins: the protein clocks of bacteriophage infections. Annu Rev Microbiol 2000; 54: 799-825.
[http://dx.doi.org/10.1146/annurev.micro.54.1.799] [PMID: 11018145]

[54]   Park T, Struck DK, Dankenbring CA, Young R. The pinholin of lambdoid phage 21: control of lysis by membrane depolarization. J Bacteriol 2007; 189(24): 9135-9.
[http://dx.doi.org/10.1128/JB.00847-07] [PMID: 17827300]

[55]   Rodríguez-Rubio L, Gutiérrez D, Martínez B, Rodríguez A, García P. Lytic activity of LysH5 endolysin secreted by Lactococcus lactis using the secretion signal sequence of bacteriocin Lcn972. Appl Environ Microbiol 2012; 78(9): 3469-72.
[http://dx.doi.org/10.1128/AEM.00018-12] [PMID: 22344638]

[56]   Höltje JV, Mirelman D, Sharon N, Schwarz U. Novel type of murein transglycosylase in *Escherichia coli*. J Bacteriol 1975; 124(3): 1067-76.
[http://dx.doi.org/10.1128/JB.124.3.1067-1076.1975] [PMID: 357]

[57]   Rodríguez-Rubio L, Gutiérrez D, Donovan DM, Martínez B, Rodríguez A, García P. Phage lytic proteins: Biotechnological applications beyond clinical antimicrobials. Crit Rev Biotechnol 2016; 36(3): 542-52.
[PMID: 25603721]

[58]   Vandamme EJ, Mortelmans K. A century of bacteriophage research and applications: impacts on biotechnology, health, ecology and the economy. J Chem Technol Biotechnol 2019; 94(2): 323-42.
[http://dx.doi.org/10.1002/jctb.5810]

[59]   Sunderland KS, Yang M, Mao C. Phage-enabled nanomedicine: From probes to therapeutics in precision medicine. Angew Chem Int Ed Engl 2017; 56(8): 1964-92.
[http://dx.doi.org/10.1002/anie.201606181] [PMID: 27491926]

[60]   García P, Martínez B, Obeso JM, Rodríguez A. Bacteriophages and their application in food safety. Lett Appl Microbiol 2008; 47(6): 479-85.
[http://dx.doi.org/10.1111/j.1472-765X.2008.02458.x] [PMID: 19120914]

[61]   Rodríguez Sauceda EN. Natural antimicrobial agent used in the preservation of fruits and vegetables. Rev Soc Cult Desar Sustent 2011; 7(1): 153-70.

[62]   Chan BK, Abedon ST, Loc-Carrillo C. Phage cocktails and the future of phage therapy. Future Microbiol 2013; 8(6): 769-83.
[http://dx.doi.org/10.2217/fmb.13.47] [PMID: 23701332]

[63]   Morozova VV, Vlassov VV, Tikunova NV. Applications of bacteriophages in the treatment of localized infections in humans. Front Microbiol 1696; 2018(9): 1-8.
[PMID: 30116226]

[64]   Gabisonia T, Loladze M, Chakhunashvili N, *et al.* New Bacteriophage Cocktail against Antibiotic Resistant *Escherichia coli.* Bull Georg Nati Acad Sci 2018; 12(3): 95-102.

[65]   Rios AC, Vila MMDC, Lima R, *et al.* Structural and functional stabilization of bacteriophage particles within the aqueous core of a W/O/W multiple emulsion: a potential biotherapeutic system for the inhalation treatment of bacterial pneumonia. Process Biochem 2018; 64: 177-92.
[http://dx.doi.org/10.1016/j.procbio.2017.09.022]

[66]   Pirnay JP, De Vos D, Verbeken G, *et al.* The phage therapy paradigm: prêt-à-porter or sur-mesure? Pharm Res 2011; 28(4): 934-7.
[http://dx.doi.org/10.1007/s11095-010-0313-5] [PMID: 21063753]

[67]   Kochetkova VA, Mamontov AS, Moskovtseva RL, *et al.* [Phagotherapy of postoperative suppurative-inflammatory complications in patients with neoplasms]. Sov Med 1989; 6(6): 23-6.
[PMID: 2799488]

[68]   Lazareva EB, Smirnov SV, Khvatov VB, *et al.* [Efficacy of bacteriophages in complex treatment of patients with burn wounds]. Antibiot Khimioter 2001; 46(1): 10-4.
[PMID: 11221078]

[69]   Dzholdoshbekov J, Sidikov B. Limphostimulation and bacteriophages in treatment of suppurative complication of diabetic foot. Вестник КРСУ 2014; 14(10): 111-3.

[70]   Weber-Dabrowska B, Zimecki M, Mulczyk M. Effective phage therapy is associated with normalization of cytokine production by blood cell cultures. Arch Immunol Ther Exp (Warsz) 2000; 48(1): 31-7.
[PMID: 10722229]

[71]   Perepanova TS, Darbeeva OS, Kotliarova GA, *et al.* The efficacy of bacteriophage preparations in treating inflammatory urologic diseases Urolog Nefrolog 1995; 5: 14-7.

[72]   Tamariz JH, Lezameta L, Guerra H. [Phagotherapy faced with *Staphylococcus aureus* methicilin resistant infections in mice]. Rev Peru Med Exp Salud Publica 2014; 31(1): 69-77.
[PMID: 24718529]

[73]   Gongze Zhao J, Bridgewater LC. Combating obesity through gut microbiome targeted bacteriophage therapy. Life Sci Undergrad Poster. Schol Arch 2017; 2: 2572-4479.

[74]   Reardon S. Phage therapy gets revitalized. Nature 2014; 510(7503): 15-6.
[http://dx.doi.org/10.1038/510015a] [PMID: 24899282]

[75]   Pastagia M, Schuch R, Fischetti VA, Huang DB. Lysins: the arrival of pathogen-directed anti-infectives. J Med Microbiol 2013; 62(Pt_10): 1506-16.

[76]   Nelson D, Loomis L, Fischetti VA. Prevention and elimination of upper respiratory colonization of mice by group A streptococci by using a bacteriophage lytic enzyme. Proc Natl Acad Sci [Internet] 2001; 98(7): 4107 LP-12.
[http://dx.doi.org/10.1073/pnas.061038398]

[77]   Modi R, Hirvi Y, Hill A, Griffiths MW. Effect of phage on survival of *Salmonella enteritidis* during manufacture and storage of cheddar cheese made from raw and pasteurized milk. J Food Prot 2001; 64(7): 927-33.
[http://dx.doi.org/10.4315/0362-028X-64.7.927] [PMID: 11456198]

[78]   Leverentz B, Conway WS, Alavidze Z, *et al.* Examination of bacteriophage as a biocontrol method for salmonella on fresh-cut fruit: a model study. J Food Prot 2001; 64(8): 1116-21.
[http://dx.doi.org/10.4315/0362-028X-64.8.1116] [PMID: 11510645]

[79]   Whichard JM, Sriranganathan N, Pierson FW. Suppression of *Salmonella* growth by wild-type and large-plaque variants of bacteriophage Felix O1 in liquid culture and on chicken frankfurters. J Food Prot 2003; 66(2): 220-5.
[http://dx.doi.org/10.4315/0362-028X-66.2.220] [PMID: 12597480]

[80]   Goode D, Allen VM, Barrow PA. Reduction of experimental Salmonella and Campylobacter contamination of chicken skin by application of lytic bacteriophages. Appl Environ Microbiol 2003; 69(8): 5032-6.
[http://dx.doi.org/10.1128/AEM.69.8.5032-5036.2003] [PMID: 12902308]

[81]   Leverentz B, Conway WS, Janisiewicz W, Camp MJ. Optimizing concentration and timing of a phage spray application to reduce *Listeria monocytogenes* on honeydew melon tissue. J Food Prot 2004; 67(8): 1682-6.
[http://dx.doi.org/10.4315/0362-028X-67.8.1682] [PMID: 15330534]

[82]   O'Flynn G, Ross RP, Fitzgerald GF, Coffey A. Evaluation of a cocktail of three bacteriophages for biocontrol of *Escherichia coli* O157:H7. Appl Environ Microbiol 2004; 70(6): 3417-24.
[http://dx.doi.org/10.1128/AEM.70.6.3417-3424.2004] [PMID: 15184139]

[83]   Sheng H, Knecht HJ, Kudva IT, Hovde CJ. Application of bacteriophages to control intestinal *Escherichia coli* O157:H7 levels in ruminants. Appl Environ Microbiol 2006; 72(8): 5359-66.
[http://dx.doi.org/10.1128/AEM.00099-06] [PMID: 16885287]

[84]   Gill JJ, Sabour PM, Leslie KE, Griffiths MW. Bovine whey proteins inhibit the interaction of *Staphylococcus aureus* and bacteriophage K J Appl Microbiol 2006; 1101: 377-86.

[85]   Garcia P, Madera C, Martinez B, Rodriguez A. Biocontrol of *Staphylococcus aureus* in curd manufacturing processes using bacteriophages. Int Dairy J 2007; 17: 1232-9.
[http://dx.doi.org/10.1016/j.idairyj.2007.03.014]

[86]   Kim KP, Klumpp J, Loessner MJ. *Enterobacter sakazakii* bacteriophages can prevent bacterial growth in reconstituted infant formula. Int J Food Microbiol 2007; 115(2): 195-203.
[http://dx.doi.org/10.1016/j.ijfoodmicro.2006.10.029] [PMID: 17196280]

[87]   Lee S, Kim MG, Lee HS, Heo S, Kwon M, Kim G. Isolation and characterization of *Listeria phages* for control of growth of *Listeria monocytogenes* in milk. Han-gug Chugsan Sigpum Hag-hoeji 2017; 37(2): 320-8.
[http://dx.doi.org/10.5851/kosfa.2017.37.2.320] [PMID: 28515656]

[88]   Leverentz B, Conway WS, Camp MJ, *et al.* Biocontrol of *Listeria monocytogenes* on fresh-cut produce by treatment with lytic bacteriophages and a bacteriocin. Appl Environ Microbiol 2003; 69(8): 4519-26.
[http://dx.doi.org/10.1128/AEM.69.8.4519-4526.2003] [PMID: 12902237]

[89]   O'Flynn G, Ross RP, Fitzgerald GF, Coffey A. Evaluation of a cocktail of three bacteriophages for biocontrol of *Escherichia coli* O157:H7. Appl Environ Microbiol 2004; 70(6): 3417-24.
[http://dx.doi.org/10.1128/AEM.70.6.3417-3424.2004] [PMID: 15184139]

[90]   Carlton RM, Noordman WH, Biswas B, de Meester ED, Loessner MJ. Bacteriophage P100 for control of *Listeria monocytogenes* in foods: genome sequence, bioinformatic analyses, oral toxicity study, and application. Regul Toxicol Pharmacol 2005; 43(3): 301-12.
[http://dx.doi.org/10.1016/j.yrtph.2005.08.005] [PMID: 16188359]

[91]   Galarce NE, Bravo JL, Robeson JP, Borie CF. Bacteriophage cocktail reduces *Salmonella enterica* serovar *Enteritidis* counts in raw and smoked salmon tissues. Rev Argent Microbiol 2014; 46(4): 333-7.
[http://dx.doi.org/10.1016/S0325-7541(14)70092-6] [PMID: 25576418]

[92]   Sulakvelidze A, Barrow P. Phage therapy in animals and agribusiness, in bacteriophages: Biology and Applications. In: Kutter E, Sulakvelidze A, Eds. Boca Raton, FL: CRC Press 2005; pp. 335-80.

[93]   Chibeu A, Agius L, Gao A, Sabour PM, Kropinski AM, Balamurugan S. Efficacy of bacteriophage LISTEX™P100 combined with chemical antimicrobials in reducing Listeria monocytogenes in cooked turkey and roast beef. Int J Food Microbiol 2013; 167(2): 208-14.
[http://dx.doi.org/10.1016/j.ijfoodmicro.2013.08.018] [PMID: 24125778]

[94]   Wagenaar JA, Van Bergen MA, Mueller MA, Wassenaar TM, Carlton RM. Phage therapy reduces *Campylobacter jejuni* colonization in broilers. Vet Microbiol 2005; 109(3-4): 275-83.
[http://dx.doi.org/10.1016/j.vetmic.2005.06.002] [PMID: 16024187]

[95]   Atterbury RJ, Van Bergen MAP, Ortiz F, *et al.* Bacteriophage therapy to reduce *salmonella* colonization of broiler chickens. Appl Environ Microbiol 2007; 73(14): 4543-9.
[http://dx.doi.org/10.1128/AEM.00049-07] [PMID: 17526794]

[96]   Borie C, Albala I, Sánchez P, *et al.* Bacteriophage treatment reduces *Salmonella* colonization of infected chickens. Avian Dis 2008; 52(1): 64-7.
[http://dx.doi.org/10.1637/8091-082007-Reg] [PMID: 18459298]

[97]   Firlieyanti AS, Connerton PL, Connerton IF. Campylobacters and their bacteriophages from chicken liver: The prospect for phage biocontrol. Int J Food Microbiol 2016; 237: 121-7.
[http://dx.doi.org/10.1016/j.ijfoodmicro.2016.08.026] [PMID: 27565524]

[98]   Grant A, Parveen S, Schwarz J, Hashem F, Vimini B. Reduction of *Salmonella* in ground chicken using a bacteriophage. Poult Sci 2017; 96(8): 2845-52.
[http://dx.doi.org/10.3382/ps/pex062] [PMID: 28371846]

[99]   Waseh S, Hanifi-Moghaddam P, Coleman R, *et al.* Orally administered P22 phage tailspike protein reduces *salmonella* colonization in chickens: prospects of a novel therapy against bacterial infections. PLoS One 2010; 5(11): e13904.
[http://dx.doi.org/10.1371/journal.pone.0013904] [PMID: 21124920]

[100] Raya RR, Varey P, Oot RA, *et al.* Isolation and characterization of a new T-even bacteriophage, CEV1, and determination of its potential to reduce *Escherichia coli* O157:H7 levels in sheep. Appl Environ Microbiol 2006; 72(9): 6405-10.
[http://dx.doi.org/10.1128/AEM.03011-05] [PMID: 16957272]

[101] García P, Martínez B, Obeso JM, Rodríguez A. Bacteriophages and their application in food safety. Lett Appl Microbiol 2008; 47(6): 479-85.
[http://dx.doi.org/10.1111/j.1472-765X.2008.02458.x] [PMID: 19120914]

[102] Zhukov-Verezhnikov NN, Peremitina LD, Berillo EA, Komissarov VP, Bardymov VM. [Therapeutic effect of bacteriophage preparations in the complex treatment of suppurative surgical diseases]. Sov Med 1978; 12(12): 64-6.
[PMID: 734488]

[103] Elbreki M, Ross RP, Hill C, O'Mahony J, McAuliffe O, Coffey A. Bacteriophages and their derivatives as biotherapeutic agents in disease prevention and treatment. J Viruses 2014; 2014: 1-20.
[http://dx.doi.org/10.1155/2014/382539]

[104] Dublanchet A, Patey O, Mazure H, Liddle M, Smithyman AM. Indications and limitations of phage therapy in human medicine: personal experience and literature review. Preprints 2018; pp. 1-30.

[105] Loc Carrillo C, Atterbury RJ, el-Shibiny A, *et al.* Bacteriophage therapy to reduce *Campylobacter jejuni* colonization of broiler chickens. Appl Environ Microbiol 2005; 71(11): 6554-63.
[http://dx.doi.org/10.1128/AEM.71.11.6554-6563.2005] [PMID: 16269681]

[106]   Butler SM, Camilli A. Going against the grain: chemotaxis and infection in *Vibrio cholerae*. Nat Rev Microbiol 2005; 3(8): 611-20.
[http://dx.doi.org/10.1038/nrmicro1207] [PMID: 16012515]

[107]   Seed KD. Battling phages: How bacteria defend against viral attack. PLoS Pathog 2015; 11(6): e1004847.
[http://dx.doi.org/10.1371/journal.ppat.1004847] [PMID: 26066799]

[108]   Azeredo J, Sutherland IW. The use of phages for the removal of infectious biofilms. Curr Pharm Biotechnol 2008; 9(4): 261-6.
[http://dx.doi.org/10.2174/138920108785161604] [PMID: 18691087]

[109]   Ventura M, Sozzi T, Turroni F, Matteuzzi D, van Sinderen D. The impact of bacteriophages on probiotic bacteria and gut microbiota diversity. Genes Nutr 2011; 6(3): 205-7.
[http://dx.doi.org/10.1007/s12263-010-0188-4] [PMID: 21484155]

[110]   Scholl D, Adhya S, Merril C. *Escherichia coli* K1's capsule is a barrier to bacteriophage T7. Appl Environ Microbiol 2005; 71(8): 4872-4.
[http://dx.doi.org/10.1128/AEM.71.8.4872-4874.2005] [PMID: 16085886]

[111]   Levin BR, Bull JJ. Population and evolutionary dynamics of phage therapy. Nat Rev Microbiol 2004; 2(2): 166-73.
[http://dx.doi.org/10.1038/nrmicro822] [PMID: 15040264]

[112]   Coffey A, Ross RP. Bacteriophage-resistance systems in dairy starter strains: molecular analysis to application. Antonie van Leeuwenhoek 2002; 82(1-4): 303-21.
[http://dx.doi.org/10.1023/A:1020639717181] [PMID: 12369198]

[113]   Terns MP, Terns RM. CRISPR-based adaptive immune systems. Curr Opin Microbiol 2011; 14(3): 321-7.
[http://dx.doi.org/10.1016/j.mib.2011.03.005] [PMID: 21531607]

[114]   Manning AJ, Kuehn MJ. Contribution of bacterial outer membrane vesicles to innate bacterial defense. BMC Microbiol 2011; 11: 258.
[http://dx.doi.org/10.1186/1471-2180-11-258] [PMID: 22133164]

[115]   Cumby N, Edwards AM, Davidson AR, Maxwell KL. The bacteriophage HK97 gp15 moron element encodes a novel superinfection exclusion protein. J Bacteriol 2012; 194(18): 5012-9.
[http://dx.doi.org/10.1128/JB.00843-12] [PMID: 22797755]

[116]   Tock MR, Dryden DT. The biology of restriction and anti-restriction. Curr Opin Microbiol 2005; 8(4): 466-72.
[http://dx.doi.org/10.1016/j.mib.2005.06.003] [PMID: 15979932]

[117]   Chopin MC, Chopin A, Bidnenko E. Phage abortive infection in lactococci: Variations on a theme. Curr Opin Microbiol 2005; 8(4): 473-9.
[http://dx.doi.org/10.1016/j.mib.2005.06.006] [PMID: 15979388]

[118]   Fineran PC, Blower TR, Foulds IJ, Humphreys DP, Lilley KS, Salmond GPC. The phage abortive infection system, ToxIN, functions as a protein-RNA toxin-antitoxin pair. Proc Natl Acad Sci USA 2009; 106(3): 894-9.
[http://dx.doi.org/10.1073/pnas.0808832106] [PMID: 19124776]

[119]   Dinsmore PK, Klaenhammer TR. Phenotypic consequences of altering the copy number of abiA, a gene responsible for aborting bacteriophage infections in Lactococcus lactis. Appl Environ Microbiol 1994; 60(4): 1129-36.
[http://dx.doi.org/10.1128/AEM.60.4.1129-1136.1994] [PMID: 16349225]

[120]   Parreira R, Ehrlich SD, Chopin MC. Dramatic decay of phage transcripts in lactococcal cells carrying the abortive infection determinant AbiB. Mol Microbiol 1996; 19(2): 221-30.
[http://dx.doi.org/10.1046/j.1365-2958.1996.371896.x] [PMID: 8825768]

[121]   Durmaz E, Higgins DL, Klaenhammer TR. Molecular characterization of a second abortive phage resistance gene present in Lactococcus lactis subsp. lactis ME2. J Bacteriol 1992; 174(22): 7463-9.
[http://dx.doi.org/10.1128/JB.174.22.7463-7469.1992] [PMID: 1429469]

[122]   Bidnenko E, Ehrlich D, Chopin MC. Phage operon involved in sensitivity to the Lactococcus lactis abortive infection mechanism AbiD1. J Bacteriol 1995; 177(13): 3824-9.
[http://dx.doi.org/10.1128/JB.177.13.3824-3829.1995] [PMID: 7601849]

[123]   Domingues S, Chopin A, Ehrlich SD, Chopin MC. The Lactococcal abortive phage infection system AbiP prevents both phage DNA replication and temporal transcription switch. J Bacteriol 2004; 186(3): 713-21.
[http://dx.doi.org/10.1128/JB.186.3.713-721.2004] [PMID: 14729697]

[124]   Durmaz E, Klaenhammer TR. Abortive phage resistance mechanism AbiZ speeds the lysis clock to cause premature lysis of phage-infected Lactococcus lactis. J Bacteriol 2007; 189(4): 1417-25.
[http://dx.doi.org/10.1128/JB.00904-06] [PMID: 17012400]

[125]   Górski A, Międzybrodzki R, Borysowski J, et al. Phage as a modulator of immune responses: practical implications for phage therapy. Adv Virus Res 2012; 83: 41-71.
[http://dx.doi.org/10.1016/B978-0-12-394438-2.00002-5] [PMID: 22748808]

[126]   Górski A, Jończyk-Matysiak E, Łusiak-Szelachowska M, Międzybrodzki R, Weber-Dąbrowska B, Borysowski J. Phage therapy in allergic disorders? Exp Biol Med (Maywood) 2018; 243(6): 534-7.
[http://dx.doi.org/10.1177/1535370218755658] [PMID: 29359577]

[127]   Ly-Chatain MH. The factors affecting effectiveness of treatment in phages therapy. Front Microbiol 2014;18(5):51; Sulakvelidze A. Alavidze Z. Morris JG. Jr. Bacteriophage therapy. Antimicrob Agents Chemother 2001; 45: 649-59.

[128]   Forthal DN, Moog C. Fc receptor-mediated antiviral antibodies. Curr Opin HIV AIDS 2009; 4(5): 388-93.
[http://dx.doi.org/10.1097/COH.0b013e32832f0a89] [PMID: 20048702]

[129]   Sulakvelidze A, Alavidze Z, Morris JG Jr. Bacteriophage therapy. Antimicrob Agents Chemother 2001; 45(3): 649-59.
[http://dx.doi.org/10.1128/AAC.45.3.649-659.2001] [PMID: 11181338]

[130]   Miedzybrodzki R, Fortuna W, Weber-Da₎browska B, Górski A. A retrospective analysis of changes in inflammatory markers in patients treated with bacterial viruses. Clin Exp Med 2009; 9(4): 303-12.
[http://dx.doi.org/10.1007/s10238-009-0044-2] [PMID: 19350363]

[131]   Van Belleghem JD, Clement F, Merabishvili M, Lavigne R, Vaneechoutte M. Pro- and anti-inflammatory responses of peripheral blood mononuclear cells induced by *Staphylococcus aureus* and *Pseudomonas aeruginosa* phages. Sci Rep 2017; 7(1): 8004.
[http://dx.doi.org/10.1038/s41598-017-08336-9] [PMID: 28808331]

[132]   Sun Y, Feng B. Inflammation response of phage-based films on titanium surface *in vitro* Faseb J 2017; 31 (Suppl 1): 657.15.

[133]   Międzybrodzki R, Świtala-Jeleń K, Fortuna W, et al. Bacteriophage preparation inhibition of reactive oxygen species generation by endotoxin-stimulated polymorphonuclear leukocytes. Virus Res 2008; 131(2): 233-42.
[http://dx.doi.org/10.1016/j.virusres.2007.09.013] [PMID: 17996972]

[134]   Górski A, Kniotek M, Perkowska-Ptasińska A, et al. Bacteriophages and transplantation tolerance. Transplant Proc 2006; 38(1): 331-3.
[http://dx.doi.org/10.1016/j.transproceed.2005.12.073] [PMID: 16504739]

[135]   Zhvania P, Hoyle NS, Nadareishvili L, Nizharadze D, Kutateladze M. Phage Therapy in a 16-Yea--Old Boy with Netherton Syndrome. Front Med (Lausanne) 2017; 4(94): 94.
[http://dx.doi.org/10.3389/fmed.2017.00094] [PMID: 28717637]

[136] Alexander C, Rietschel ET. Bacterial lipopolysaccharides and innate immunity. J Endotoxin Res 2001; 7(3): 167-202.
[PMID: 11581570]

[137] Miernikiewicz P, Kłopot Λ, Soluch R, *et al.* T4 phage tail adhesin Gp12 counteracts LPS-induced inflammation *in vivo*. Front Microbiol 2016; 7(1112): 1112.
[http://dx.doi.org/10.3389/fmicb.2016.01112] [PMID: 27471503]

[138] Krut O, Bekeredjian-Ding I. Contribution of the immune response to phage therapy. J Immunol 2018; 200(9): 3037-44.
[http://dx.doi.org/10.4049/jimmunol.1701745] [PMID: 29685950]

[139] Dąbrowska K, Miernikiewicz P, Piotrowicz A, *et al.* Immunogenicity studies of proteins forming the T4 phage head surface. J Virol 2014; 88(21): 12551-7.
[http://dx.doi.org/10.1128/JVI.02043-14] [PMID: 25142581]

[140] Pyun KH, Ochs HD, Wedgwood RJ, Yang XQ, Heller SR, Reimer CB. Human antibody responses to bacteriophage phi X 174: sequential induction of IgM and IgG subclass antibody. Clin Immunol Immunopathol 1989; 51(2): 252-63.
[http://dx.doi.org/10.1016/0090-1229(89)90024-X] [PMID: 2522846]

[141] Rubinstein A, Mizrachi Y, Bernstein L, *et al.* Progressive specific immune attrition after primary, secondary and tertiary immunizations with bacteriophage phi X174 in asymptomatic HIV-1 infected patients. AIDS 2000; 14(4): F55-62.
[http://dx.doi.org/10.1097/00002030-200003100-00004] [PMID: 10770533]

[142] Majewska J, Beta W, Lecion D, *et al.* Oral application of T4 phage induces weak antibody production in the gut and in the blood. Viruses 2015; 7(8): 4783-99.
[http://dx.doi.org/10.3390/v7082845] [PMID: 26308042]

[143] Robertson K, Furukawa Y, Underwood A, Black L, Liu JL. Deletion of the Hoc and Soc capsid proteins affects the surface and cellular uptake properties of bacteriophage T4 derived nanoparticles. Biochem Biophys Res Commun 2012; 418(3): 537-40.
[http://dx.doi.org/10.1016/j.bbrc.2012.01.061] [PMID: 22285187]

CHAPTER 5

Subtractive Genomics Approaches: Towards Anti-Bacterial Drug Discovery

Fatima Shahid, Muhammad Shehroz, Tahreem Zaheer and **Amjad Ali[*]**

Atta-ur-Rahman School of Applied Biosciences (ASAB), National University of Sciences and Technology (NUST), Islamabad, Pakistan

Abstract: Pathogenic bacteria are evolving at a much faster rate and have the ability to acquire new antibacterial resistance patterns. The most common pathogenic bacteria are now becoming increasingly resistant to available antibiotics. The CDC has suggested to find alternative therapeutics to combat the growing antimicrobial resistance. Thanks to technological development in sequencing platforms and sophisticated bioinformatics pipelines, it now easier to analyze large-scale genomic data and propose alternative and novel treatment options. Subtractive genomics is one such approach that mines whole genomic DNA for identification of potential drug target(s). This strategy employs various computational filters using databases and online servers to screen and prioritize certain candidate proteins. Each filter analyzes the whole proteome of bacteria under study in a step-wise manner. Initially, strain-specific paralogous and host-specific homologous sequences are subtracted from the bacterial proteome to remove duplicates and prevent cytotoxicity and autoimmunity related challenges. The sorted proteome is further refined to identify essential genes involved in crucial metabolic pathways of the pathogen and thus can be used as targets for treatment interventions. Functional annotation is carried out to elucidate the involvement of these proteins in important cellular processes, metabolic pathway, and subcellular location analyses are carried out for finding the probable cellular location of the candidate proteins in the cell. Proteins with certain physicochemical properties like favorable molecular weight, hydrophobicity, and pI are rendered fine drug targets, thus filter. Importantly, the scrutinized proteins are screened against FDA approved DrugBank to identify their druggability potential. Finally, molecular docking analyses of the novel druggable targets with already present drugs are carried out. Only then, the prioritized candidate proteins can prove to be promising candidates for novel drug design and development.

Keywords: Cytoplasmic proteins, Drug targets, Membrane proteins, Metabolic pathways, Proteome, Subtractive proteomics.

---

[*] **Corresponding author Amjad Ali:** Atta-ur-Rahman School of Applied Biosciences (ASAB), National University of Sciences and Technology (NUST), Islamabad, Pakistan; Tel: +92 51 90856138; E-mail: amjaduni@gmail.com

Atta-ur-Rahman and M. Iqbal Choudhary (Eds.)

INTRODUCTION

Comparative and subtractive genomics approach, together with metabolic-pathway analysis provide a potent regime to categorize the set of proteins that are essential for the pathogen's existence but are not present in the host [1]. Subtracting host genome from the set of pathogen essential genes assists in finding non-human homologous protein candidates which guarantee no interaction of drugs with host proteins [2]. Subtraction in its literal terms means removed from bottom, taking a smaller yet important chunk from a larger dataset. Conversely, comparative genomics approach focuses on choosing proteins that are highly conserved among a number of species and interpreting them as promising targets. Subtractive genomics is an approach where the genomic dataset is analyzed and a smaller chunk under observation is subtracted and analyzed for its likely results. Using innovative bioinformatics tools that have been integrated with genomics, proteomics, and metabolomics may support the identification of putative drug targets against pathogens causing deadly infectious diseases [3]. After the target(s) have been predicted, *in silico* virtual screening of different chemical databases could generate fresh opportunities to choose and design the finest inhibitors [4].

Characteristics of an Ideal Drug Target

A candidate that fulfils the following criteria can be referred to as an ideal drug target.

  i. It must be involved in the pathogenesis of the organism under study or significant for its survival.
 ii. It should be structurally druggable; possess the power to bind small molecules (inhibitors).
iii. It should be functionally and structurally characterized to assist the study of small molecular inhibition via already established assays
 iv. It should be different from already known drug targets against which FDA have approved drugs, in order to escape the toxicity of cross-resistance [5].

Both wet lab and dry lab studies can assist drug target prediction, however, computational biology aided methods are preferred as they cut down cost, save time and resources.

Significance of Drug Target Identification

For the past few years, Drug target discovery has been the fundamental emphasis in both the research and development sector as well as in the pharmaceutical industry. Choosing the precise drug targets is required for the fruitful development, testing, and marketing of drugs [6].

Literature indicates that therapeutic drug targets belong to approximately 130 different protein families but mainly confine to G-protein-coupled receptors, enzymes, nuclear hormone receptors, certain transporters, as well as ion channels [7].

Prediction of putative targets in pathogens can significantly aid in developing innovative drug candidates against known and new targets or determining novel targets for existing drugs. Nevertheless, the experimental methods for this are very costly, laborious and challenging.

Late phase drug approval-failures are contributing to the increasing economic strain. This has pushed scientists to optimize their drug target identification regime to accelerate success rates.

Although it is essential to adjust drugs according to efficacy, pharmacokinetics, and toxicity, however, it should be ensured that they modulate the appropriate target, to begin with.

Unfortunately, several drugs fail to give the promising results either due of their poor efficacy or toxicity issues, while dealing with large populations. Undoubtedly, minor changes can lead to significant enhancements to already practiced schemes. However, drug candidate optimization cannot help with these problems if the prevalence of the target is low among the focused patient population. Alongside, the improved success rates of drug approval by regulatory authorities significantly rely upon picking the most promising target timely.

The best targets are the one strongly associated with the disease under study, having a well-established function in pathology plus they can be detected in high numbers/amount among the concerned patient population. Selecting the optimum target effectively curbs the anticipated disease pathway while leaving all other related pathways unaffected to produce minimal or no side effects.

Subtractive Genomics Based Efforts for Drug Target Identification

Drug target prediction efforts are initiated at the end of the previous century, probably started with drug targets prediction in pathogens utilizing the 10 publicly available complete genome sequences [2]. To date, drug target identification using *in silico* regime has been quite successful as it has yielded a large number of targets against several pathogens. This process mostly involves comparative genomics and DEG is a key component of the entire scheme [8]. Nevertheless, certain strain-specific, as well as species-specific and novel targets, have also been predicted [9]. While the major focus of this framework is metabolic pathways linked to cytoplasmic and membrane-associated proteins, some studies have only focused on cytoplasmic entities and used membrane related proteins along with secretome for vaccine target identification [10]. Normally, only pathogen unique pathways are selected but some studies have described otherwise [9]. It has been reported that targets belonging to pathogen unique pathways are around 60-70% common in all genotypes while 30-40% are strain or genus-specific. Yet, to attack a pathogen after the entire screening process, non-host homologous proteins are preferred targets [8]. Extensive computational studies have been carried out regarding various human and animal infecting pathogens. Some of them that showed significant results are briefly discussed here.

Recently, 16 strains of the zoonotic pathogen *Leptospira* were screened by Gupta *et al.* using target identification tool (TiD) followed by comparative genomic approach and metabolic pathway analysis to identify 8 broad spectrum novel drug targets [11]. The Target-pathogen database was developed by Sosa *et al.* in 2018 and used to prioritize drug targets in *Leishmania major* and nine other human pathogens based on essentiality, druggablity, structural and functional significance [12]. Spore forming *Clostridium botulinum* has become a major threat to the human race. Using drugs against this deadly pathogen has detrimental effects like bursting of cells and leading to worse neurological symptoms. Hence a study was conducted by Ahmed *et al.* to predict bacterial essential genes that prove to be bactericidal in case of *C. botulinum.* For mitigating botulism a computational framework was exploited to screen out 131 antibacterial targets on the basis of their evolutionary status, essentiality and low percentage homology with human host and gut flora. These can be further explored for their effectiveness in wet lab *C. botulinum* 131 targets [13]. Likewise, putative drug targets have been predicted against *Helicobacter pylori, Leptospira interrogans, Acinetobacter baumannii, Klebsiella pneumonia, Providencia stuartii, Trypanosoma cruzi, Shigella flexneri, Schistosoma manosoni, Leishmania major* and many others [10, 14 - 21].

Beside human hosts, drug targets have also been predicted against animal pathogens using comparative genomics frame works. *Corynebacterium pseudotuberculosis* (*Cp*) responsible for goat and sheep disease, the Caseous lymphadenitis. The pathogenesis of this disease was not widely explored and needed to study for development proper drugs against these infections. In order to tackle this veterinary pathogen, *in silico* subtractive genomic approach was applied by using four strains. Resultantly, 6 targets were identified and subjected to virtual screening [8]. Later, an integrated structure based *in silico* approach was implemented to evaluate the druggability and physiochemical nature of pathogen proteins that resulted in prediction of 31 putative drug targets for targeting bacterium [22].

In 2016, a total of 13 drug targets were identified in Dichelobacter nodosus using subtractive genomics approach [23], while recently in 2019 subtractive genomics was employed against *Clostridium botulinum, Mycobacterium tuberculosis, Brucella abortus* strain 2308, and *Salmonella typhi* [24 - 27].

Approaches Used for Promising Drug Target Prediction

Subtractive genomics involves various reduction/screening steps to predict putative therapeutic targets. These steps need to be amalgamated in a framework that can offer the entire antibacterial regime on the same platform. Hence in 1998, Bruccoleri *et al.* developed a user-friendly approach that enabled users to specify the input genomes and worked on the principle of essentiality and genome conservation to facilitate efficient *in silico* target discovery [28]. Later, to automate the entire process, FindTarget was introduced. It operated by using BLASTp to compare proteomes however it has challenges in performing the whole procedure [29]. As an improvement T-iDT tool was developed to predict bacterial essential genes that were not homologues to human hosts. Nevertheless, this tool was devoid of pathway analysis filter [30]. This is followed by, mGenomeSubtractor which is an integrated tool that offered multiple filters like essentiality, virulence, and species-specific target identification [31]. We believe, there is room for improvement in the existing pipelines and efforts are required to form and comprehensive *in silico* pipeline for target prediction, nevertheless target validation will yet to be done through appropriate experimental studies. The schematic workflow of drug target prediction is presented in Fig. (**1**), highlighting the important steps and stages in drug designing and development process.

DrugSol and its Utility

After thorough literature survey, we have come up with the idea of integrating the below-mentioned filters to design a framework called **DrugSol** (providing a smart solution for alternative drug targets prediction). It will automate the *in silico* drug target prediction process exploiting the genomes (proteomes) of challenging bacterial pathogens. The pipeline will take protein multi-FASTA (amino acid) files as input that will be processed through a series of established tools, databases and algorithms. The individual steps are discussed here in brief.

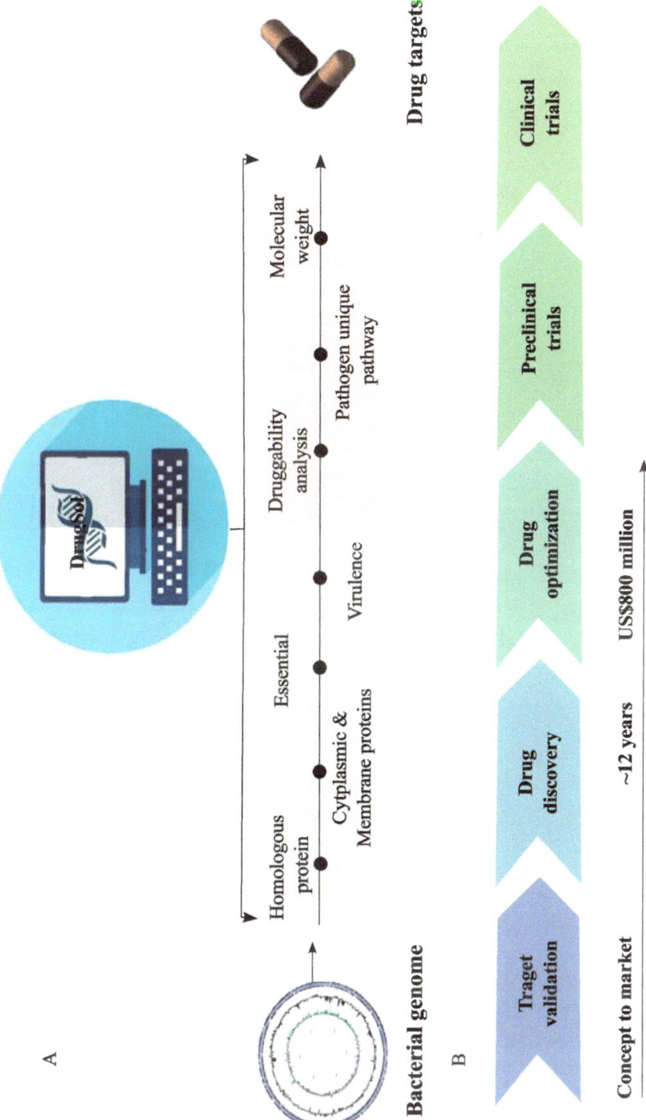

Fig. (1). The scheme for prediction and validation of potential drug targets **A**) DrugSol, our in-house pipeline (unpublished) is employed here which integrating all the filters elaborated in this chapter for predict novel targets for the FDA approved drugs **B**) steps in experimental validation of the prioritized drug targets till their commercialization, the whole process may take about 12-15 years.

Non-host Homologues

The accessibility of the human genome sequence has simplified the drug discovery process. Readily available human genome can be searched for similarities with the pathogen's shortlisted proteins by employ BLAST or other suitable algorithms. A bacterial gene/protein exhibiting minimal resemblance with the human host is regarded as a good target to be dealt with drug [32]. In the era of personalized medicine, it is however recommended to use the best reference genome for a given population.

Subcellular Localization

It is usually believed that protein function is linked to its subcellular localization because the surrounding environment significantly contribute to and influence the protein functions. Subcellular localization of pathogens' proteins is a vital element for the identification of suitable drug targets in biological studies. Both cytoplasmic and membrane proteins have been pronounced as the fine drug targets as suggested by experimental reported and the literature [33]. In this context, CELLO2GO has emerged as a readily available, online system to screen subcellular localization of the query protein [34].

Essentiality

The idea of non-host homologous proteomic target identification emphases on bacteria essential proteins. These are the proteins that play a vital role in growth, development, adaptability and viability of the pathogen. Targeting such proteins ensures extermination of the pathogen. The database of essential genes (DEG) is a comprehensive repository of genes manifesting essential functions across a vast majority of organisms. Comparative genomics and subtractive proteomics approaches employ DEG as a key component of target identification scheme to filter essential genes and proteins [35].

Virulence

In the modern era, pathogenic bacterial strains are a major cause of global disease outbreaks. Over the last few years, bacterial pathogenesis has been intensely studied to obtain better insights into disease mechanisms at a cellular level. Reportedly, many pathogens produce virulence factors that influence the host immune system. They can lead to host cell lysis and stimulate tissue destruction, while in some cases they might inhibit the process of complement activation, inhibit neutrophil function and hinder phagocytosis. Several studies elucidating the mechanisms of action, structural and functional properties of virulence factors have paved the way to get better insights into anti-virulence strategies. Virulence Factor Databae (VFDB), a database that has collectively stored virulence factors from pathogens, has emerged as a comprehensive repository for all virulence factors from medically challenging pathogens [36].

Annotation

Uniprot (universal protein resource) is a comprehensive repository that is freely available and provides thorough information about protein sequence and function. Integrated information from his database can be readily used to annotate the protein under study [37].

Druggability Potential Evaluation

Proteins that exhibit around 80% or more matched percentage when searched against targets for to FDA approved drugs present in DrugBank are termed as druggable targets and their ability to modulate a target is termed as druggability [38]. DrugBank is a highly annotated, free, online resource that groups comprehensive drug data with wide-ranging drug targets and detailed knowledge of mechanisms of drug action. It has extensively facilitated *in silico* drug target discovery, paved ways towards drug design, simplified drug and ligand docking, enabled easy drug metabolism and outcome prediction, and enlightened scientists about possible drug interactions and their consequences [39].

Analyses of Metabolic Pathways

It is necessary to discover and evaluate the biological processes in which the putative drug targets participate. This enables us to identify choke points reactions. Supposedly, blocking these reactions can trigger an increase in certain toxic metabolite concentration inside the cell or lead to deficiency of some vital compound, rendering genes and proteins associated with these reactions pharmacokinetically significant [22]. KEGG Automatic Annotation Server (KAAS) offers high performance functional annotation of genes obtained through BLAST evaluations against KEGG database. As a result of this analysis, KEGG Orthology (KO) and KEGG pathways are obtained [40].

OUR CONTRIBUTION

Sequence Acquisition

The protein sequences of *Neisseria gonorrhoeae* strain FA 1090 (reference strain) were retrieved from NCBI GenBank. The proteome is comprised of 1886 proteins that were subjected to subtractive processing with certain established rules and parameters.

Human Homology Filter

The initial step was executed by finding non-human homologs. This step was mandatory to elute proteins that were similar to host proteins in order to circumvent chances of autoimmunity. A total of 1886 proteins present in the reference sequence were subjected to BLASTp against RefSeq using percentage identity cutoff >35%, a Bit Score >100 and E-Value < 0000.1. Resultantly, 1668 proteins were found to be non- human homologs. Strict criteria of BLASTp filters non homologous proteins which are considered safe targets (as explained in Non host homologues section). Non-human homology bearing proteins also prevent the chances of autoimmunity and adverse reactions.

Subcellular Localization

The hence filtered 1668 proteins were subjected to further protein screening by using CELLO2GO. As a result, 687 proteins were found to be a part of cytoplasm while 338 were membrane proteins. Protein prioritization according to specific subcellular localizations substantially assisted in drug target identification as eluting inapt pathogenic proteins for targeting reduces the overall process cost and time.

Essentiality

Next, 1025 proteins in the selected subcellular locations were checked for essentiality using DEG. BLASTp was performed by using E-value <0.0001 and Bit score >100 to rule out non-essential proteins. Among them, 543 proteins were found to be involved in essential metabolic pathways of the pathogen and were attractive entities to be targeted by drugs. Essential proteins required for survival of pathogens are generally conserved. Hence, they are considered as promising drug targets.

Virulence

In this next step, the filtered proteins (543) were checked through VFDB for virulence potential analysis. Only 146 proteins fulfilled all the above-mentioned criteria were additionally found to be virulent BlastP considering an E-value <0.0001.

Annotated

Among 146 proteins, only 126 candidate virulent proteins were functionally annotated and then subjected to further analysis, such as druggability analysis.

Druggability Potential Evaluation

Druggability potential of the screened proteins was accessed and only 21 proteins that showed high matched frequencies with targets of FDA approved drugs, they are found to be drugable and further explored.

Analyses of Metabolic Pathways

The concluding step in the drug target prediction was to check the involvement of shortlisted proteins in certain essential metabolic processes. Proteins that participated in human, as well as pathogenic pathways, were discarded and finally the 11 pathogen associated unique proteins were filtered.

Physiochemical properties

The 11 proteins were further examined for physiochemical characteristics using Expasy ProtParam to identify their amino acid composition, instability index, theoretical pI, estimated half-life, GRAVY index (grand average of hydropathicity). These 11 proteins were: acyl-ACP--UDP-N-acetylglucosamine O-acyltransferase, GlnA, tryptophan synthase subunit alpha, RNA polymerase sigma factor RpoH, thioredoxin-disulfide reductase, RNA polymerase sigma factor RpoD, anthranilate phosphoribosyltransferase, dihydropteroate synthase, multidrug efflux RND transporter periplasmic adaptor subunit MtrC, penicillin-binding protein 2, and LysR family transcriptional regulator OxyR. Among these proteins only 5 proteins were found to be stable and had favourable GRAVy index. The detailed information of these proteins can be seen in Table (**1**).

Table 1. The detailed information about 11 pathogen-associated unique proteins.

Sr. No.	Protein Name		KEGG Orthology	Pathways	pI	Mol Weight	GRAVY
1551|sp|B4RR10|LPXA_NEIG2YP_208836.1	acyl-ACP--UDP-N-acetylglucosamine O-acyltransferase		ko00540	Lipopolysaccharide biosynthesis	6.13	28170.9	-0.096
			ko01100	Metabolic pathways			
			ko01503	Cationic antimicrobial peptide (CAMP) resistance			
234|sp|Q5F9Y6|TRPA_NEIG1YP_207413.1	tryptophan synthase subunit alpha [*Neisseria gonorrhoeae*]		K01695		5.05	27992.2	0.113
			ko04727	GABAergic synapse			
			ko00260	Glycine, serine and threonine metabolism			
			ko00400	Phenylalanine, tyrosine and tryptophan biosynthesis			
			ko01100	Metabolic pathways			
			ko01110	Biosynthesis of secondary metabolites			
530|sp|P80892|TRXB_ALIFSYP_207723.1	thioredoxin-disulfide reductase	K00384	ko00450	Selenocompound metabolism	5.15	33654.1	-0.106
880|sp|P52325|RPOD_NEIGOYP_208094.1	RNA polymerase sigma factor RpoD [*Neisseria gonorrhoeae*]		K03086	None	4.88	73680.3	-0.602

(Table 1) cont.....

Sr. No.	Protein Name		KEGG Orthology	Pathways	pI	Mol Weight	GRAVY
1159|sp|Q51161|DHPS_NEIMBYP_208404.1	dihydropteroate synthase	K00796	ko00790	Folate biosynthesis	5.44	30379.8	-0.037
1175|sp|P43505|MTRC_NEIGOYP_208425.1	multidrug efflux RND transporter periplasmic adaptor subunit MtrC [*Neisseria gonorrhoeae*]		ko01100	Metabolic pathways	8.75	42757.6	-0.062
			ko01501	beta-Lactam resistance			
			ko01503	Cationic antimicrobial peptide (CAMP) resistance			

Pros and Cons of *in silico* Drug Target Mining

Subtractive genomics-based framework has the potential to the entire bacterial pathogen proteome promptly and predicts putative drug target proteins. This can help saving in the total project costs and time, as it competently reduces the false-positive protein hits. It can also reduce the total reagent and animal cost of the study. The final results are independent of the universal set of rules and depend only on the applied filters and the input [41]. The filter may be made stringent and enhanced as per the researcher desire and requirement, this may affect the prediction in either way. The complete pathogen and host genomes/proteome are required for the implementation of subtractive genomic approach. If one of them is not attainable the process becomes less effective or impracticable. Moreover, the flexibility of proteins under study and their molecular conformation may hamper precise predictions. Even though the drug targets are ought to effective for human hosts, nevertheless animal models are required for prior testing and applications. A major species barrier exists between humans and model animals that need to be addressed for better results [42].

Success Stories

Choice of an appropriate drug target leads to fruitful results in clinical testing and formulation of effective new drugs. Several studies have been carried out to approximate the number of drug targets and some databases, namely DrugBank and TTD (therapeutic drug target database), have been developed for this purpose as well. In 2009, a study reported 156 putative drug targets that were devoid of a drug at that time [43]. After a thorough examination of their structure, sequence physiochemical properties and comparison with human host profiles, the 41 putative drug targets were ought to show clinically promising results. Out of these 41 targets, 16 reached Phase 3 clinical trials. The subsequent evaluation led to shortlisting of 10 candidates that have produced Food and Drug Administration approved drugs formulation. Additionally, neutral endopeptidase (one of the putative target) when joined with an already existing approved target, angiotensin II receptor, led to the formulation of a renowned FDA approved combination drug sacubitril/valsartan [44].

CONSENT FOR PUBLICATION

Not applicable.

CONFLICT OF INTEREST

The author declares that there is no conflict of interest in this chapter.

ACKNOWLEDGEMENTS

Declared none.

REFERENCES

[1]　Mondal SI, Ferdous S, Jewel NA, *et al.* Identification of potential drug targets by subtractive genome analysis of *Escherichia coli* O157:H7: an *in silico* approach. Adv Appl Bioinform Chem 2015; 8: 49-63.
[http://dx.doi.org/10.2147/AABC.S88522] [PMID: 26677339]

[2]　Galperin MY, Koonin EV. Searching for drug targets in microbial genomes. Curr Opin Biotechnol 1999; 10(6): 571-8.
[http://dx.doi.org/10.1016/S0958-1669(99)00035-X] [PMID: 10600691]

[3]　Koonin EV, Tatusov RL, Galperin MY. Beyond complete genomes: from sequence to structure and function. Curr Opin Struct Biol 1998; 8(3): 355-63.
[http://dx.doi.org/10.1016/S0959-440X(98)80070-5] [PMID: 9666332]

[4]　Lavecchia A, Di Giovanni C. Virtual screening strategies in drug discovery: a critical review. Curr Med Chem 2013; 20(23): 2839-60.
[http://dx.doi.org/10.2174/09298673113209990001] [PMID: 23651302]

[5]　Holman AG, Davis PJ, Foster JM, Carlow CK, Kumar S. Computational prediction of essential genes in an unculturable endosymbiotic bacterium, Wolbachia of Brugia malayi. BMC Microbiol 2009; 9(1): 243.
[http://dx.doi.org/10.1186/1471-2180-9-243] [PMID: 19943957]

[6]　Drews J. Drug discovery: a historical perspective science 2000; 287(5460): 1960-4.

[7]　Imming P, Sinning C, Meyer A. Drugs, their targets and the nature and number of drug targets. Nat Rev Drug Discov 2006; 5(10): 821-34.
[http://dx.doi.org/10.1038/nrd2132] [PMID: 17016423]

[8]　Barh D, Jain N, Tiwari S, *et al.* A novel comparative genomics analysis for common drug and vaccine targets in *Corynebacterium pseudotuberculosis* and other CMN group of human pathogens. Chem Biol Drug Des 2011; 78(1): 73-84.
[http://dx.doi.org/10.1111/j.1747-0285.2011.01118.x] [PMID: 21443692]

[9]　Barh D, Kumar A. *In silico* identification of candidate drug and vaccine targets from various pathways in *Neisseria gonorrhoeae*. In silico Biol (Gedrukt) 2009; 9(4): 225-31.
[http://dx.doi.org/10.3233/ISB-2009-0399] [PMID: 20109152]

[10]　Dutta A, Singh SK, Ghosh P, Mukherjee R, Mitter S, Bandyopadhyay D. *In silico* identification of potential therapeutic targets in the human pathogen *Helicobacter pylori*. In silico biology 2006; 6(1,2): 43-7.

[11]　Gupta R, Pradhan D, Jain AK, Rai CS. TiD: Standalone software for mining putative drug targets from

bacterial proteome. Genomics 2017; 109(1): 51-7.
[http://dx.doi.org/10.1016/j.ygeno.2016.11.005] [PMID: 27856224]

[12]   Sosa EJ, Burguener G, Lanzarotti E, *et al.* Target-Pathogen: a structural bioinformatic approach to prioritize drug targets in pathogens. Nucleic Acids Res 2018; 46(D1): D413-8.
[http://dx.doi.org/10.1093/nar/gkx1015] [PMID: 29106651]

[13]   Muhammad SA, Ahmed S, Ali A, *et al.* Prioritizing drug targets in Clostridium botulinum with a computational systems biology approach. Genomics 2014; 104(1): 24-35.
[http://dx.doi.org/10.1016/j.ygeno.2014.05.002] [PMID: 24837790]

[14]   Kim HU, Kim TY, Lee SY. Genome-scale metabolic network analysis and drug targeting of multi-drug resistant pathogen Acinetobacter baumannii AYE. Mol Biosyst 2010; 6(2): 339-48.
[http://dx.doi.org/10.1039/B916446D] [PMID: 20094653]

[15]   Raman K, Yeturu K, Chandra N. targetTB: a target identification pipeline for *Mycobacterium tuberculosis* through an interactome, reactome and genome-scale structural analysis. BMC Syst Biol 2008; 2(1): 109.
[http://dx.doi.org/10.1186/1752-0509-2-109] [PMID: 19099550]

[16]   Amineni U, Pradhan D, Marisetty H. *In silico* identification of common putative drug targets in Leptospira interrogans. J Chem Biol 2010; 3(4): 165-73.
[http://dx.doi.org/10.1007/s12154-010-0039-1] [PMID: 21572503]

[17]   Georrge JJ, Umrania V. *In silico* identification of putative drug targets in Klebsiella pneumonia MGH78578. Indian Journal of Biotechnology 2011; 10(4): 432-9.

[18]   Reguera RM, Calvo-Álvarez E, Álvarez-Velilla R, Balaña-Fouce R. Target-based *vs.* phenotypic screenings in Leishmania drug discovery: A marriage of convenience or a dialogue of the deaf? Int J Parasitol Drugs Drug Resist 2014; 4(3): 355-7.
[http://dx.doi.org/10.1016/j.ijpddr.2014.05.001] [PMID: 25516847]

[19]   Caffrey CR, Rohwer A, Oellien F, *et al.* A comparative chemogenomics strategy to predict potential drug targets in the metazoan pathogen, Schistosoma mansoni. PLoS One 2009; 4(2): e4413.
[http://dx.doi.org/10.1371/journal.pone.0004413] [PMID: 19198654]

[20]   Arora N, Banerjee AK, Murty US. *In silico* characterization of Shikimate Kinase of Shigella flexneri: a potential drug target. Interdiscip Sci 2010; 2(3): 280-90.
[http://dx.doi.org/10.1007/s12539-010-0012-2] [PMID: 20658341]

[21]   Alves-Ferreira M, Guimarães ACR, Capriles PV, Dardenne LE, Degrave WM. A new approach for potential drug target discovery through *in silico* metabolic pathway analysis using *Trypanosoma cruzi* genome information. Mem Inst Oswaldo Cruz 2009; 104(8): 1100-10.
[http://dx.doi.org/10.1590/S0074-02762009000800006] [PMID: 20140370]

[22]   Radusky LG, Hassan S, Lanzarotti E, *et al.* An integrated structural proteomics approach along the druggable genome of *Corynebacterium pseudotuberculosis* species for putative druggable targets. BMC Genomics 2015; 16(5) (Suppl. 5): S9.
[http://dx.doi.org/10.1186/1471-2164-16-S5-S9] [PMID: 26041381]

[23]   Acharya A, Garg LC. Drug target identification and prioritization for treatment of ovine foot rot: an *In silico* approach. Int J Genomics 2016; 2016: 7361361.

[24]   Sudha R, Katiyar A, Katiyar P, Singh H, Prasad P. Identification of potential drug targets and vaccine candidates in Clostridium botulinum using subtractive genomics approach. Bioinformation 2019; 15(1): 18-25.
[http://dx.doi.org/10.6026/97320630015018] [PMID: 31359994]

[25]   Saravanan S, Shylaja G. Genome subtraction to identify the novel therapeutic targets in *Mycobacterium tuberculosis*. Drug Invention Today 2019; 12(8): 1620-4.

[26]   Mahmud A, Khan MT, Iqbal A. Identification of novel drug targets for humans and potential vaccine targets for cattle by subtractive genomic analysis of *Brucella abortus* strain 2308. Microb Pathog

2019; 137: 103731.
[http://dx.doi.org/10.1016/j.micpath.2019.103731] [PMID: 31509762]

[27] Mukherjee S, Gangopadhay K, Mukherjee SB. Identification of potential new vaccine candidates in *Salmonella* typhi using reverse vaccinology and subtractive genomics-based approach. bioRxiv 2019; 521518.

[28] Bruccoleri RE, Dougherty TJ, Davison DB. Concordance analysis of microbial genomes. Nucleic Acids Res 1998; 26(19): 4482-6.
[http://dx.doi.org/10.1093/nar/26.19.4482] [PMID: 9742253]

[29] Chetouani F, Glaser P, Kunst F. FindTarget: software for subtractive genome analysis. Microbiology 2001; 147(Pt 10): 2643-9.
[http://dx.doi.org/10.1099/00221287-147-10-2643] [PMID: 11577143]

[30] Singh NK, Selvam SM, Chakravarthy P. T-iDT : tool for identification of drug target in bacteria and validation by *Mycobacterium tuberculosis*. In silico Biol (Gedrukt) 2006; 6(6): 485-93.
[PMID: 17518759]

[31] Shao Y, He X, Harrison EM, Tai C, Ou H-Y, Rajakumar K, *et al.* mGenomeSubtractor: a web-based tool for parallel *in silico* subtractive hybridization analysis of multiple bacterial genomes Nucleic acids research 2010; 38(suppl_2): .reviews2002.1- reviews2002.10.

[32] Pertsemlidis A, Fondon JW. Having a BLAST with bioinformatics (and avoiding BLASTphemy). Genome biology 2001; 2(10): reviews2002.1- reviews2002.10.

[33] Hasan MA, Khan MA, Sharmin T, Hasan Mazumder MH, Chowdhury AS. Identification of putative drug targets in Vancomycin-resistant *Staphylococcus aureus* (VRSA) using computer aided protein data analysis. Gene 2016; 575(1): 132-43.
[http://dx.doi.org/10.1016/j.gene.2015.08.044] [PMID: 26319513]

[34] Yu C-S, Cheng C-W, Su W-C, *et al.* CELLO2GO: a web server for protein subCELlular LOcalization prediction with functional gene ontology annotation. PLoS One 2014; 9(6): e99368.
[http://dx.doi.org/10.1371/journal.pone.0099368] [PMID: 24911789]

[35] Zhang R, Lin Y. DEG 5.0, a database of essential genes in both prokaryotes and eukaryotes. Nucleic acids research 2008; 37 (1): D455-8.

[36] Chen L, Yang J, Yu J, Yao Z, Sun L, Shen Y, *et al.* VFDB: a reference database for bacterial virulence factors. Nucleic acids research 2005; 33(1): D325-D8.

[37] Bairoch A, Apweiler R, Wu CH, Barker WC, Boeckmann B, Ferro S, *et al.* The universal protein resource (UniProt) Nucleic acids research 2005; 33 (1): D154-D9.

[38] Hossain T, Kamruzzaman M, Choudhury TZ, Mahmood HN, Nabi A, Hosen M. Application of the subtractive genomics and molecular docking analysis for the identification of novel putative drug targets against *Salmonella enterica* subsp. *enterica serovar* Poona BioMed research international 2017; 2017

[39] Wishart DS, Knox C, Guo AC, *et al.* DrugBank: A comprehensive resource for *in silico* drug discovery and exploration. Nucleic acids research 2006; 34 (1): D668-D72.
[http://dx.doi.org/10.1093/nar/gkj067]

[40] Aoki KF, Kanehisa M. Using the KEGG database resource. Cur proto bioinform 2005; 11(1): 12. 1-1.. 54.
[http://dx.doi.org/10.1002/0471250953.bi0112s11]

[41] Ekins S, Mestres J, Testa B. *In silico* pharmacology for drug discovery: applications to targets and beyond. Br J Pharmacol 2007; 152(1): 21-37.
[http://dx.doi.org/10.1038/sj.bjp.0707306] [PMID: 17549046]

[42] Barh D, Tiwari S, Jain N, Ali A, Santos AR, Misra AN, *et al. In silico* subtractive genomics for target identification in human bacterial pathogens. Drug Dev Res 2011; 72(2): 162-77.

[http://dx.doi.org/10.1002/ddr.20413]

[43]   Zhu F, Han L, Zheng C, *et al.* What are next generation innovative therapeutic targets? Clues from genetic, structural, physicochemical, and systems profiles of successful targets. J Pharmacol Exp Ther 2009; 330(1): 304-15.
[http://dx.doi.org/10.1124/jpet.108.149955] [PMID: 19357322]

[44]   Zhu F, Li XX, Yang SY, Chen YZ. Clinical success of drug targets prospectively predicted by *in silico* study. Trends Pharmacol Sci 2018; 39(3): 229-31.
[http://dx.doi.org/10.1016/j.tips.2017.12.002] [PMID: 29295742]

CHAPTER 6

Recent Advances in the Discovery of Antimicrobials through Metagenomics

Daljeet Singh Dhanjal, Reena Singh[*] **and Chirag Chopra**[*]

School of Bioengineering and Biosciences, Lovely Professional University, Phagwara, Punjab, India

Abstract: Natural products obtained from the microbes have been reported as substitutes to contemporary drugs obtained from plants. With the increasing need for new therapies, new natural products are being explored using the traditional methods. As only a small fraction of microbes can be cultured in the laboratory, many microbes continue to remain unexplored for their ability to synthesize secondary metabolites. In the past few decades, the reduced cost of DNA sequencing and developments in computational tools have made the Metagenomic Approach effective and popular. Uncultured microbes can be studied through bioprospecting of the unexplored geographical niches. Moreover, Bioinformatics tools have enabled us to find the gene clusters that, in metagenomics, imply the real potential of finding novel open reading frames (ORFs). Screening of genomes for secondary metabolite-genes like non-ribosomal peptide synthases (NRPS) and polyketide synthases (PKS), has resulted in the discovery of new or previously known metabolites. Technological advancement and innovations in the culture-independent approach have allowed us to explore novel chemistries from environmental samples to identify the molecules of therapeutic value. This chapter will discuss the methods for identifying secondary metabolite genes from the genome, and the new approaches for functional metagenomic screening toward the discovery of antimicrobials. Moreover, insights into this approach will be provided to generate opportunities to explore natural products for combating the global demand for novel antibiotics.

Keywords: Antimicrobial, Bioinformatics, Bioprospecting, Metagenomics, Mining, Multi-Drug Resistance, Non-Ribosomal Peptide Synthases, Polyketide Synthases, Secondary Metabolite-Regulated Expression, Substrate-Induced Gene Expression.

[*] **Corresponding authors Reena Singh & Chirag Chopra:** School of Bioengineering and Biosciences, Lovely Professional University, Phagwara, Punjab, India; Tel: +91 96220 22616; E-mails: chirag.18298@lpu.co.in; reena.19408@lpu.co.in

INTRODUCTION

Infectious diseases are the primary cause of morbidity and mortality globally. Human intervention and massive usage of antimicrobial compounds have contributed to the progression of drug-resistance in microorganism [1, 2]. As a result, microorganisms are becoming resistant to multiple drugs, making the treatment difficult and expensive and are becoming a worldwide threat [3]. The multi-drug resistant (MDR) microbial species include *Acinetobacter, Escherichia coli*, Klebsiella pneumoniae, Salmonella spp., Shigella spp., *Staphylococcus aureus*, Streptococcus pneumoniae, and *Neisseria gonorrhoeae* [4]. Some reports have stated that *N. gonorrhoeae* is evolving and becoming resistant to broad-spectrum drugs cephalosporin and fluoroquinolones. It has also been classified as the priority pathogen by the world health organization (WHO) [5]. On the other hand, various synthetic medicines like aspirin, diclofenac, and Ibuprofen are readily available in the market and widely used for treating different diseases. However, their association with minor side-effects like headaches and back pain and severe side-effects like toxicity, breathlessness and haemorrhage are grave matters of concern. These challenges have caused a shift towards the exploration of natural products [6, 7].

Nature provides a generous niche for a large variety of medicinal plants, marine and terrestrial organisms and microbes, from which new antimicrobial agents can be obtained [8]. Different microbes produce a diverse variety of structurally different compounds. Such compounds obtained from microbes as penicillin, gentamicin, omegamycin, and streptomycin, have encouraged the discovery of newer and better compounds, that can act as sedatives, pain killers, heart stimulators, and show anti-cancer activity [9]. A definitive characteristic of any medicine, whether man-made or natural is that it should be effective, non-toxic, target-specific, non-mutagenic, non-irritant and stable [10]. These variations in chemical structures of compounds help us in developing new compounds as well as scaffolds, which can help us to meet the demand and need of new drugs for treating critical human diseases [11].

Culture-dependent approaches have enabled the discovery of new bioactive molecules but are limited by the fact that many microbes continue to remain unexplored and uncultivable [12]. As a result, a large variety of microbes is expected to stay elusive if we rely only on the traditional culture-dependent approach [13]. Thus, to have better insights into the microbes, metagenomics has emerged as a valuable tool to unearth most unexplored microbes. We can now understand the diverse biochemical pathways of uncultured microbes and surpass the limitations of culture-dependent approaches [14]. The approaches used in bioprospecting the metagenomes for useful genes or ORFs have bene summarized in Fig. (**1**). Proximally-located genes generally encode the enzymes involved in the biosynthesis of metabolites. These genes together form a cluster called the biosynthetic gene cluster (BGC). Metagenomics entails the construction of metagenomic libraries, their screening, and recognising these biosynthetic gene clusters [15]. The researchers using this approach, thereby, highlight the importance of new habitats in the exploration of untapped microbes that produce useful antimicrobial compounds having lesser side-effects [16, 17]. Mining of the metagenomes for BGCs has given us non-ribosomal peptide synthetases (NRPSs), polyketide synthetases (PKSs) and NRPS-PKS complexes through robust screening of the potent antimicrobial producers producing diverse antimicrobial compounds [18].

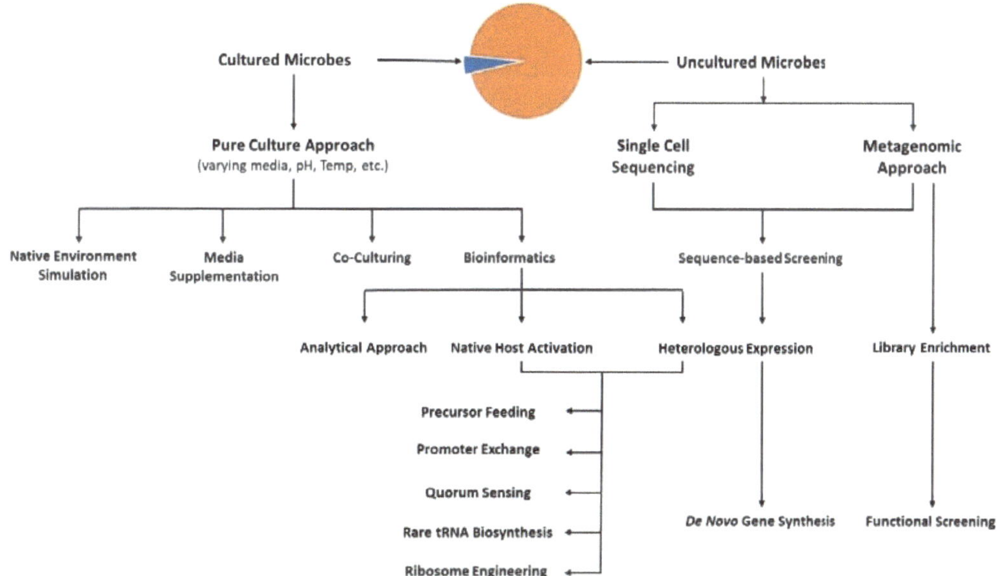

Fig. (1). Diagrammatic illustration of Approaches for Microbiome Mining.

MAJOR MODULAR ENZYMES AND THEIR ASSOCIATED DOMAINS

Bacteria are the primary producers of secondary metabolites which exhibit antimicrobial activities. These compounds are synthesised by modular enzymes like NRPS and PKS [19]. The diversity of PKS and NRPS explains the diversity of secondary metabolites [20].

Non-ribosomal Peptide Synthetases (NRPS)

Generally, the length of a non-ribosomal peptide is 2-45 amino acids, and their diversity is due to different combinations formed by amino acids, including *N*-

methylated amino acids [21]. These diverse NRPSs have a modular organization and are composed of three functional domains:

a. Adenylation domain, which performs the function of selection and adenylation of amino acids;
b. Peptidyl carrier protein domain (PCP), which catalyses the formation of covalent bonds between the amino acids; and
c. Condensation domain, that performs the catalytic function for elongation of the peptide [22].

Further, different domains may also be present, which work like tailoring-enzymes. These domains include cyclases, glycosyltransferases, methyltransferases, oxygenases, and racemases, for modifying the structure of secondary metabolites [23]. The list of different domains and their function in the synthesis of secondary metabolites is summarised in Table **1**.

Table 1. List of Functional Domains involved in Secondary Metabolites.

Domain	Containing Protein	Function	Reference(s)
Acyltransferase	PKS	• Selection of acyl-CoA substrate • Activation of acyl-CoA *via* acylation • Binding to the acyl carrier protein	[24]
Acyl carrier protein (Thiolation)	PKS	• Binding to acyl-CoA substrate	[24]
Adenylation	NRPS	• Selection of amino acid • Binding of amino acid to PCP	[25]
Acyl carrier protein synthase	PKS	• Catalyze the conversion reaction of apo-ACP (inactive) to holo-ACP (active)	[26]
Condensation domain	NRPS	• Helps in peptide bond formation	[25]
Cyclization Domain	NRPS	• Helps in peptide bond formation • Catalyzes the cyclisation reaction	[25]
Coenzyme A ligase	NRPS	• Catalyzes the ligation reaction of acyl groups with CoA	[27]
Dehydratase	PKS	• Helps in dehydration reaction of β-hydroxy carbonyl to a C=C bond	[24]
Enoylreductase	PKS	• Reduces the double bond	[24]
Epimerization domain	NRPS	• Helps in flipping stereo-chemistry	[28]
Enoyl CoA hydratase	NRPS	• Helps in hydration of double bond on acyl-CoA	[29]

Domain	Containing Protein	Function	Reference(s)
FkbH – like domain	PKS	• Incorporation of "scarce" extender units • Transferring of glyceryl moiety to an ACP	[30]
Ketosynthase	PKS	• Helps in catalyzing the condensation reaction	[24]
Ketoreductase	PKS	• Reduces the β-keto group to an OH group	[24]
O/N/C methyltransferase	NRPS	• Addition of methyl group to carbon, nitrogen, and oxygen	[25]
Peptidyl carrier protein (thiolation)	NRPS	• Helps in the binding of amino acid	[25]
Thioesterase	NRPS	• Helps in releasing the full-length chain • Catalyzes the macro-cyclisation reaction	[31]
Terminal reductase domain	NRPS	• Catalyzes the process of reductive release from NRPS or PKS assembly lines	[32]
X-domain	NRPS	• Recruiting the targeted P450 oxygenase • Binding of P450 oxygenase to NRPS bound peptide for cross-linking of the side chain in glycopeptides	[33]

Polyketide Synthases (PKS)

Various microbial secondary metabolites have been classified as polyketides. Polyketides are compounds that are synthesized by a diverse class of multi-domain enzymes called polyketide synthases (PKSs) [34]. The compounds are known to display several bioactivities. PKSs are large proteins and work as assembly lines, and the different component subunits of this assembly line are referred to as "modules". Generally, PKS modules are made of three functional domains, namely:

a. Acyl-transferase domain (AT), which performs the function in activating, binding of specific substrates (*e.g.* CoA-activated acyl group);
b. Acyl-carrier protein domain (ACP), and
c. Ketosynthase domain (KS), which catalyzes the condensation and de-carboxylation reaction between acyl-CoA (substrate) and the elongating polyketide chain [35].

Further, functional group modifications are done via tailoring-domains like dehydratase (DH), enoyl reductase (ER), and keto-reductase (KR) as illustrated in Table **1**. A thioesterase domain (TE) performs the role in the termination of the assembly line. Moreover, an alternative mechanism involves trans-AT domain performing a similar function of TE. Here, the genes encoding AT domains are not present within the module but somewhere else within the gene cluster [36].

The sheer diversity of the products and the several industrial applications of these products make PKSs potential biotechnological targets. PKSs are versatile proteins whose structure shows remarkable diversity and yet share common functionality enough to belong to the same class [37]. The PKSs are further classified into three different categories based on differences in the arrangement of synthetic modules.

Type I PKSs

This category of PKSs is composed of diverse, non-iteratively acting modules present on one or more proteins that successively assemble to produce the final compound. Moreover, each module executes only one elongation step. The acyl-carrier protein domain is used for substrate activation [38]. The type I PKSs are further divided into two sub-classes *viz.* the iterative type I PKSs and the modular type I PKSs. The iterative type I PKSs repeatedly use their modules in a cyclic manner to generate the final product. An example of the iterative type I PKS is the fatty acid synthase complex of humans. The iterative type I PKSs have been further classified into three subtypes known as highly-reducing (HR-PKS), partially reducing (PR-PKS) and non- reducing (NR-PKS).

The modular type I PKSs are diverse, and except for their conserved AT domain (responsible for chain-extension), they do not use their domain in a cyclin manner. The most studied example of the modular type I PKS is the erythromycin synthase complex. Since these are modular PKSs, their further classification is also logical, depending on the combination of subunits present in the complex (AT+KS+ACP or AT+KS+ACP+KR and many more) [39].

Type II PKSs

These clusters of PKS are composed of the same core structure domains like ACP, AT and KS, but irrespective of the modular structure of these clusters, each gene encodes a mono-functioning catalytic domain. These PKSs synthesize oxidized aromatic compounds [40].

Type III PKSs

They work as homodimeric enzymes and catalyze the condensation reaction. This category differs from type II PKSs in that the type III PKS modules directly act on the Acyl-CoA (substrate) iteratively and lack the substrate-binding domain ACP [41].

Some researchers suggest that the PKSs can form hybrid clusters with FASs (Fatty acid synthases) and NRPSs (Non-ribosomal Peptide Synthases). Remarkably, these biosynthetic pathways share homology in their basic chemistry, which allows these modules to cross-talk and synthesize a hybrid molecule [42]. Moreover, the synthesized hybrid molecules can incorporate unusual amino acids apart from the 20 usual amino acids [43].

Other Molecules

Other bacterial secondary metabolites that work as antibiotics are Ribosomally-synthesized and Post-translationally-modified Peptides (RiPPs). Although the final products show high variation in size and structure, all RiPPs are synthesized *via* the same biosynthesis mechanism. These synthesized peptides are precursors as they contain the leader as well as the core peptide [44]. Later, the processing of RiPPs takes place *via* modifying enzymes like cyclases, dehydratases, and methylases. In the end, the leader peptide is proteolytically digested for releasing the core peptide. A few essential classes of RiPPs are linear azo-containing peptides (LAPs), lanti-peptides, lasso-peptides, and thiopeptides [45]. Furthermore, bacterial terpenes often referred to as terpenoids with antibiotic activity, have also been discovered [46].

EXPLORATION OF NEW HABITATS

Nature beholds untold secrets, for thousands of years it has been providing us with bioactive compounds of pharmacological importance and continues to do so. Microbes are the biological factories that synthesize useful molecules and inhabit diverse ecosystems like soil, sediments, marine, hot springs, the artic. They can live in symbiosis with animals and plants (example, endophytic microorganisms) [20, 47, 48]. In 1940, the discovery of antibiotics like penicillin, actinomycin, chloramphenicol, and streptomycin highlighted the potential of soil-borne microbes in pharmaceutical industries [49]. These discoveries also marked the beginning of research on antimicrobials derived from microorganisms. The sources of these antimicrobials range from bacteria and fungi to highly specialized genera of Archaea and Myxobacteria. Although the science of metagenomics came decades later, the research on microbial antimicrobials had already provided numerous antibiotics. As it turns out, there is an excellent potential for the identification of antibiotic-production genes from metagenomes. The production of the secondary metabolites varies with the geographical location of the metagenomic sample. Research done by Reddy et al. showed that the biosynthetic gene sequences show diversity in samples from different locations. This fact indicates a huge number of such genes in the biosphere [50].

Moreover, recent studies have provided evidence about the association of environmental factors with variations in PKSs or NRPSs of microbes isolated from different geographical niches and have established a relationship between biosynthetic domain-composition with changes in latitude/longitude [51]. However, with the use of conventional approaches, we are only able to isolate a handful of microbes. More than 90% of the microbes remain hidden as they are unculturable through standard practices [10]. The advent of the metagenomic approach revealed that the uncultured microbes contain many unknown BGCs and moved the focus from actinobacteria to other microbes like cyanobacteria, marine archaea, symbiotic fungi and proteobacteria [52, 53]. For example, Asenjonamides A–C, belonging to the β-diketone polyketides, were synthesized by *Streptomyces asenjonii* KNN 42.f isolated from the hyper-arid soil of Atacama Desert [54]. In 1992, Gold stated that "the microbes exist in all locations where they can survive". He also advocated further that there is no place on earth, which is free from microbes [55]. Deducing from these studies, the assessment of microbial diversity and exploration of new habitats for discovering the novel bioactive molecules is needed. It is not only sustainable for human healthcare but also provides better insights into the rich microbial world.

Extreme Environment: A Niche for Novel Strains

Every microbial species has its self-chemotype, and to discover new antimicrobials, we must have a better understanding of the genome as well as the metabolome of the new species [56]. The chances of discovering a novel microbial species are better if the samples are collected from extreme environments having extreme temperature, extreme pressure, high radiation, high salinity, limited nutrients and having unusually high/low pH [57]. The microbes residing in such environments are adapted to survive and reproduce under the said harsh environmental conditions. They can synthesize small molecules possessing useful biological activities, such as melanin for protection from UV radiation and extreme temperatures, polyol-compounds as well as sugar molecules to bear osmotic stress and maintain turgor pressure and membrane structure [58]. Since microbes from extreme environments are exposed to harsh conditions which are not experienced by mesophilic microbes, it is likely that the compounds they produce are explicitly for survival and reproducing in such conditions [59]. Microbes in the extreme environments seem to be promising candidates for isolating new bioactive molecules, as evident from increasing reports about the discovery of new compounds from extreme environments [60, 61]. Marthiapeptide A, a cyclic peptide compound, was obtained from

Marinactinospora thermotolerans SCSIO 00652, which was isolated from deep-sea sediments of the South China Sea [62]. Abyssomicin C, member of the spirotetronate class I was isolated from Verrucosispora strain AB 18-032, which was isolated from Japanese sea sediments [63]. Halocin C8, an antimicrobial compound was obtained from the halophilic archaea isolated from chotts, dry salt lakes, salt flat and sebkha of Algerian Sahara (hypersaline environment) [64]. Three rhamnolipids having antimicrobial activity were isolated from *Pseudomonas* strain BNT1, isolated from the different microbial strain-isolates of Rosa Sea, Antarctica [65]. Gene for palmitoylputrescine, an antibiotic was screened from the metagenomic DNA isolated from a Bromeliad tank water collected from Costa Rica [66]. In contrast, the gene for an isocyanide-containing antibiotic was also screened from the soil metagenome [67]. These studies highlight and present these extreme environments as a promising resource for extensive research on the production of biologically active products like anti-bacterial, anti-fungal, anti-tumor, and antioxidant compounds.

ROLE OF METAGENOMICS IN EXPLORATION OF UNCULTURED MICROBES

Till date, about 90% of microbes have remained uncultured under *in-vitro* conditions as per the 16S rRNA (ribosomal RNA) data. Therefore, novel approaches are required to tap into the vast diversity of microbes producing various natural products and surpass the limitation of conventional culture-dependent approach [68]. Metagenomics is an approach that involves the extraction and sequencing of environmental DNA from different environmental samples. Most importantly, this field has grown exponentially in the last few years, and its techniques are now routinely used [69]. This approach, combined with traditional culture-dependent approaches serves to unravel the unknown microbial population from different habitats [70]. The gene clusters of NRPSs and PKSs of interest are used for designing probes for high-throughput screening of the genes for natural products which include various antibiotics, antifungal and immunosuppressants [71]. This part focusses on the recent developments in the metagenomics approach and procedures used to explore genes producing new secondary metabolites.

1. The workflow of the Metagenomic Approach

Generally, there are two main strategies used in the metagenomic approach. The first one is based on the functional screening of environmental DNA library [72]. The clones in the library are screened based on information like visually noticeable reporter activity, bioassays, enzyme-assays or advanced screening methods using biosensors [17]. Environmental samples are collected from diverse ecological and geographical regions, natural habitats or extreme environment [73, 74].

Further, the environmental DNA (eDNA) is extracted either by direct or indirect extraction methods. The direct methods are those in which the cell lysis is performed directly on the environmental sample, without any intermittent step to separate the cells. The lysis solution is directly mixed with the environmental sample, followed by purification of the DNA. The indirect methods first separate the cells from the rest of the sample, and then the cell lysis step follows. The indirect method involves blending and ion-exchange matrices. The extracted eDNA is then cloned and ligated into a shuttle vector and transferred into a heterologous host for creating the metagenomic library [10, 75]. In function-based screening, the metagenomic library is assessed for observable phenotypic changes, heterologous complementation, METREX (**Met**abolite-**R**egulated **EX**pression) or SIGEX (**S**ubstrate-**I**nduced **G**ene **EX**pression) [76]. The pigment, indirubin having an antibacterial activity was isolated from the metagenomic library of forest soil of Jindong Valley, Korea by using function-based screening [77]. Sequence-based screening involves screening during polymerase chain reaction in which specific BGC sequences are used for amplification followed by sequencing. Sequence tags of DNA are then organised through phylogenetic trees, and their biosynthetic origin is determined by comparing it with reference database entries [78]. Based on the sequence similarity with the known BGCs; potential BGCs could be identified from the environmental sample.

Moreover, *in-silico* determination of targeted BGCs and successive heterologous gene expression can be used to identify novel antimicrobial compounds [73]. Further, BGCs can be reassembled *in-silico*. The metagenomic library constructed *via* this approach harbours BGCs resembling the *in-silico* constructed BGC of interest, and the sequence data is analysed for specific sequences of interest. Both approaches follow similar steps-

a. assembling and amending of novel BGCs for heterologous expression in the targeted host,
b. production of natural product in the targeted host and
c. structure elucidation of the natural product by high-throughput techniques [79].

Per the recent studies conducted on polyketide BGCs cloned directly from the soil, two antibiotics, *i.e.* Fasamycin A and B were discovered which inhibits the FabF activity in FASII (Fatty Acid Biosynthesis Type II) pathway [80]. The discovery of antibiotics from the culture-independent approach has repeatedly proven that this method has the potential to provide access to various novel antimicrobial compounds with different modes of action compared to the antimicrobials currently in use. The two methods, *i.e.* classical functional-based screening and targeted sequence-based screening, which are employed in metagenomic studies, are summarised in a workflow as illustrated in Fig. (2).

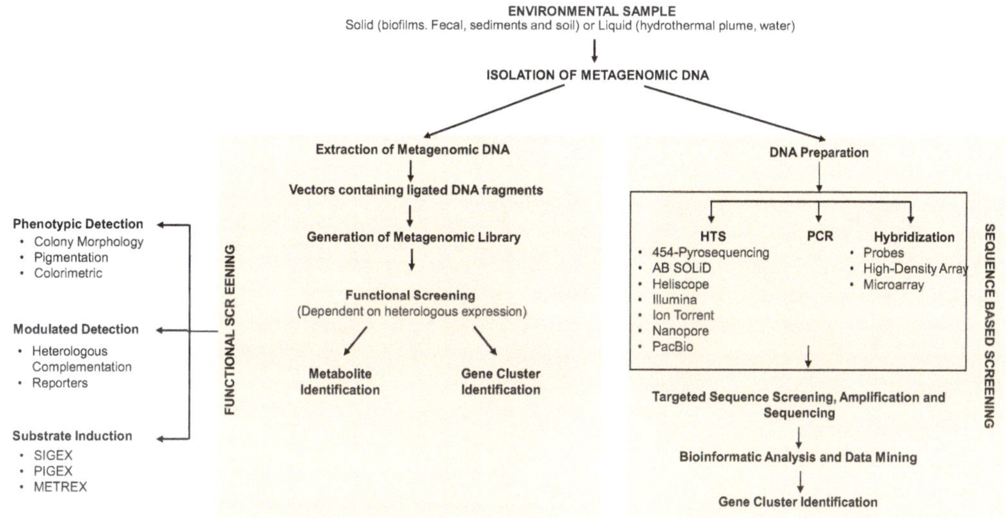

Fig. (2). Systemic workflow of metagenomic approach.

2. Direct Metagenomic Screening based on Function

Function-based metagenomic screening involves DNA isolation from the microbial population to explore the function of encoded proteins. This process involves the cloning of fragmented eDNA, expression of genes in the surrogate host, and assessment of enzyme activities. This approach enables us to discover new enzymes whose functions cannot be predicted based on sequence only [81]. The information gathered from the function-based approach is further used to annotate genes and genomes obtained by metagenomics approach, which is based on sequence [82]. This approach is not exclusively dependent on structural changes such as altered chromatographic patterns, which attributes to identifying new bioactive molecules [83]. Another approach is the top agar overlay method, which assesses the growth inhibition of pathogenic microbes [84].

Further, advanced approaches involve biosensor/reporter-based screens like METREX and SIGEX. In METREX approach, we screen the quorum sensing inhibitors which bind at transcriptional activator regions such as LuxR, which induces the expression of the targeted gene and initiates the accumulation of GFP

(Green Fluorescent Protein). The accumulated GFP serves as the reporting signal for targeted clones, thus showing communication [85]. On the other hand, SIGEX shows the expression of a catabolic gene in the presence of the substrate [86]. These two methods help us to explore new genes or gene products which remain unknown *via* the sequence-based approach as no prior knowledge is available for that gene or gene product. However, to date, very few antimicrobial agents have been discovered by function-based metagenomics like Indigo, Indirubin, *N*-acyltyrosines, turbomycin A, and violacein [77, 78, 87, 88].

3. Sequence-based Metagenomic Screening

The main feature which differentiates the sequence-based and function-based screening are that we do not need a heterologous expression for identifying the clone of interest in the sequence-based approach. Instead, it requires a targeted gene cluster of interest *via* sequence analysis [89]. Thus, genomic information is collected without culturing the microbes in *in-vitro* conditions [90]. High-throughput sequencing (HTS) has helped us in identifying BGCs in some genomes and small endobiont metagenomes. Thus, this approach can be used to determine the degree of diversity of the microbial species present in a sample [91]. The large size and complexity of soil metagenomes have restricted its usage for exploration. If we sequence the tagged amplicons from these soil metagenomes and gather information, there is a potential of bioprospecting large metagenomes containing an estimated over 20,000 unique species [92]. These sequences may further contain novel BGCs sequence tags. This makes sense, after all, the sequence tags that may be used for screening would have some conservation because a majority of these tags would identify NRPSs and PKSs [92, 93]. Moreover, the assessment of microbial diversity is convenient as no assemblage of the genome is required, and we can directly infer the information related to the ecology of microbes from the existing sample [94]. Therefore, most discoveries made using this approach have used degenerate PCR primers. The degenerate primers amplify the conserved BGCs of interest. Thus, the complex mixture of amplicons having various conserved fragments from potent BGCs obtained from environmental samples defines the term NPSTs (Natural Product Sequence Tags) [95].

In contrast to high-throughput sequencing (HTS), the available data involves small stretches of DNA and thus obstructs the identification of novel BGCs. Such smaller genomic reads are assembled using clustering algorithms to form the metagenome-assembled clusters. The protein sequences are taken as the input along with the metagenomic reads. The input protein sequences are mapped with metagenomic reads to generate contiguous stretches of DNA. These sequences are then assembled by aligning the contigs and eliminating common sequences [96]. Also, tools like MetaCAA allow generation of metagenome-assembled genomes (MAGs). MetaCAA uses a sequential clustering algorithm, in which the metagenome reads are clustered into smaller groups, followed by alignment and assembly of the clusters to form the contiguous sequences. The contigs and the unassembled reads are then combined to generate the larger "assembled" genome [97]. Tools like anti-SMASH (Antibiotics and Secondary Metabolite Analysis Shell; https://antismash.secondary metabolites.org/#!/start) utilise such metagenome assemblies as input for the prediction of gene clusters, non-ribosomal peptides and RiPP BGCs [98]. On the other hand, tools based on the phylogenetic relationships of sequence tags like eSNAPD (**S**urveyor of **NA**tural **P**roduct **D**iversity) and NaPDoS (**Na**tural **P**roduct **Do**main **S**eeker) aid us in searching both close and distantly related species from big datasets [99, 100]. eSNAPD is curated by the Rockefeller University and is a web-server providing the tool for analysis of the metagenomic libraries and bacterial culture collections for BGCs. For this analysis, the server requires two inputs. The first input is the amplicon sequence data or library barcodes of the Illumina or 454 amplicons. The second input file is a simple text file containing the illumine tag sequence, sequencing primers and the library code. The input sequence is refined by identification of sequences like the BGCs for characterized known molecules. For refinement, the input environmental DNA sequences are aligned with the databases such as Genbank using the BLAST (Basic Local Alignment Search Tool) program. For the similarity search, eSNAPD matches the input sequences with fourteen different domains of NRPSs and PKSs. The best results are defined by the BLAST e-value (expectation value).

On the other hand, NaPDoS is a tool that identifies the sequences of the C and KS domains from the input sequences. NaPDoS accepts both protein and nucleotides as input. Within the nucleotide sequences, the user can input the amplicon data, assembled contigs or the whole genome sequence. From the input sequences, NaPDoS trims-out the C and KS domain sequences, followed by a BLAST search as well construction of the phylogenetic. The final output gives the domain identification along with a prediction of the natural compounds that may be produced by the members of the environmental sample. Recent advancements have enabled the use of hosts of different phylogenetic backgrounds for heterologous gene expression such as myxobacteria, for the biosynthesis of natural products [101, 102]. However, sequence-based metagenomic screening has enabled us to identify antimicrobials like arimetamycin A, clarepoxcins A-E, landepoxcins A-B, malacidins A-B, and tetarimycin A [79, 103 - 105].

4. Sequence Advancement: Potential of Single-Cell Genomics and High-Throughput Sequencing

Advancement in high-throughput sequencing has made the cost of whole-genome sequencing affordable. Therefore, development of techniques for isolation of DNA from a single cell, transcriptome, and whole genome amplification, and genome sequencing of a single cell can potentially allow high-resolution analysis and open new prospects for genetic analysis [106]. In metagenomics, sequencing of single-cell microbe enables identification of new phyla and allows us to gain insights into the genetics of non-culturable microbes [107]. Another advantage of single-cell genomics is that this approach reduces the complexity of genomic signals. In this process, three WGA (Whole Genome Amplification) methods are the most commonly used viz. DOP-PCR (Degenerate-Oligonucleotide-Primed PCR – a purely PCR dependent approach), MDA (Multiple Displacement Amplification- isothermal based approach) and combination of both like MALBAC (Multiple Annealing and Looping Based Amplification Cycles) [108]. These approaches have increased the coverage of identification of novel BGCs exhibiting antibacterial, antifungal and cytotoxic activity. The Apratoxin A has been identified based on MDA and sequence-based screening of the metagenomic library [109]. High-throughput techniques like DNA-microarray, SNP array and HTS are commonly used for obtaining single-cell WGA. Among these, HTS has numerous advantages such as evaluation of each amplified nucleotide from the cell and identification of several mutations, the precision of results, and identification and differentiation of structural variations within a genome through read-pair mapping [110].

MINING OF GENOMES: CURRENT SCENARIO AND FUTURE POTENTIAL

In 2002, the whole-genome sequence of *Streptomyces coelicolor* A3, a model microbe was published, which provided new information about this well-characterized strain in the context of secondary metabolites [111]. Previously, it was known to produce actinorhodin, a calcium-dependent antibiotic, methylenomycin, and undecylprodigiosin [112 - 115]. However, later in 2011, the development of antiSMASH allowed us to identify novel BGCs, which was evident from its potential in exploring the unknown metabolites [116]. Thus, we focus on the envision of genome mining that how BGCs can drive natural product discovery.

1. Prediction of Biosynthetic Gene Cluster (BGC) and their targeted activation

Due to advances in sequencing technology, we can unravel the hidden information about the microbes. More than 19,000 complete sequences of microbes have been published, and more than 200,000 permanent drafts are now available in the Genomes Online Database (https://gold.jgi.doe.gov/) [117]. Further, analysis of the available data revealed that there is far more information about BGCs embedded in the genome of microbes than the numbers of isolated natural products, providing us with the essence that a large number of natural products have remained unexplored till date [118, 119]. Nowadays, different experiments that are conducted for analyzing the BGCs are mainly dependent on the *in-silico* analysis of the microbial genome [120]. Both NRPS-precursors and PKS-assembly lines can now be predicted using various computational tools like anti-SMASH, ARTS (Antibiotic Resistance Target Seeker), NRPSpredictor2, PRISM4, SEARCHPKS and more as described in Table **2** [121]. The predictions based on computational analysis of the unexplored natural products, are based on biosynthetic genes and serve as powerful tools for subsequent analyses like genomic-metabolomic correlation. Also, structure elucidation solely based on *in-silico* analysis is quite reliable [122].

On the other hand, knocking out or targeted activation of BGCs also needs computational analysis for the selection of the BGCs [123]. Numerous online tools have been developed to categorize the new compounds in specific families by correlating BGCs of NRPSs and RiPPs with the obtained data [124]. Now, BGCs are also accessed for resistance genes present near the biosynthetic genes, which provide the information about their mode of action *via* tools like ARTS and PRISM3 [125, 126]. Anti-SMASH is a tool for identification of metabolite gene-clusters and well as a comparison of gene clusters in different genomic sequences. The input for anti-SMASH is the assembled metagenome sequence in standard formats, based on which it gives the prediction analysis of NRPSs as well as PKSs. The ARTS server is a multi-utility server that provides the users with an automated server for carrying out anti-SMASH analysis, prediction of antibiotic targets as well as resistance genes. The NRPSpredictor2 is an online web-server designed for predicting the specificity of the adenylation domain of NRPSs. Its utility comes from the fact that there is a huge diversity of the adenylation domain specificities, which determines the amino acid residue to be incorporated on the non-ribosomally synthesized peptide. In the NRPSpredictor2, an input query of an adenylation domain is matched with a trained set of adenylation domain sequences to yield the potential substrate specificities. PRISM is an online tool used for prediction of BGCs using the microbial genome sequence as an input. The output also provides the structures of the proteins that could be biosynthetic enzymes. One of the resistance genes associated with BGCs has been reported in which the spectinomycin synthesis gene has similar domains as in DNA methylase (N-6 adenine-specific DNA methylases and N-4 cytosine-specific DNA methylases) that confer the aminoglycoside-resistance to *Streptomyces spectabilis* [127]. Hence, the selection of BGCs in the proximity of resistance genes found in the gene clusters, confirms the potential for the identification of new antibiotics.

Table 2. List of Computational Prediction Tools and Database for mining Secondary Metabolites BGCs.

Tools	Web Address	BGCA	BGC Db	BGCBP	DA	GM	M	NRP Db	RBMP	RDS	RiPPA	sgRNA	References
antiSMASH 4	http://antismash.secondarymetabolites.org	√			√	√							[98]
antiSMASH database	http://antismash-db.secondarymetabolites.org		√										[128]
ARTS	http://arts.ziemertlab.com					√							[126]
BAGEL 3	http://bagel.molgenrug.nl/					√							[129]
CASSIS	https://sbi.hki-jena.de/cassis/cassis.php			√									[130]
CRISPy-web	http://crispy.secondarymetabolites.org											√	[131]
eSNaPD v2	http://esnapd2.rockefeller.edu					√							[100]
FunGeneClusterS	https://fungiminions.shinyapps.io/FunGeneClusterS			√									[132]
fungiSMASH	http://fungismash.secondarymetabolites.org	√			√	√							[98]
GNP	http://magarveylab.ca/gnp						√						[133]
GRAPE/GARLIC	https://magarveylab.ca/gast/					√							[134, 135]
MIBiG	http://mibig.secondarymetabolites.org		√							√			[136]
NaPDoS	http://napdos.ucsd.edu					√							[99]
NORINE	http://bioinfo.lifl.fr/NRP							√					[137]
NP.searcher	http://dna.sherman.lsi.umich.edu/				√	√							[138]
NRPSpredictor	http://nrps.informatik.uni-tuebingen.de				√								[139]
plantiSMASH	http://plantismash.secondarymetabolites.org	√				√							[140]
PRISM 3	http://magarveylab.ca/prism	√			√	√							[125]
RODEO	http://www.ripprodeo.org					√					√		[141]
SBSPKS v2/SEARCHPKS	http://202.54.226.228/~pksdb/sbspks_updated/master.html		√		√								[142]
Smile2Monomers	http://bioinfo.lifl.fr/norine/smiles2monomers.jsp								√				[143]
SMURF	http://www.jcvi.org/smurf					√							[144]

BGCA – BGC Analysis; BGC Db – BGC Database; BGCBP – BGC Boundary Prediction; DA – Domain Analysis; GM – Genome Mining; M – Metabolomics; NRP Db – Non-ribosomal Peptide Database; RBMP – Retro-biosynthetic Monomer Prediction; RDS - Reference Data Set; RiPPA - RiPP Analysis; sgRNA – sgRNA design

2. Genetic Manipulations of the Biosynthetic Machinery for the Discovery of New Antimicrobials

Genetic manipulation of antimicrobial-producing strains is challenging, as they contain various BGCs which on modification may alter other metabolic pathways [145]. The available literature has a few cases involving modification of one of the biosynthetic genes, producing a known compound in the host *via* gene knockdown. The need for such a knock-down is justified because different metabolites are expressed in different concentrations. As a result, the more abundant metabolites can mast the bioactivities of the rarer ones [146]. There are instances of research that prove the efficacy of selective knockdown in discovering novel metabolites. As an example, the new amexanthomycins A–J were also discovered by knocking out of *rifA* gene encoding the synthesis of rifampicin in *Amycolatopsis mediterranei* strain S699 [147].

Further, transcription regulators present near the BGCs of known antimicrobials have significant potential on the expression of secondary metabolite [148]. Some of these regulators act as activators or repressors, but, replacing the natural promoter with a conditional one can lead to activation or inhibition of priority BGCs [149]. For example, rpoB mutation in *Bacillus subtilis* resulted in the overexpression of 3,3'-neotrehalosediamine, an amino-sugar antibiotic [150]. In contrast, the two novel anguicyclinone metabolites UVM6 and rabelomycin were isolated through the disruption of tetR repressor surrounded by two silent BGCs in *Streptomyces* sp [151]. Discovery of the antibiotic thienamycin from *Streptomyces cattleya* was achieved from ThnI regulator gene of the LTTR (LysR-type transcriptional regulator) family, working as an activator of thienamycin (β-lactam antibiotic) biosynthesis [152]. On the other hand, swapping the native promoter with an inducible one upregulates the expression of first BGCs of the operon, which can thus be stringently controlled by regulating the activation of the promoter [153]. For example, the introduction of *ermE* promoter in PKS-NRPS type I (hybrid) operon upregulated the production of polycyclic tetramate macrolactam 6-*epi*-alteramide A [154]. In the knock-out mutant, without any stimulation, no metabolite was produced, but the same could be achieved upon addition of inducible promoter for overexpression of metabolites [155]. Considering the strategies as mentioned above, we need to have better knowledge about the operon structure and the metabolic profile reported by precise detection system like high-resolution MS (Mass Spectrometry) to detect the minute concentration of the targeted mass [156].

The native, modified and synthetic promoters are required to increase the yield of natural products. Now, research groups are focusing on increasing the number of new promoters in promoter libraries. These findings favor and unlock the real potential of this approach for better regulation of genes in the near future [157]. For an organism with larger genome size, the heterologous gene expression is lesser. Per the observations made in one report, strains with small genomes face the challenge of heterologous expression for studying gene-function and metabolic changes in-detail and correlating it with targeted manipulation within the strain [158]. Thus, to overcome these obstructions, secondary metabolite gene clusters and insertion sequences (unnecessary genomic segments) are removed to improve the genetic stability and lessen the burden on metabolic machinery [159]. For example, deletion of four endogenous BGCs from *S. coelicolor* strain M145 and the addition of point mutations into *rpoB* and *rpsL* genes increased the expression of biosynthetic genes. The introduction of actinorhodin (*rpoB* and *rpsL* genes) gene cluster drastically increased the antibiotic production when compared to the parental strain [160]. After the success of this approach with small genomes, it is now possible to use these genomes for studying the heterologous gene expression of BGCs discovered by metagenomic approach and silent BGCs expression obtained from different strains [161].

3. Different Mechanisms of Activation of Silent BGCs

Several BGCs that synthesize antimicrobials remain unnoticed because of very less concentration of the product and are designated as cryptic or silent BGCs. Currently, two strategies are used to access these silent BGCs [148]. The first one involves the optimization of growth conditions, different small-molecule inducers, trace metals, and epigenetic modifications, and the second approach involves targeted genome sequencing, notably for regulatory genes. Systematic variation in growth conditions like the addition of chemical elicitors, co-cultivation, temperature, and pH has been reported to upregulate expression of BGCs [162]. Variation in the chemical composition of media and culturing time promotes the production of secondary metabolites. For example, limiting concentration of iron elicits the production of antibiotic lugdunin from *Staphylococcus lugdunensis,* which was previously reported as silent under *in-vitro* conditions. During the co-culturing of *S. griseus* and *S. tanashiensis,* the siderophore desferrioxamine E synthesized by *S. griseus* promotes the growth of *S. tanashiensis* [163, 164]. Rare earth metals have been reported to elicit the cryptic metabolite production in *Streptomyces* spp [165]. However, innovative strategies like iChip (isolation chip) allow recovery of about 50% of the microbes residing in an environmental sample [166]. iChip provides a multicellular scaffold containing minute diffusion chambers. Each diffusion chamber is inoculated with a dilution of the environmental sample that s mixed with an agar solution. After seeding of the chamber, the chip is returned to the original environment from which the dilutions are prepared (burying in the soil or suspension in water stream). This allows the growth of the microorganisms in the chip. The use of iChip led to the discovery of lassomycin, an antibiotic having anti-TB activity and teixobactin, an antibacterial compound [167]. The production of novel metabolites at the industrial scale is still under evaluation.

Certain studies have provided evidence that antibiotics like gentamicin, streptomycin, and rifamycin upregulate the expression of BGCs in which the ribosomal proteins and RNA polymerase have been mutated [168]. Mutation in specific repressors causes activation of cryptic or silent BGCs, because of which two new aminoglycosides were isolated from *Streptomyces sp.* strain PGA64 [169]. In recent years, chromatin remodeling used for regulating the gene expression of eukaryotes has now been used on the microbial genomes successfully [170]. Silent BGCs can also be easily located within the tightly packed heterochromatin regions *via* epigenetic modification (DNA/histone methylation and acetylation) and chromatin remodeling, as they induce the expression of silent BGCs [171]. Till date, no natural products have been discovered by using this approach. However, variation in expression of the biosynthetic gene was observed although in most of the cases expression was very low.

ANTIBIOTIC AND BIOACTIVE COMPOUNDS DISCOVERED THROUGH METAGENOMIC APPROACH

Isolation of Turbomycin A and B, Indirubin, and N-acyltyrosine antibiotics from the metagenomic library has proven the prospect of metagenomic approach in exploring new antimicrobial compounds [77, 88, 172]. In 2013, the research provided evidence of *Bor* gene cluster belonging to a rare family of indolotryptoline compounds and was isolated from soil. The Bor gene products have an anti-cancerous property and show prominent effects on cancer cell lines [173]. In addition to these studies, the metagenomic approach has shed some light on the microbial biodiversity and prompted research for exploring the bioactive compounds of medical importance [10]. Both homology-based and function-based approaches are used for screening and isolating the novel bioactive compounds through heterologous gene expression. However, these approaches have limitations, that the expression vectors might not express specific gene clusters [174]. Thus, the development of better expression systems is required to enhance the selectivity, sensitivity, specificity, and efficacy of gene expression, which would fundamentally increase the value of metagenomics. METREX (metabolite-regulated EXpression), a uniquely designed system which involves GFP expression in the host under a conditional promoter, generates fluorescence leading to the identification of the target gene on interaction with the metabolite of interest. Even, small segments of compounds have been recognised by this approach [16].

Moreover, continuous developments in sequencing techniques and bioinformatics tools have made the sequence-based metagenomic approach more targeted and useful for the discovery of antimicrobial and bioactive compounds [175]. The decreasing cost of sequencing genomic or metagenomic DNA has enabled scientists to investigate the microbial community at a large scale [176]. Borchet *et al.* (2016) chose the subunits of NRPS and PKS domains for investigating the microbial diversity of different sponge species [177]. The results revealed the presence of NRPSs or PKSs of microbial origin, implying a vast repository of bioactive molecules. Further, better knowledge of these antimicrobial biosynthetic pathways has led to the development of various bioinformatics tools like antiSMASH, eSNAPD, and PRISM, that can predict the presence of the gene of interest [175]. Integration of these tools with new heterologous expression systems and pathway engineering methods will pave a new way to produce novel antimicrobials. List of information regarding the antimicrobial compounds identified by metagenomic approach is provided in Table **3**.

Table 3. Systematic summary of antimicrobials discovered by the metagenomic approach.

Antimicrobial	Environment	Country	Method	References
Argolaphos A and B	Soil	USA	SBS	[178]
Arimetamycin A	Soil	USA	SBS	[103]
Arixanthomycins A	Soil	USA	SBS	[179]
Ascidiacyclamide	Marine Invertebrate	Australia	ABS	[180]
Beta-lactamases	Topsoil	Alaska	FBS	[181]
Bisucaberin	Deep-Sea Sediment	East China	ABS	[182]
Borregomycin A	Dessert Soil	USA	SBS	[173]
Bryostatins	Marine Invertebrate	USA	SBS	[183]
Calixanthomycin A	Desert soil	USA	SBS	[184]
Calyculin A	Marine Sponge	Japan	SBS	[185]
Clarepoxin D	Soil	USA	SBS	[79]
Deoxyviolacein	Soil	USA	FBS	[78]
Difluostatin A	Sea Sediment	South China	SBS	[186]
Enterocin	Marine Sediment	Fiji	FBS	[187]
Enterobactin	Soil	USA	FBS	[188]
Erdacin	Soil	USA	FBS	[189]
Erdasporine A	Soil	USA	SBS	[190]
Fasamycins A and B	Topsoil	USA	ABS	[80]
Fluostatin F-H	Soil	USA	ABS	[191]
Hydroxysporine	Soil	USA	SBS	[192]
Indirubin	Topsoil	Korea	FBS	[77]
Isocyanide -containing antibiotic	Soil	USA	FBS	[67]
Lactocillin	human gut microbiome	USA	SBS	[193]
Landepoxin A	Soil	USA	SBS	[79]
Landomycin E	Soil	USA	SBS	[194]

(Table 3) cont.....

Antimicrobial	Environment	Country	Method	References
Lazarimide A	Soil	USA	SBS	[195]
Long-chain N-acyltyrosine antibiotics	Soil and Water	The USA and the Republic of Costa Rica	ABS	[172]
The long-chain fatty acid enol ester compound	Soil	USA	FBS	[196]
Long-chain *N*-acyl tryptophan	Soil	USA	FBS	[197]
Long-chain *N*-acyl arginine	Soil	USA	FBS	[197]
Malacidin A and B	Dessert Soil	USA	ABS	[105]
Minimide	Marine Invertebrate	USA	ABS	[198]
Onnamide A	Marine Sponge	Indonesia	SBS	[199]
Palmitoylputrescine	Water	Republic of Costa Rica	ABS	[66]
Patellamide D	Marine Invertebrate	Australia	ABS	[180]
Pederin	Terrestrial lichen	Europe	SBS	[200]
Reductasporine	Soil	USA	SBS	[192]
Sulfo-glycopeptide compounds	Desert Soil	USA	SBS	[201]
Taromycin A	Marine Sediment	USA	SBS	[202]
Tetarimycin A	Soil	USA	SBS	[104]
Terragine	Topsoil	Canada	ABS	[203]
Trisulfo-teicoplanin	Soil	USA	SBS	[204]
Turbomycin A and B	Topsoil	USA	ABS	[88]
Ulithiacyclamide	Marine invertebrate	Fiji, Palau, Solomon island	SBS	[205]
Utahmycins A and B	Soil	USA	SBS	[206]
Vibrioferrin	Tidal-flat Sediment	Japan	FBS	[207]
Violacein	Soil	Australia	FBS	[208]
Zn-coproporphyrin III	Marine Sponge	Japan	FBS	[209]

*SBS - Sequence-Based Screening; ABS – Activity-Based Screening, FBS – Functional-Based Screening

CONCLUSION AND FUTURE PERSPECTIVES

Metagenomics is a prolific approach for unearthing the natural products showing valuable bioactivities and unique chemical characteristics. As the majority of microbes producing secondary metabolites remain unexplored because of being non-cultivable, characterizing BGCs and their machinery is important, and the role of analytical chemistry (for identifying and characterization of new compounds) is indispensable.

In the past few decades, the focus on the isolation of natural products from culturable microbes has moved from extensively studied locations to relatively-unexplored habitats with the varied environment. This shift has had a massive influence on the discovery of novel secondary metabolites with sufficient bioactivity even though a large number of unexplored habitats await exploration. Moreover, developments in techniques of genomics provided extensive insights into BGCs in the genome of microbes in comparison to the number of secondary metabolites obtained under standard *in-vitro* conditions. These findings demonstrate that culturing novel strains for lesser compounds devalues their real potential.

Technologies like iChip have provided the platform for robust and high-throughput isolation of unculturable microbes, as discussed above. Such technology-driven culture-dependent approaches are recommendable for natural product discovery. In the past decade, the field of genomics has tremendously developed through innovative methods for exploring diversity as well as the distribution of BGCs encoding for novel antimicrobial at the gene level. Thus, to overcome these obstructions of a traditional isolation procedure and to explore the uncultured microbes, different metagenomics approaches seem to be an amicable solution. Deep insights into the organization of BGCs combined with the affordability of whole genome sequencing and development of prediction tools for elucidating the structure of natural products have together strengthened this research field to explore novel compounds. BGCs obtained from cultured and non-cultured microbes can further be analyzed through heterologous gene expression by cloning the BGCs and restructuring them. Therefore, by combining different methods of recombinant DNA technology, we can expand the diversity of natural chemicals *via the* production of newer and better metabolites and increasing the expression of downregulated BGCs. Regardless of the development in the field of genomics, we must not forget that sequence-based approaches need the support of analytical chemistry and microbial technology for isolation, identification, and production of compounds. For the field of analytical chemistry, different bioinformatics tools have been developed for easy and robust analysis. Nowadays, natural products research involving the field of applied analytical chemistry is focused on the retro-biosynthetic logic to link secondary metabolites with its respective BGCs. Therefore, we need to further develop the microbial culturing techniques to fully utilize the real potential of these techniques to discover new antimicrobials. Even improvement in any one of the three disciplines will cause a synergistic effect when effectively used in combination with other techniques. The exchange of information and a combination of different techniques of analytical chemistry, microbiology, and molecular biology will help us to get the deep insight into unexplored natural product reservoir and exploit it to full potential.

Advancements in the field of molecular and synthetic biology have drastically altered the approaches to discover natural products. Exponentially increasing genomic information of culturable microbes has led to the development of targeted approaches to access silent BGCs. Although, the therapeutic products discovered from culturable microbes represent only the tip of the iceberg of microbiomes. Whole Genome Sequencing has provided the means for by-passing the traditional barriers involved in drug discovery and allow us to access the BGCs of the environmental microbiome. Single-cell sequencing has also reduced the problems associated with sequence assembly, as this approach provides the complete sequence of the genome of one cell. The success of the metagenomic approach could be increased multiple folds if we overcame two significant obstacles: high-throughput functional screening and efficient heterologous expression. In the recent years, considerable advances have been made on both obstructions, but further progress is needed to make the screening, and heterologous expression approaches more effective, cheaper and less labor-intensive, which can reduce the overall time for gene discovery and annotation. Such progress will be a great achievement in the expedition for natural products of therapeutic importance.

CONSENT FOR PUBLICATION

Not applicable.

CONFLICT OF INTEREST

The authors confirm that this chapter content has no conflict of interest.

ACKNOWLEDGEMENTS

Declared none.

REFERENCES

[1]   Franco BE, Altagracia Martínez M, Sánchez Rodríguez MA, Wertheimer AI. The determinants of the antibiotic resistance process. Infect Drug Resist 2009; 2: 1-11.
[http://dx.doi.org/10.2147/idr.s4899] [PMID: 21694883]

[2]   Prestinaci F, Pezzotti P, Pantosti A. Antimicrobial resistance: a global multifaceted phenomenon. Pathog Glob Health 2015; 109(7): 309-18.
[http://dx.doi.org/10.1179/2047773215Y.0000000030] [PMID: 26343252]

[3]   Hayashi MA, Bizerra FC, Da Silva PI Jr. Antimicrobial compounds from natural sources. Front Microbiol 2013; 4: 195.
[http://dx.doi.org/10.3389/fmicb.2013.00195] [PMID: 23874329]

[4]   Dahal RH, Chaudhary DK. Microbial Infections and Antimicrobial Resistance in Nepal: Current Trends and Recommendations. Open Microbiol J 2018; 12: 230-42.
[http://dx.doi.org/10.2174/1874285801812010230] [PMID: 30197696]

[5]   Suay-García B, Pérez-Gracia MT. Future prospects for neisseria gonorrhoeae treatment. Antibiotics (Basel) 2018; 7(2): E49.
[http://dx.doi.org/10.3390/antibiotics7020049] [PMID: 29914071]

[6]   Cooper ZD. Adverse Effects of Synthetic Cannabinoids: Management of Acute Toxicity and Withdrawal. Curr Psychiatry Rep 2016; 18(5): 52.
[http://dx.doi.org/10.1007/s11920-016-0694-1] [PMID: 27074934]

[7]   Chatterjee A, Bandyopadhyay SK. Herbal Remedy: An Alternate Therapy of Nonsteroidal Anti-Inflammatory Drug Induced Gastric Ulcer Healing. Ulcers 2014; 2014: 1-13.
[http://dx.doi.org/10.1155/2014/361586]

[8]   Cragg GM, Newman DJ. Natural product drug discovery in the next millennium. Pharm Biol 2001; 39 (Suppl. 1): 8-17.
[http://dx.doi.org/10.1076/phbi.39.s1.8.0009] [PMID: 21554167]

[9]   Clardy J, Fischbach MA, Currie CR. The natural history of antibiotics. Curr Biol 2009; 19(11): R437-41.
[http://dx.doi.org/10.1016/j.cub.2009.04.001] [PMID: 19515346]

[10]   Dhanjal DS, Sharma D. Microbial metagenomics for industrial and environmental bioprospecting: The unknown envoy. In: Singh J, Sharma D, Kumar G, Sharma NR, Eds. Microbial Bioprospecting for Sustainable Development. Singapore: Springer Singapore 2018; pp. 327-52.

[11]   Yuan H, Ma Q, Ye L, Piao G. The traditional medicine and modern medicine from natural products. Molecules 2016; 21(5): E559.
[http://dx.doi.org/10.3390/molecules21050559] [PMID: 27136524]

[12]   Miao V, Davies J. Metagenomics and Antibiotic Discovery from Uncultivated Bacteria. In: Epstein S, Ed. Uncultivated Microorg. 1ˢᵗ ed. Berlin, Heidelberg: Springer 2008; 10: pp. 217-36.
[http://dx.doi.org/10.1007/978-3-540-85465-4_8]

[13]   Dhanjal DS, Chopra C, Anand P, Chopra RS. Accessing the microbial diversity of sugarcane fields from Gujjarwal village, Ludhiana and their molecular identification. Res J Pharm Technol 2017; 10: 3439-42.
[http://dx.doi.org/10.5958/0974-360X.2017.00612.6]

[14]   Miller IJ, Chevrette MG, Kwan JC. Interpreting microbial biosynthesis in the genomic age: Biological and practical considerations. Mar Drugs 2017; 15(6): 165.
[http://dx.doi.org/10.3390/md15060165] [PMID: 28587290]

[15]   Kimura N. Metagenomic approaches to understanding phylogenetic diversity in quorum sensing. Virulence 2014; 5(3): 433-42.
[http://dx.doi.org/10.4161/viru.27850] [PMID: 24429899]

[16]   Bashir Y, Pradeep Singh S, Kumar Konwar B. Metagenomics: An Application Based Perspective. Zhongguo Shengwuzhipinxue Zazhi 2014; 2014: 1-7.
[http://dx.doi.org/10.1155/2014/146030]

[17]   Neelakanta G, Sultana H. The Use of Metagenomic Approaches to Analyze Changes in Microbial Communities. Microbiol Insights 2013; 6: MBI.S10819.
[http://dx.doi.org/10.4137/MBI.S10819]

[18]   Müller CA, Oberauner-Wappis L, Peyman A, Amos GCA, Wellington EMH, Berg G. Mining for nonribosomal peptide synthetase and polyketide synthase genes revealed a high level of diversity in the Sphagnum bog metagenome. Appl Environ Microbiol 2015; 81(15): 5064-72.
[http://dx.doi.org/10.1128/AEM.00631-15] [PMID: 26002894]

[19]   Crits-Christoph A, Diamond S, Butterfield CN, Thomas BC, Banfield JF. Novel soil bacteria possess diverse genes for secondary metabolite biosynthesis. Nature 2018; 558(7710): 440-4.
[http://dx.doi.org/10.1038/s41586-018-0207-y] [PMID: 29899444]

[20]   Loureiro C, Medema MH, van der Oost J, Sipkema D. Exploration and exploitation of the environment for novel specialized metabolites. Curr Opin Biotechnol 2018; 50: 206-13.
[http://dx.doi.org/10.1016/j.copbio.2018.01.017] [PMID: 29454184]

[21]   Du L, Lou L. PKS and NRPS release mechanisms. Nat Prod Rep 2010; 27(2): 255-78.
[http://dx.doi.org/10.1039/B912037H] [PMID: 20111804]

[22]   Drake EJ, Miller BR, Shi C, *et al.* Structures of two distinct conformations of holo-non-ribosomal peptide synthetases. Nature 2016; 529(7585): 235-8.
[http://dx.doi.org/10.1038/nature16163] [PMID: 26762461]

[23]   Walsh CT, Chen H, Keating TA, *et al.* Tailoring enzymes that modify nonribosomal peptides during and after chain elongation on NRPS assembly lines. Curr Opin Chem Biol 2001; 5(5): 525-34.
[http://dx.doi.org/10.1016/S1367-5931(00)00235-0] [PMID: 11578925]

[24]   Gokhale RS, Sankaranarayanan R, Mohanty D. Versatility of polyketide synthases in generating metabolic diversity. Curr Opin Struct Biol 2007; 17(6): 736-43.
[http://dx.doi.org/10.1016/j.sbi.2007.08.021] [PMID: 17935970]

[25]   Hur GH, Vickery CR, Burkart MD. Explorations of catalytic domains in non-ribosomal peptide synthetase enzymology. Nat Prod Rep 2012; 29(10): 1074-98.
[http://dx.doi.org/10.1039/c2np20025b] [PMID: 22802156]

[26]   Chan DI, Vogel HJ. Current understanding of fatty acid biosynthesis and the acyl carrier protein. Biochem J 2010; 430(1): 1-19.
[http://dx.doi.org/10.1042/BJ20100462] [PMID: 20662770]

[27]   Koetsier MJ, Jekel PA, Wijma HJ, Bovenberg RAL, Janssen DB. Aminoacyl-coenzyme A synthesis catalyzed by a CoA ligase from Penicillium chrysogenum. FEBS Lett 2011; 585(6): 893-8.
[http://dx.doi.org/10.1016/j.febslet.2011.02.018] [PMID: 21334330]

[28]   Stein DB, Linne U, Hahn M, Marahiel MA. Impact of epimerization domains on the intermodular transfer of enzyme-bound intermediates in nonribosomal peptide synthesis. ChemBioChem 2006; 7(11): 1807-14.
[http://dx.doi.org/10.1002/cbic.200600192] [PMID: 16952189]

[29]   Agnihotri G, Liu HW. Enoyl-CoA hydratase. reaction, mechanism, and inhibition. Bioorg Med Chem 2003; 11(1): 9-20.
[http://dx.doi.org/10.1016/S0968-0896(02)00333-4] [PMID: 12467702]

[30]   Chan YA, Podevels AM, Kevany BM, Thomas MG. Biosynthesis of polyketide synthase extender units. Nat Prod Rep 2009; 26(1): 90-114.
[http://dx.doi.org/10.1039/B801658P] [PMID: 19374124]

[31]   Weissman KJ. Genetic engineering of modular PKSs: from combinatorial biosynthesis to synthetic biology. Nat Prod Rep 2016; 33(2): 203-30.
[http://dx.doi.org/10.1039/C5NP00109A] [PMID: 26555805]

[32]   Barajas JF, Phelan RM, Schaub AJ, *et al.* Comprehensive structural and biochemical analysis of the terminal myxalamid reductase domain for the engineered production of primary alcohols. Chem Biol 2015; 22(8): 1018-29.
[http://dx.doi.org/10.1016/j.chembiol.2015.06.022] [PMID: 26235055]

[33]   Haslinger K, Peschke M, Brieke C, Maximowitsch E, Cryle MJ. X-domain of peptide synthetases recruits oxygenases crucial for glycopeptide biosynthesis. Nature 2015; 521(7550): 105-9.
[http://dx.doi.org/10.1038/nature14141] [PMID: 25686610]

[34]   Helfrich EJN, Piel J. Biosynthesis of polyketides by trans-AT polyketide synthases. Nat Prod Rep

2016; 33(2): 231-316.
[http://dx.doi.org/10.1039/C5NP00125K] [PMID: 26689670]

[35]   Robbins T, Liu YC, Cane DE, Khosla C. Structure and mechanism of assembly line polyketide synthases. Curr Opin Struct Biol 2016; 41: 10-8.
[http://dx.doi.org/10.1016/j.sbi.2016.05.009] [PMID: 27266330]

[36]   Piel J. Biosynthesis of polyketides by trans-AT polyketide synthases. Nat Prod Rep 2010; 27(7): 996-1047.
[http://dx.doi.org/10.1039/b816430b] [PMID: 20464003]

[37]   Shen B, Thorson JS. Expanding nature's chemical repertoire through metabolic engineering and biocatalysis. Curr Opin Chem Biol 2012; 16(1-2): 99-100.
[http://dx.doi.org/10.1016/j.cbpa.2012.03.006] [PMID: 22464247]

[38]   Cheng YQ, Coughlin JM, Lim SK, Shen B. Type I polyketide synthases that require discrete acyltransferases. Methods Enzymol 2009; 459: 165-86.
[http://dx.doi.org/10.1016/S0076-6879(09)04608-4] [PMID: 19362640]

[39]   Keatinge-Clay AT. The structures of type I polyketide synthases. Nat Prod Rep 2012; 29(10): 1050-73.
[http://dx.doi.org/10.1039/c2np20019h] [PMID: 22858605]

[40]   Hertweck C, Luzhetskyy A, Rebets Y, Bechthold A. Type II polyketide synthases: gaining a deeper insight into enzymatic teamwork. Nat Prod Rep 2007; 24(1): 162-90.
[http://dx.doi.org/10.1039/B507395M] [PMID: 17268612]

[41]   Yu D, Xu F, Zeng J, Zhan J. Type III polyketide synthases in natural product biosynthesis. IUBMB Life 2012; 64(4): 285-95.
[http://dx.doi.org/10.1002/iub.1005] [PMID: 22362498]

[42]   Masschelein J, Mattheus W, Gao LJ, *et al.* A PKS/NRPS/FAS hybrid gene cluster from Serratia plymuthica RVH1 encoding the biosynthesis of three broad spectrum, zeamine-related antibiotics. PLoS One 2013; 8(1): e54143.
[http://dx.doi.org/10.1371/journal.pone.0054143] [PMID: 23349809]

[43]   Du L, Sánchez C, Shen B. Hybrid peptide-polyketide natural products: biosynthesis and prospects toward engineering novel molecules. Metab Eng 2001; 3(1): 78-95.
[http://dx.doi.org/10.1006/mben.2000.0171] [PMID: 11162234]

[44]   Arnison PG, Bibb MJ, Bierbaum G, *et al.* Ribosomally synthesized and post-translationally modified peptide natural products: overview and recommendations for a universal nomenclature. Nat Prod Rep 2013; 30(1): 108-60.
[http://dx.doi.org/10.1039/C2NP20085F] [PMID: 23165928]

[45]   Ortega MA, van der Donk WA. New insights into the biosynthetic logic of ribosomally synthesized and post-translationally modified peptide natural products. Cell Chem Biol 2016; 23(1): 31-44.
[http://dx.doi.org/10.1016/j.chembiol.2015.11.012] [PMID: 26933734]

[46]   Cane DE, Ikeda H. Exploration and mining of the bacterial terpenome. Acc Chem Res 2012; 45(3): 463-72.
[http://dx.doi.org/10.1021/ar200198d] [PMID: 22039990]

[47]   Monciardini P, Iorio M, Maffioli S, Sosio M, Donadio S. Discovering new bioactive molecules from microbial sources. Microb Biotechnol 2014; 7(3): 209-20.
[http://dx.doi.org/10.1111/1751-7915.12123] [PMID: 24661414]

[48]   Penesyan A, Kjelleberg S, Egan S. Development of novel drugs from marine surface associated microorganisms. Mar Drugs 2010; 8(3): 438-59.
[http://dx.doi.org/10.3390/md8030438] [PMID: 20411108]

[49]   Bérdy J. Bioactive microbial metabolites. J Antibiot (Tokyo) 2005; 58(1): 1-26.
[http://dx.doi.org/10.1038/ja.2005.1] [PMID: 15813176]

[50]   Reddy BVB, Kallifidas D, Kim JH, Charlop-Powers Z, Feng Z, Brady SF. Natural product biosynthetic gene diversity in geographically distinct soil microbiomes. Appl Environ Microbiol 2012; 78(10): 3744-52.
[http://dx.doi.org/10.1128/AEM.00102-12] [PMID: 22427492]

[51]   Lemetre C, Maniko J, Charlop-Powers Z, Sparrow B, Lowe AJ, Brady SF. Bacterial natural product biosynthetic domain composition in soil correlates with changes in latitude on a continent-wide scale. Proc Natl Acad Sci USA 2017; 114(44): 11615-20.
[http://dx.doi.org/10.1073/pnas.1710262114] [PMID: 29078342]

[52]   Handelsman J. Metagenomics: Application of genomics to uncultured microorganisms. Microbiol Mol Biol Rev 2004; 68(4): 669-85.
[http://dx.doi.org/10.1128/MMBR.68.4.669-685.2004] [PMID: 15590779]

[53]   Schloss PD, Handelsman J. Metagenomics for studying unculturable microorganisms: Cutting the Gordian knot. Genome Biol 2005; 6(8): 229.
[http://dx.doi.org/10.1186/gb-2005-6-8-229] [PMID: 16086859]

[54]   Abdelkader MSA, Philippon T, Asenjo JA, *et al.* Asenjonamides A-C, antibacterial metabolites isolated from Streptomyces asenjonii strain KNN 42.f from an extreme-hyper arid Atacama Desert soil. J Antibiot (Tokyo) 2018; 71(4): 425-31.
[http://dx.doi.org/10.1038/s41429-017-0012-0] [PMID: 29362461]

[55]   Gold T. The deep, hot biosphere. Proc Natl Acad Sci USA 1992; 89(13): 6045-9.
[http://dx.doi.org/10.1073/pnas.89.13.6045] [PMID: 1631089]

[56]   Fields FR, Lee SW, McConnell MJ. Using bacterial genomes and essential genes for the development of new antibiotics. Biochem Pharmacol 2017; 134: 74-86.
[http://dx.doi.org/10.1016/j.bcp.2016.12.002] [PMID: 27940263]

[57]   Poli A, Finore I, Romano I, Gioiello A, Lama L, Nicolaus B. Microbial diversity in extreme marine habitats and their biomolecules. Microorganisms 2017; 5(2): 25.
[http://dx.doi.org/10.3390/microorganisms5020025] [PMID: 28509857]

[58]   Robinson CH. Cold adaptation in Arctic and Antarctic fungi. New Phytol 2001; 151: 341-53.
[http://dx.doi.org/10.1046/j.1469-8137.2001.00177.x]

[59]   Rampelotto PH. Extremophiles and extreme environments. Life (Basel) 2013; 3(3): 482-5.
[http://dx.doi.org/10.3390/life3030482] [PMID: 25369817]

[60]   Lewin A, Wentzel A, Valla S. Metagenomics of microbial life in extreme temperature environments. Curr Opin Biotechnol 2013; 24(3): 516-25.
[http://dx.doi.org/10.1016/j.copbio.2012.10.012] [PMID: 23146837]

[61]   Di Donato P, Buono A, Poli A, *et al.* Exploring marine environments for the identification of extremophiles and their enzymes for sustainable and green bioprocesses. Sustain 2018; 11(1): 149.
[http://dx.doi.org/10.3390/su11010149]

[62]   Zhou X, Huang H, Chen Y, *et al.* Marthiapeptide A, an anti-infective and cytotoxic polythiazole cyclopeptide from a 60 L scale fermentation of the deep sea-derived Marinactinospora thermotolerans SCSIO 00652. J Nat Prod 2012; 75(12): 2251-5.
[http://dx.doi.org/10.1021/np300554f] [PMID: 23215246]

[63]   Bister B, Bischoff D, Ströbele M, *et al.* Abyssomicin C-A polycyclic antibiotic from a marine Verrucosispora strain as an inhibitor of the p-aminobenzoic acid/tetrahydrofolate biosynthesis pathway. Angew Chem Int Ed Engl 2004; 43(19): 2574-6.
[http://dx.doi.org/10.1002/anie.200353160] [PMID: 15127456]

[64]   Quadri I, Hassani II, l'Haridon S, Chalopin M, Hacène H, Jebbar M. Characterization and antimicrobial potential of extremely halophilic archaea isolated from hypersaline environments of the Algerian Sahara. Microbiol Res 2016; 186-187: 119-31.
[http://dx.doi.org/10.1016/j.micres.2016.04.003] [PMID: 27242149]

[65]   Tedesco P, Maida I, Palma Esposito F, *et al*. Antimicrobial activity of monoramnholipids produced by bacterial strains isolated from the Ross Sea (Antarctica). Mar Drugs 2016; 14(5): E83.
[http://dx.doi.org/10.3390/md14050083] [PMID: 27128927]

[66]   Brady SF, Clardy J. Palmitoylputrescine, an antibiotic isolated from the heterologous expression of DNA extracted from bromeliad tank water. J Nat Prod 2004; 67(8): 1283-6.
[http://dx.doi.org/10.1021/np0499766] [PMID: 15332842]

[67]   Brady SF, Clardy J. Cloning and heterologous expression of isocyanide biosynthetic genes from environmental DNA. Angew Chem Int Ed Engl 2005; 44(43): 7063-5.
[http://dx.doi.org/10.1002/anie.200501941] [PMID: 16206308]

[68]   Streit WR, Schmitz RA. Metagenomics--the key to the uncultured microbes. Curr Opin Microbiol 2004; 7(5): 492-8.
[http://dx.doi.org/10.1016/j.mib.2004.08.002] [PMID: 15451504]

[69]   Tringe SG, Rubin EM. Metagenomics: DNA sequencing of environmental samples. Nat Rev Genet 2005; 6(11): 805-14.
[http://dx.doi.org/10.1038/nrg1709] [PMID: 16304596]

[70]   Wang Y, Chen Y, Zhou Q, *et al*. A culture-independent approach to unravel uncultured bacteria and functional genes in a complex microbial community. PLoS One 2012; 7(10): e47530.
[http://dx.doi.org/10.1371/journal.pone.0047530] [PMID: 23082176]

[71]   Liu X, Ashforth E, Ren B, *et al*. Bioprospecting microbial natural product libraries from the marine environment for drug discovery. J Antibiot (Tokyo) 2010; 63(8): 415-22.
[http://dx.doi.org/10.1038/ja.2010.56] [PMID: 20606699]

[72]   Brady SF. Construction of soil environmental DNA cosmid libraries and screening for clones that produce biologically active small molecules. Nat Protoc 2007; 2(5): 1297-305.
[http://dx.doi.org/10.1038/nprot.2007.195] [PMID: 17546026]

[73]   Lok C. Mining the microbial dark matter. Nature 2015; 522(7556): 270-3.
[http://dx.doi.org/10.1038/522270a] [PMID: 26085253]

[74]   Liu J, Hua ZS, Chen LX, *et al*. Correlating microbial diversity patterns with geochemistry in an extreme and heterogeneous environment of mine tailings. Appl Environ Microbiol 2014; 80(12): 3677-86.
[http://dx.doi.org/10.1128/AEM.00294-14] [PMID: 24727268]

[75]   Batra N, Bhatia S, Behal A, Singh J, Joshi A. Metagenomic research: Methods and ecological applications. In: Nelson KE, Ed. Encyclopedia of Metagenomics. Boston, MA: Springer 2013; pp. 1-11.

[76]   Simon C, Daniel R. Metagenomic analyses: past and future trends. Appl Environ Microbiol 2011; 77(4): 1153-61.
[http://dx.doi.org/10.1128/AEM.02345-10] [PMID: 21169428]

[77]   Lim HK, Chung EJ, Kim JC, *et al*. Characterization of a forest soil metagenome clone that confers indirubin and indigo production on *Escherichia coli*. Appl Environ Microbiol 2005; 71(12): 7768-77.
[http://dx.doi.org/10.1128/AEM.71.12.7768-7777.2005] [PMID: 16332749]

[78]   Brady SF, Chao CJ, Handelsman J, Clardy J. Cloning and heterologous expression of a natural product biosynthetic gene cluster from eDNA. Org Lett 2001; 3(13): 1981-4.
[http://dx.doi.org/10.1021/ol015949k] [PMID: 11418029]

[79]   Owen JG, Charlop-Powers Z, Smith AG, *et al*. Multiplexed metagenome mining using short DNA sequence tags facilitates targeted discovery of epoxyketone proteasome inhibitors. Proc Natl Acad Sci USA 2015; 112(14): 4221-6.
[http://dx.doi.org/10.1073/pnas.1501124112] [PMID: 25831524]

[80]   Feng Z, Chakraborty D, Dewell SB, Reddy BVB, Brady SF. Environmental DNA-encoded antibiotics

fasamycins A and B inhibit FabF in type II fatty acid biosynthesis. J Am Chem Soc 2012; 134(6): 2981-7.
[http://dx.doi.org/10.1021/ja207662w] [PMID: 22224500]

[81]   Uchiyama T, Miyazaki K. Functional metagenomics for enzyme discovery: challenges to efficient screening. Curr Opin Biotechnol 2009; 20(6): 616-22.
[http://dx.doi.org/10.1016/j.copbio.2009.09.010] [PMID: 19850467]

[82]   Lam KN, Cheng J, Engel K, Neufeld JD, Charles TC. Current and future resources for functional metagenomics. Front Microbiol 2015; 6: 1196.
[http://dx.doi.org/10.3389/fmicb.2015.01196] [PMID: 26579102]

[83]   Craig JW, Chang FY, Kim JH, Obiajulu SC, Brady SF. Expanding small-molecule functional metagenomics through parallel screening of broad-host-range cosmid environmental DNA libraries in diverse proteobacteria. Appl Environ Microbiol 2010; 76(5): 1633-41.
[http://dx.doi.org/10.1128/AEM.02169-09] [PMID: 20081001]

[84]   Perron GG, Whyte L, Turnbaugh PJ, *et al.* Functional characterization of bacteria isolated from ancient arctic soil exposes diverse resistance mechanisms to modern antibiotics. PLoS One 2015; 10(3): e0069533.
[http://dx.doi.org/10.1371/journal.pone.0069533] [PMID: 25807523]

[85]   Williamson LL, Borlee BR, Schloss PD, Guan C, Allen HK, Handelsman J. Intracellular screen to identify metagenomic clones that induce or inhibit a quorum-sensing biosensor. Appl Environ Microbiol 2005; 71(10): 6335-44.
[http://dx.doi.org/10.1128/AEM.71.10.6335-6344.2005] [PMID: 16204555]

[86]   Ferrer M, Beloqui A, Timmis KN, Golyshin PN. Metagenomics for mining new genetic resources of microbial communities. J Mol Microbiol Biotechnol 2009; 16(1-2): 109-23.
[http://dx.doi.org/10.1159/000142898] [PMID: 18957866]

[87]   Brady SF, Chao CJ, Clardy J. New natural product families from an environmental DNA (eDNA) gene cluster. J Am Chem Soc 2002; 124(34): 9968-9.
[http://dx.doi.org/10.1021/ja0268985] [PMID: 12188643]

[88]   Gillespie DE, Brady SF, Bettermann AD, *et al.* Isolation of antibiotics turbomycin a and B from a metagenomic library of soil microbial DNA. Appl Environ Microbiol 2002; 68(9): 4301-6.
[http://dx.doi.org/10.1128/AEM.68.9.4301-4306.2002] [PMID: 12200279]

[89]   Culligan EP, Sleator RD, Marchesi JR, Hill C. Metagenomics and novel gene discovery: promise and potential for novel therapeutics. Virulence 2014; 5(3): 399-412.
[http://dx.doi.org/10.4161/viru.27208] [PMID: 24317337]

[90]   Handelsman J. Metagenomics and Microbial Communities. Encycl Life Sci. Chichester, UK: John Wiley & Sons, Ltd 2007.

[91]   Shokralla S, Spall JL, Gibson JF, Hajibabaei M. Next-generation sequencing technologies for environmental DNA research. Mol Ecol 2012; 21(8): 1794-805.
[http://dx.doi.org/10.1111/j.1365-294X.2012.05538.x] [PMID: 22486820]

[92]   Frisli T, Haverkamp THA, Jakobsen KS, Stenseth NC, Rudi K. Estimation of metagenome size and structure in an experimental soil microbiota from low coverage next-generation sequence data. J Appl Microbiol 2013; 114(1): 141-51.
[http://dx.doi.org/10.1111/jam.12035] [PMID: 23039191]

[93]   Giddings L-A, Newman DJ. Bioactive Compounds from Extremophiles. Cham: Springer 2015; pp. 1-47.

[94]   Hiraoka S, Yang CC, Iwasaki W. Metagenomics and bioinformatics in microbial ecology: Current status and beyond. Microbes Environ 2016; 31(3): 204-12.
[http://dx.doi.org/10.1264/jsme2.ME16024] [PMID: 27383682]

[95]   Hug JJ, Bader CD, Remškar M, Cirnski K, Müller R. Concepts and methods to access novel

antibiotics from actinomycetes. Antibiotics (Basel) 2018; 7(2): E44.
[http://dx.doi.org/10.3390/antibiotics7020044] [PMID: 29789481]

[96]   Sim M, Kim J. Metagenome assembly through clustering of next-generation sequencing data using protein sequences. J Microbiol Methods 2015; 109: 180-7.
[http://dx.doi.org/10.1016/j.mimet.2015.01.002] [PMID: 25572018]

[97]   Reddy RM, Mohammed MH, Mande SS. MetaCAA: A clustering-aided methodology for efficient assembly of metagenomic datasets. Genomics 2014; 103(2-3): 161-8.
[http://dx.doi.org/10.1016/j.ygeno.2014.02.007] [PMID: 24607570]

[98]   Blin K, Wolf T, Chevrette MG, *et al.* antiSMASH 4.0-improvements in chemistry prediction and gene cluster boundary identification. Nucleic Acids Res 2017; 45(W1): W36-41.
[http://dx.doi.org/10.1093/nar/gkx319] [PMID: 28460038]

[99]   Ziemert N, Podell S, Penn K, Badger JH, Allen E, Jensen PR. The natural product domain seeker NaPDoS: a phylogeny based bioinformatic tool to classify secondary metabolite gene diversity. PLoS One 2012; 7(3): e34064.
[http://dx.doi.org/10.1371/journal.pone.0034064] [PMID: 22479523]

[100]   Reddy BV, Milshteyn A, Charlop-Powers Z, Brady SF. eSNaPD: a versatile, web-based bioinformatics platform for surveying and mining natural product biosynthetic diversity from metagenomes. Chem Biol 2014; 21(8): 1023-33.
[http://dx.doi.org/10.1016/j.chembiol.2014.06.007] [PMID: 25065533]

[101]   Thakur P, Chopra C, Anand P, Dhanjal DS, Chopra RS. Myxobacteria: Unraveling the potential of a unique microbiome niche. In: Singh J, Sharma D, Kumar G, Sharma NR, Eds. Microbial Bioprospecting for Sustainable Development. Springer Singapore 2018; pp. 137-63.

[102]   Ongley SE, Bian X, Neilan BA, Müller R. Recent advances in the heterologous expression of microbial natural product biosynthetic pathways. Nat Prod Rep 2013; 30(8): 1121-38.
[http://dx.doi.org/10.1039/c3np70034h] [PMID: 23832108]

[103]   Kang HS, Brady SF, Arimetamycin A. Arimetamycin A: Improving clinically relevant families of natural products through sequence-guided screening of soil metagenomes. Angew Chem Int Ed Engl 2013; 52(42): 11063-7.
[http://dx.doi.org/10.1002/anie.201305109] [PMID: 24038656]

[104]   Kallifidas D, Kang HS, Brady SF. Tetarimycin A, an MRSA-active antibiotic identified through induced expression of environmental DNA gene clusters. J Am Chem Soc 2012; 134(48): 19552-5.
[http://dx.doi.org/10.1021/ja3093828] [PMID: 23157252]

[105]   Hover BM, Kim SH, Katz M, *et al.* Culture-independent discovery of the malacidins as calcium-dependent antibiotics with activity against multidrug-resistant Gram-positive pathogens. Nat Microbiol 2018; 3(4): 415-22.
[http://dx.doi.org/10.1038/s41564-018-0110-1] [PMID: 29434326]

[106]   Zhang J, Chiodini R, Badr A, Zhang G. The impact of next-generation sequencing on genomics. J Genet Genomics 2011; 38(3): 95-109.
[http://dx.doi.org/10.1016/j.jgg.2011.02.003] [PMID: 21477781]

[107]   de Fátima Alves L, Westmann CA, Lovate GL, *et al.* metagenomic approaches for understanding new concepts in microbial science. Int J Genomics 2018; 2018: 2312987.

[108]   Wang Y, Navin NE. Advances and applications of single-cell sequencing technologies. Mol Cell 2015; 58(4): 598-609.
[http://dx.doi.org/10.1016/j.molcel.2015.05.005] [PMID: 26000845]

[109]   Grindberg RV, Ishoey T, Brinza D, *et al.* Single cell genome amplification accelerates identification of the apratoxin biosynthetic pathway from a complex microbial assemblage. PLoS One 2011; 6(4): e18565.
[http://dx.doi.org/10.1371/journal.pone.0018565] [PMID: 21533272]

[110] Macaulay IC, Voet T. Single cell genomics: advances and future perspectives. PLoS Genet 2014; 10(1): e1004126.
[http://dx.doi.org/10.1371/journal.pgen.1004126] [PMID: 24497842]

[111] Bentley SD, Chater KF, Cerdeño-Tárraga AM, *et al.* Complete genome sequence of the model actinomycete Streptomyces coelicolor A3(2). Nature 2002; 417(6885): 141-7.
[http://dx.doi.org/10.1038/417141a] [PMID: 12000953]

[112] Lakey JH, Lea EJA, Rudd BAM, Wright HM, Hopwood DA. A new channel-forming antibiotic from Streptomyces coelicolor A3(2) which requires calcium for its activity. J Gen Microbiol 1983; 129(12): 3565-73.
[http://dx.doi.org/10.1099/00221287-129-12-3565] [PMID: 6321633]

[113] Rudd BAM, Hopwood DA. A pigmented mycelial antibiotic in Streptomyces coelicolor: control by a chromosomal gene cluster. J Gen Microbiol 1980; 119(2): 333-40.
[http://dx.doi.org/10.1099/00221287-119-2-333] [PMID: 7229612]

[114] Tsao SW, Rudd BAM, He XG, Chang CJ, Floss HG. Identification of a red pigment from Streptomyces coelicolor A3(2) as a mixture of prodigiosin derivatives. J Antibiot (Tokyo) 1985; 38(1): 128-31.
[http://dx.doi.org/10.7164/antibiotics.38.128] [PMID: 3972724]

[115] Wright LF, Hopwood DA. Actinorhodin is a chromosomally-determined antibiotic in Streptomyces coelicolar A3(2). J Gen Microbiol 1976; 96(2): 289-97.
[http://dx.doi.org/10.1099/00221287-96-2-289] [PMID: 993778]

[116] Medema MH, Blin K, Cimermancic P, *et al.* antiSMASH: rapid identification, annotation and analysis of secondary metabolite biosynthesis gene clusters in bacterial and fungal genome sequences. Nucleic Acids Res 2011; 39(Web Server issue): W339-46.
[http://dx.doi.org/10.1093/nar/gkr466] [PMID: 21672958]

[117] Li P, Guo Z, Tang W, Chen Y. Activation of three natural product biosynthetic gene clusters from *Streptomyces lavendulae* CGMCC 4.1386 by a reporter-guided strategy. Synth Syst Biotechnol 2018; 3(4): 254-60.
[http://dx.doi.org/10.1016/j.synbio.2018.10.010] [PMID: 30417141]

[118] Harvey AL, Edrada-Ebel R, Quinn RJ. The re-emergence of natural products for drug discovery in the genomics era. Nat Rev Drug Discov 2015; 14(2): 111-29.
[http://dx.doi.org/10.1038/nrd4510] [PMID: 25614221]

[119] Medema MH, Fischbach MA. Computational approaches to natural product discovery. Nat Chem Biol 2015; 11(9): 639-48.
[http://dx.doi.org/10.1038/nchembio.1884] [PMID: 26284671]

[120] Vallenet D, Calteau A, Cruveiller S, *et al.* MicroScope in 2017: an expanding and evolving integrated resource for community expertise of microbial genomes. Nucleic Acids Res 2017; 45(D1): D517-28.
[http://dx.doi.org/10.1093/nar/gkw1101] [PMID: 27899624]

[121] Blin K, Kim HU, Medema MH, Weber T. Recent development of antiSMASH and other computational approaches to mine secondary metabolite biosynthetic gene clusters. Brief Bioinform 2019; 20(4): 1103-13.
[http://dx.doi.org/10.1093/bib/bbx146] [PMID: 29112695]

[122] Covington BC, McLean JA, Bachmann BO. Comparative mass spectrometry-based metabolomics strategies for the investigation of microbial secondary metabolites. Nat Prod Rep 2017; 34(1): 6-24.
[http://dx.doi.org/10.1039/C6NP00048G] [PMID: 27604382]

[123] Reen FJ, Romano S, Dobson ADW, O'Gara F. The sound of silence: Activating silent biosynthetic gene clusters in marine microorganisms. Mar Drugs 2015; 13(8): 4754-83.
[http://dx.doi.org/10.3390/md13084754] [PMID: 26264003]

[124] Weber T, Kim HU. The secondary metabolite bioinformatics portal: Computational tools to facilitate

synthetic biology of secondary metabolite production. Synth Syst Biotechnol 2016; 1(2): 69-79.
[http://dx.doi.org/10.1016/j.synbio.2015.12.002] [PMID: 29062930]

[125] Skinnider MA, Merwin NJ, Johnston CW, Magarvey NA. PRISM 3: expanded prediction of natural
product chemical structures from microbial genomes. Nucleic Acids Res 2017; 45(W1): W49-54.
[http://dx.doi.org/10.1093/nar/gkx320] [PMID: 28460067]

[126] Alanjary M, Kronmiller B, Adamek M, *et al.* The Antibiotic Resistant Target Seeker (ARTS), an
exploration engine for antibiotic cluster prioritization and novel drug target discovery. Nucleic Acids
Res 2017; 45(W1): W42-8.
[http://dx.doi.org/10.1093/nar/gkx360] [PMID: 28472505]

[127] Kim KR, Kim TJ, Suh JW. The gene cluster for spectinomycin biosynthesis and the aminoglycoside-
resistance function of spcM in Streptomyces spectabilis. Curr Microbiol 2008; 57(4): 371-4.
[http://dx.doi.org/10.1007/s00284-008-9204-y] [PMID: 18663525]

[128] Blin K, Medema MH, Kottmann R, Lee SY, Weber T. The antiSMASH database, a comprehensive
database of microbial secondary metabolite biosynthetic gene clusters. Nucleic Acids Res 2017;
45(D1): D555-9.
[http://dx.doi.org/10.1093/nar/gkw960] [PMID: 27924032]

[129] van Heel AJ, de Jong A, Montalbán-López M, Kok J, Kuipers OP. BAGEL3: Automated identification
of genes encoding bacteriocins and (non-)bactericidal posttranslationally modified peptides. Nucleic
Acids Res 2013; 41(W1): W448-53.
[http://dx.doi.org/10.1093/nar/gkt391] [PMID: 23677608]

[130] Wolf T, Shelest V, Nath N, Shelest E. CASSIS and SMIPS: promoter-based prediction of secondary
metabolite gene clusters in eukaryotic genomes. Bioinformatics 2016; 32(8): 1138-43.
[http://dx.doi.org/10.1093/bioinformatics/btv713] [PMID: 26656005]

[131] Blin K, Pedersen LE, Weber T, Lee SY. CRISPy-web: An online resource to design sgRNAs for
CRISPR applications. Synth Syst Biotechnol 2016; 1(2): 118-21.
[http://dx.doi.org/10.1016/j.synbio.2016.01.003] [PMID: 29062934]

[132] Vesth TC, Brandl J, Andersen MR. FunGeneClusterS: Predicting fungal gene clusters from genome
and transcriptome data. Synth Syst Biotechnol 2016; 1(2): 122-9.
[http://dx.doi.org/10.1016/j.synbio.2016.01.002] [PMID: 29062935]

[133] Johnston CW, Skinnider MA, Wyatt MA, *et al.* An automated Genomes-to-Natural Products platform
(GNP) for the discovery of modular natural products. Nat Commun 2015; 6: 8421.
[http://dx.doi.org/10.1038/ncomms9421] [PMID: 26412281]

[134] Johnston CW, Skinnider MA, Dejong CA, *et al.* Assembly and clustering of natural antibiotics guides
target identification. Nat Chem Biol 2016; 12(4): 233-9.
[http://dx.doi.org/10.1038/nchembio.2018] [PMID: 26829473]

[135] Dejong CA, Chen GM, Li H, *et al.* Polyketide and nonribosomal peptide retro-biosynthesis and global
gene cluster matching. Nat Chem Biol 2016; 12(12): 1007-14.
[http://dx.doi.org/10.1038/nchembio.2188] [PMID: 27694801]

[136] Medema MH, Kottmann R, Yilmaz P, *et al.* Minimum Information about a Biosynthetic Gene cluster.
Nat Chem Biol 2015; 11(9): 625-31.
[http://dx.doi.org/10.1038/nchembio.1890] [PMID: 26284661]

[137] Pupin M, Esmaeel Q, Flissi A, Dufresne Y, Jacques P, Leclère V. Norine: A powerful resource for
novel nonribosomal peptide discovery. Synth Syst Biotechnol 2016; 1(2): 89-94.
[http://dx.doi.org/10.1016/j.synbio.2015.11.001] [PMID: 29082924]

[138] Li MHT, Ung PMU, Zajkowski J, Garneau-Tsodikova S, Sherman DH. Automated genome mining for
natural products. BMC Bioinformatics 2009; 10: 185.
[http://dx.doi.org/10.1186/1471-2105-10-185] [PMID: 19531248]

[139] Röttig M, Medema MH, Blin K, Weber T, Rausch C, Kohlbacher O. NRPSpredictor2--a web server

for predicting NRPS adenylation domain specificity. Nucleic Acids Res 2011; 39(2): W362-7.
[http://dx.doi.org/10.1093/nar/gkr323] [PMID: 21558170]

[140] Kautsar SA, Suarez Duran HG, Blin K, Osbourn A, Medema MH. plantiSMASH: automated identification, annotation and expression analysis of plant biosynthetic gene clusters. Nucleic Acids Res 2017; 45(W1): W55-63.
[http://dx.doi.org/10.1093/nar/gkx305] [PMID: 28453650]

[141] Tietz JI, Schwalen CJ, Patel PS, *et al.* A new genome-mining tool redefines the lasso peptide biosynthetic landscape. Nat Chem Biol 2017; 13(5): 470-8.
[http://dx.doi.org/10.1038/nchembio.2319] [PMID: 28244986]

[142] Khater S, Gupta M, Agrawal P, *et al.* SBSPKSv2: structure-based sequence analysis of polyketide synthases and non-ribosomal peptide synthetases. Nucleic Acids Res 2017; 45(W1): W72-9.
[http://dx.doi.org/10.1093/nar/gkx344] [PMID: 28460065]

[143] Dufresne Y, Noé L, Leclère V, Pupin M. Smiles2Monomers: a link between chemical and biological structures for polymers. J Cheminform 2015; 7: 62.
[http://dx.doi.org/10.1186/s13321-015-0111-5] [PMID: 26715946]

[144] Khaldi N, Seifuddin FT, Turner G, *et al.* SMURF: Genomic mapping of fungal secondary metabolite clusters. Fungal Genet Biol 2010; 47(9): 736-41.
[http://dx.doi.org/10.1016/j.fgb.2010.06.003] [PMID: 20554054]

[145] Genilloud O. Mining actinomycetes for novel antibiotics in the omics era: Are we ready to exploit this new paradigm? Antibiotics (Basel) 2018; 7(4): E85.
[http://dx.doi.org/10.3390/antibiotics7040085] [PMID: 30257490]

[146] Romano S, Jackson SA, Patry S, Dobson ADW. Extending the "one strain many compounds" (OSMAC) principle to marine microorganisms. Mar Drugs 2018; 16(7): E244.
[http://dx.doi.org/10.3390/md16070244] [PMID: 30041461]

[147] Li X, Wu X, Zhu J, Shen Y. Amexanthomycins A-J, pentangular polyphenols produced by Amycolatopsis mediterranei S699ΔrifA. Appl Microbiol Biotechnol 2018; 102(2): 689-702.
[http://dx.doi.org/10.1007/s00253-017-8648-z] [PMID: 29181568]

[148] Baral B, Akhgari A, Metsä-Ketelä M. Activation of microbial secondary metabolic pathways: Avenues and challenges. Synth Syst Biotechnol 2018; 3(3): 163-78.
[http://dx.doi.org/10.1016/j.synbio.2018.09.001] [PMID: 30345402]

[149] Zhang MM, Qiao Y, Ang EL, Zhao H. Using natural products for drug discovery: the impact of the genomics era. Expert Opin Drug Discov 2017; 12(5): 475-87.
[http://dx.doi.org/10.1080/17460441.2017.1303478] [PMID: 28277838]

[150] Inaoka T, Takahashi K, Yada H, Yoshida M, Ochi K. RNA polymerase mutation activates the production of a dormant antibiotic 3,3′-neotrehalosadiamine via an autoinduction mechanism in Bacillus subtilis. J Biol Chem 2004; 279(5): 3885-92.
[http://dx.doi.org/10.1074/jbc.M309925200] [PMID: 14612444]

[151] Metsä-Ketelä M, Ylihonko K, Mäntsälä P. Partial activation of a silent angucycline-type gene cluster from a rubromycin β producing Streptomyces sp. PGA64. J Antibiot (Tokyo) 2004; 57(8): 502-10.
[http://dx.doi.org/10.7164/antibiotics.57.502] [PMID: 15515887]

[152] Rodríguez M, Méndez C, Salas JA, Blanco G. Transcriptional organization of ThnI-regulated thienamycin biosynthetic genes in Streptomyces cattleya. J Antibiot (Tokyo) 2010; 63(3): 135-8.
[http://dx.doi.org/10.1038/ja.2009.133] [PMID: 20094070]

[153] Wang W, Yang T, Li Y, *et al.* Development of a Synthetic Oxytetracycline-Inducible Expression System for Streptomycetes Using de Novo Characterized Genetic Parts. ACS Synth Biol 2016; 5(7): 765-73.
[http://dx.doi.org/10.1021/acssynbio.6b00087] [PMID: 27100123]

[154] Myronovskyi M, Luzhetskyy A. Native and engineered promoters in natural product discovery. Nat

Prod Rep 2016; 33(8): 1006-19.
[http://dx.doi.org/10.1039/C6NP00002A] [PMID: 27438486]

[155] Newman DJ, Cragg GM. Natural Products as Sources of New Drugs from 1981 to 2014. J Nat Prod 2016; 79(3): 629-61.
[http://dx.doi.org/10.1021/acs.jnatprod.5b01055] [PMID: 26852623]

[156] Bachmann BO, Van Lanen SG, Baltz RH. Microbial genome mining for accelerated natural products discovery: is a renaissance in the making? J Ind Microbiol Biotechnol 2014; 41(2): 175-84.
[http://dx.doi.org/10.1007/s10295-013-1389-9] [PMID: 24342967]

[157] Gilman J, Love J. Synthetic promoter design for new microbial chassis. Biochem Soc Trans 2016; 44(3): 731-7.
[http://dx.doi.org/10.1042/BST20160042] [PMID: 27284035]

[158] Lieder S, Nikel PI, de Lorenzo V, Takors R. Genome reduction boosts heterologous gene expression in Pseudomonas putida. Microb Cell Fact 2015; 14: 23.
[http://dx.doi.org/10.1186/s12934-015-0207-7] [PMID: 25890048]

[159] Wang B, Lv Y, Li X, Lin Y, Deng H, Pan L. Profiling of secondary metabolite gene clusters regulated by LaeA in Aspergillus niger FGSC A1279 based on genome sequencing and transcriptome analysis. Res Microbiol 2018; 169(2): 67-77.
[http://dx.doi.org/10.1016/j.resmic.2017.10.002] [PMID: 29054463]

[160] Gomez-Escribano JP, Bibb MJ. Engineering Streptomyces coelicolor for heterologous expression of secondary metabolite gene clusters. Microb Biotechnol 2011; 4(2): 207-15.
[http://dx.doi.org/10.1111/j.1751-7915.2010.00219.x] [PMID: 21342466]

[161] Rigali S, Anderssen S, Naômé A, van Wezel GP. Cracking the regulatory code of biosynthetic gene clusters as a strategy for natural product discovery. Biochem Pharmacol 2018; 153: 24-34.
[http://dx.doi.org/10.1016/j.bcp.2018.01.007] [PMID: 29309762]

[162] Okada BK, Seyedsayamdost MR. Antibiotic dialogues: induction of silent biosynthetic gene clusters by exogenous small molecules. FEMS Microbiol Rev 2017; 41(1): 19-33.
[http://dx.doi.org/10.1093/femsre/fuw035] [PMID: 27576366]

[163] Yamanaka K, Oikawa H, Ogawa HO, *et al.* Desferrioxamine E produced by Streptomyces griseus stimulates growth and development of Streptomyces tanashiensis. Microbiology 2005; 151(Pt 9): 2899-905.
[http://dx.doi.org/10.1099/mic.0.28139-0] [PMID: 16151202]

[164] Missineo A, Di Poto A, Geoghegan JA, *et al.* IsdC from Staphylococcus lugdunensis induces biofilm formation under low-iron growth conditions. Infect Immun 2014; 82(6): 2448-59.
[http://dx.doi.org/10.1128/IAI.01542-14] [PMID: 24686057]

[165] Tanaka Y, Hosaka T, Ochi K. Rare earth elements activate the secondary metabolite-biosynthetic gene clusters in Streptomyces coelicolor A3(2). J Antibiot (Tokyo) 2010; 63(8): 477-81.
[http://dx.doi.org/10.1038/ja.2010.53] [PMID: 20551989]

[166] Sherpa RT, Reese CJ, Montazeri Aliabadi H. Application of iChip to grow "uncultivable" microorganisms and its impact on antibiotic discovery. J Pharm Pharm Sci 2015; 18(3): 303-15.
[http://dx.doi.org/10.18433/J30894] [PMID: 26517134]

[167] Piddock LJV. Teixobactin, the first of a new class of antibiotics discovered by iChip technology? J Antimicrob Chemother 2015; 70(10): 2679-80.
[http://dx.doi.org/10.1093/jac/dkv175] [PMID: 26089440]

[168] Hosaka T, Ohnishi-Kameyama M, Muramatsu H, *et al.* Antibacterial discovery in actinomycetes strains with mutations in RNA polymerase or ribosomal protein S12. Nat Biotechnol 2009; 27(5): 462-4.
[http://dx.doi.org/10.1038/nbt.1538] [PMID: 19396160]

[169] Guo F, Xiang S, Li L, *et al.* Targeted activation of silent natural product biosynthesis pathways by

reporter-guided mutant selection. Metab Eng 2015; 28: 134-42.
[http://dx.doi.org/10.1016/j.ymben.2014.12.006] [PMID: 25554073]

[170] Riechmann JL. Transcriptional regulation: a genomic overview. Arabidopsis Book 2002; 1: e0085.
[http://dx.doi.org/10.1199/tab.0085] [PMID: 22303220]

[171] Javaid N, Choi S. Acetylation- and methylation-related epigenetic proteins in the context of their targets. Genes (Basel) 2017; 8(8): E196.
[http://dx.doi.org/10.3390/genes8080196] [PMID: 28783137]

[172] Brady SF, Chao CJ, Clardy J. Long-chain N-acyltyrosine synthases from environmental DNA. Appl Environ Microbiol 2004; 70(11): 6865-70.
[http://dx.doi.org/10.1128/AEM.70.11.6865-6870.2004] [PMID: 15528554]

[173] Chang FY, Brady SF. Discovery of indolotryptoline antiproliferative agents by homology-guided metagenomic screening. Proc Natl Acad Sci USA 2013; 110(7): 2478-83.
[http://dx.doi.org/10.1073/pnas.1218073110] [PMID: 23302687]

[174] Banik JJ, Brady SF. Recent application of metagenomic approaches toward the discovery of antimicrobials and other bioactive small molecules. Curr Opin Microbiol 2010; 13(5): 603-9.
[http://dx.doi.org/10.1016/j.mib.2010.08.012] [PMID: 20884282]

[175] Tortorella E, Tedesco P, Palma Esposito F, *et al.* Antibiotics from deep-sea microorganisms: Current discoveries and perspectives. Mar Drugs 2018; 16(10): E355.
[http://dx.doi.org/10.3390/md16100355] [PMID: 30274274]

[176] Forbes JD, Knox NC, Ronholm J, Pagotto F, Reimer A. Metagenomics: The next culture-independent game changer. Front Microbiol 2017; 8: 1069.
[http://dx.doi.org/10.3389/fmicb.2017.01069] [PMID: 28725217]

[177] Borchert E, Jackson SA, O'Gara F, Dobson ADW. Diversity of natural product biosynthetic genes in the microbiome of the deep sea sponges Inflatella pellicula, Poecillastra compressa, and Stelletta normani. Front Microbiol 2016; 7: 1027.
[http://dx.doi.org/10.3389/fmicb.2016.01027] [PMID: 27446062]

[178] Ju KS, Gao J, Doroghazi JR, *et al.* Discovery of phosphonic acid natural products by mining the genomes of 10,000 actinomycetes. Proc Natl Acad Sci USA 2015; 112(39): 12175-80.
[http://dx.doi.org/10.1073/pnas.1500873112] [PMID: 26324907]

[179] Kang HS, Brady SF. Arixanthomycins A-C: Phylogeny-guided discovery of biologically active eDNA-derived pentangular polyphenols. ACS Chem Biol 2014; 9(6): 1267-72.
[http://dx.doi.org/10.1021/cb500141b] [PMID: 24730509]

[180] Long PF, Dunlap WC, Battershill CN, Jaspars M. Shotgun cloning and heterologous expression of the patellamide gene cluster as a strategy to achieving sustained metabolite production. ChemBioChem 2005; 6(10): 1760-5.
[http://dx.doi.org/10.1002/cbic.200500210] [PMID: 15988766]

[181] Allen HK, Moe LA, Rodbumrer J, Gaarder A, Handelsman J. Functional metagenomics reveals diverse beta-lactamases in a remote Alaskan soil. ISME J 2009; 3(2): 243-51.
[http://dx.doi.org/10.1038/ismej.2008.86] [PMID: 18843302]

[182] Fujita MJ, Kimura N, Yokose H, Otsuka M. Heterologous production of bisucaberin using a biosynthetic gene cluster cloned from a deep sea metagenome. Mol Biosyst 2012; 8(2): 482-5.
[http://dx.doi.org/10.1039/C1MB05431G] [PMID: 22051782]

[183] Sudek S, Lopanik NB, Waggoner LE, *et al.* Identification of the putative bryostatin polyketide synthase gene cluster from "Candidatus Endobugula sertula", the uncultivated microbial symbiont of the marine bryozoan Bugula neritina. J Nat Prod 2007; 70(1): 67-74.
[http://dx.doi.org/10.1021/np060361d] [PMID: 17253852]

[184] Kang HS, Brady SF. Mining soil metagenomes to better understand the evolution of natural product structural diversity: pentangular polyphenols as a case study. J Am Chem Soc 2014; 136(52): 18111-9.

[http://dx.doi.org/10.1021/ja510606j] [PMID: 25521786]

[185]   Wakimoto T, Egami Y, Nakashima Y, *et al.* Calyculin biogenesis from a pyrophosphate protoxin produced by a sponge symbiont. Nat Chem Biol 2014; 10(8): 648-55.
[http://dx.doi.org/10.1038/nchembio.1573] [PMID: 24974231]

[186]   Yang C, Huang C, Zhang W, Zhu Y, Zhang C. Heterologous Expression of Fluostatin Gene Cluster Leads to a Bioactive Heterodimer. Org Lett 2015; 17(21): 5324-7.
[http://dx.doi.org/10.1021/acs.orglett.5b02683] [PMID: 26465097]

[187]   Bonet B, Teufel R, Crüsemann M, Ziemert N, Moore BS. Direct capture and heterologous expression of Salinispora natural product genes for the biosynthesis of enterocin. J Nat Prod 2015; 78(3): 539-42.
[http://dx.doi.org/10.1021/np500664q] [PMID: 25382643]

[188]   Rusnak F, Sakaitani M, Drueckhammer D, Reichert J, Walsh CT. Biosynthesis of the *Escherichia coli* siderophore enterobactin: sequence of the entF gene, expression and purification of EntF, and analysis of covalent phosphopantetheine. Biochemistry 1991; 30(11): 2916-27.
[http://dx.doi.org/10.1021/bi00225a027] [PMID: 1826089]

[189]   King RW, Bauer JD, Brady SF. An environmental DNA-derived type II polyketide biosynthetic pathway encodes the biosynthesis of the pentacyclic polyketide erdacin. Angew Chem Int Ed Engl 2009; 48(34): 6257-61.
[http://dx.doi.org/10.1002/anie.200901209] [PMID: 19621341]

[190]   Chang FY, Ternei MA, Calle PY, Brady SF. Discovery and synthetic refactoring of tryptophan dimer gene clusters from the environment. J Am Chem Soc 2013; 135(47): 17906-12.
[http://dx.doi.org/10.1021/ja408683p] [PMID: 24171465]

[191]   Feng Z, Kim JH, Brady SF. Fluostatins produced by the heterologous expression of a TAR reassembled environmental DNA derived type II PKS gene cluster. J Am Chem Soc 2010; 132(34): 11902-3.
[http://dx.doi.org/10.1021/ja104550p] [PMID: 20690632]

[192]   Chang FY, Ternei MA, Calle PY, Brady SF. Targeted metagenomics: finding rare tryptophan dimer natural products in the environment. J Am Chem Soc 2015; 137(18): 6044-52.
[http://dx.doi.org/10.1021/jacs.5b01968] [PMID: 25872030]

[193]   Donia MS, Cimermancic P, Schulze CJ, *et al.* A systematic analysis of biosynthetic gene clusters in the human microbiome reveals a common family of antibiotics. Cell 2014; 158(6): 1402-14.
[http://dx.doi.org/10.1016/j.cell.2014.08.032] [PMID: 25215495]

[194]   Matseliukh BP, Tymoshenko SH, Bambura OI, Kopeĭko OP. [Screening and characteristics of regulators of landomycin E biosynthesis in Streptomyces globisporus]. Mikrobiol Z 2011; 73(5): 16-20. [Screening and characteristics of regulators of landomycin E biosynthesis in Streptomyces globisporus].
[PMID: 22164695]

[195]   Montiel D, Kang HS, Chang FY, Charlop-Powers Z, Brady SF. Yeast homologous recombination-based promoter engineering for the activation of silent natural product biosynthetic gene clusters. Proc Natl Acad Sci USA 2015; 112(29): 8953-8.
[http://dx.doi.org/10.1073/pnas.1507606112] [PMID: 26150486]

[196]   Brady SF, Clardy J. Synthesis of long-chain fatty acid enol esters isolated from an environmental DNA clone. Org Lett 2003; 5(2): 121-4.
[http://dx.doi.org/10.1021/ol0267681] [PMID: 12529120]

[197]   Brady SF, Clardy J. N-acyl derivatives of arginine and tryptophan isolated from environmental DNA expressed in *Escherichia coli*. Org Lett 2005; 7(17): 3613-6.
[http://dx.doi.org/10.1021/ol0509585] [PMID: 16092832]

[198]   Donia MS, Ruffner DE, Cao S, Schmidt EW. Accessing the hidden majority of marine natural products through metagenomics. ChemBioChem 2011; 12(8): 1230-6.

[http://dx.doi.org/10.1002/cbic.201000780] [PMID: 21542088]

[199] Kurnia NM, Uria AR, Kusnadi Y, Dinawati L, Zilda DS, Hadi TA, *et al.* Metagenomic Survey of Potential Symbiotic Bacteria and Polyketide Synthase Genes in an Indonesian Marine Sponge. Hayati J Biosci 2017; 24: 6-15.
[http://dx.doi.org/10.1016/j.hjb.2017.04.004]

[200] Kampa A, Gagunashvili AN, Gulder TAM, *et al.* Metagenomic natural product discovery in lichen provides evidence for a family of biosynthetic pathways in diverse symbioses. Proc Natl Acad Sci USA 2013; 110(33): E3129-37.
[http://dx.doi.org/10.1073/pnas.1305867110] [PMID: 23898213]

[201] Owen JG, Reddy BVB, Ternei MA, *et al.* Mapping gene clusters within arrayed metagenomic libraries to expand the structural diversity of biomedically relevant natural products. Proc Natl Acad Sci USA 2013; 110(29): 11797-802.
[http://dx.doi.org/10.1073/pnas.1222159110] [PMID: 23824289]

[202] Yamanaka K, Reynolds KA, Kersten RD, *et al.* Direct cloning and refactoring of a silent lipopeptide biosynthetic gene cluster yields the antibiotic taromycin A. Proc Natl Acad Sci USA 2014; 111(5): 1957-62.
[http://dx.doi.org/10.1073/pnas.1319584111] [PMID: 24449899]

[203] Wang GYS, Graziani E, Waters B, *et al.* Novel natural products from soil DNA libraries in a streptomycete host. Org Lett 2000; 2(16): 2401-4.
[http://dx.doi.org/10.1021/ol005860z] [PMID: 10956506]

[204] Banik JJ, Brady SF. Cloning and characterization of new glycopeptide gene clusters found in an environmental DNA megalibrary. Proc Natl Acad Sci USA 2008; 105(45): 17273-7.
[http://dx.doi.org/10.1073/pnas.0807564105] [PMID: 18987322]

[205] Donia MS, Fricke WF, Ravel J, Schmidt EW. Variation in tropical reef symbiont metagenomes defined by secondary metabolism. PLoS One 2011; 6(3): e17897.
[http://dx.doi.org/10.1371/journal.pone.0017897] [PMID: 21445351]

[206] Bauer JD, King RW, Brady SF. Utahmycins a and B, azaquinones produced by an environmental DNA clone. J Nat Prod 2010; 73(5): 976-9.
[http://dx.doi.org/10.1021/np900786s] [PMID: 20387794]

[207] Fujita MJ, Kimura N, Sakai A, Ichikawa Y, Hanyu T, Otsuka M. Cloning and heterologous expression of the vibrioferrin biosynthetic gene cluster from a marine metagenomic library. Biosci Biotechnol Biochem 2011; 75(12): 2283-7.
[http://dx.doi.org/10.1271/bbb.110379] [PMID: 22146715]

[208] Pemberton JM, Vincent KM, Penfold RJ. Cloning and heterologous expression of the violacein biosynthesis gene cluster from Chromobacterium violaceum. Curr Microbiol 1991; 22: 355-8.
[http://dx.doi.org/10.1007/BF02092154]

[209] He R, Wakimoto T, Takeshige Y, *et al.* Porphyrins from a metagenomic library of the marine sponge Discodermia calyx. Mol Biosyst 2012; 8(9): 2334-8.
[http://dx.doi.org/10.1039/c2mb25169h] [PMID: 22735778]

CHAPTER 7

Phyto-Nano-Antimicrobials: Synthesis, Characterization, Discovery, and Advances

Pankaj Satapathy[1], S. Aishwarya[1], M. Rashmi Shetty[1], N. Akshaya Simha[1], G. Dhanapal[1], R. Aishwarya Shree[1], Antara Biswas[1], K. Kounaina[2], Anirudh G. Patil[1], M.G. Avinash[3], Aishwarya T. Devi[4], Shubha Gopal[3], M.N. Nagendra Prasad[4], S.M. Veena[5], S.P. Hudeda[2], K. Muthuchelian[1], Sunil S. More[1], Govindappa Melappa[6,*] and Farhan Zameer[1,*]

[1] *School of Basic and Applied Sciences, Department of Biological Sciences, Dayananda Sagar University, Shavige Malleshwara Hills, Kumaraswamy Layout, Bengaluru - 560 111, Karnataka, India*

[2] *Department of Dravyaguna, JSS Ayurvedic Medical College, Lalithadripura, Mysuru - 570 028, Karnataka, India*

[3] *Department of Studies in Microbiology, University of Mysore, Manasagangotri, Mysuru - 560 006, Karnataka, India*

[4] *Department of Biotechnology, JSS Science and Technology University, JSS Research Foundation, SJCE Campus, Manasagangotri, Mysore - 560 006, Karnataka, India*

[5] *Department of Biotechnology, Sapthagiri Engineering College, Bengaluru - 560 057, Karnataka, India*

[6] *Department of Botany, Davangere University,Shivagangothri, Davangere - 577 007, Karnataka, India*

Abstract: Nanotechnology has brought a revolution to the world of science and medicine. With time, the dependency on nanotechnological advancement is increasing. Synthesis of nano-scale modulators is a significant domain of focus that employs crude formulations, retro-synthesized, and pure chemicals, mostly from herbal sources with lesser side effects. However, all these methods suffer from drawbacks and limitations. For an eco-friendly nanoparticle synthesis, green chemistry has evolved with a tangential approach for the synthesis of metals (Au, Ag) and metal oxides (ZnO, CuO, TiO). Green synthesis uses plant extracts (leaves, stem, shoot) and microbes (bacteria, fungi, yeast) as reducing intermediate for the production of nanoparticles.

* **Corresponding author Farhan Zameer:** Assistant Professor in Biochemistry, School of Basic and Applied Sciences, Department of Biological Sciences, Dayananda Sagar University, Shavige MalleshwaraHills, Kumaraswamy Layout, Bengaluru-560 111, Karnataka, India; Tel: 0091-9844576378; E-mail: farhanzameeruom@gmail.com

* **Co-Corresponding author Govindappa Melappa:** Department of Botany, Davangere University, Shivagangothri, Davangere-577 007, Karnataka, India; Tel: 0091-7338601980; E-mail: dravidateja07@gmail.com

The advantage of these extracts lies within the phenolic constitutes of aldehydes, ketones, proteins, and other biomolecules that implicate the reduction of the nanoparticles.

These green synthesized nanoparticles have high efficacy ranging from anti-bacterial, anti-fungal, and wide applications in medicine. In this chapter, we discuss the methods of green synthesis, their applications, and prospects. The current chapter will pave the way for future applications and better means for the synthesis of nanoparticles leading into a newer direction with varied recognition in nano-life sciences.

Keywords: Antibacterial, Antifungal, Gold, Green Synthesis, Metal oxides, Metal, Nanomaterials, Nanoparticles, Particle diameter, Particle size, Quantum dots, Silver.

INTRODUCTION

Nanotechnology has changed the world with revolutionary thinking and methods that were not imaginable. This revolution has brought much new technology to the industry like CNT (Carbon nanotubes), QDs (Quantum dots), Graphene, and their composites. These inventions have a variety of uses and are involved in the day to day life. Nanotechnology has become an integral part of life, which is inseparable from us. To obtain nanomaterial of the desired shape, size, and functions, various fundamental synthesis approaches like top-down and bottom-up are used. To achieve this, methods like etching, milling, and sputtering are used. The use of the bottom-up approach has gained popularity in which nanomaterials are derived from simpler molecules. The methods used are chemical vapor deposition, Sol-gel processes, spray pyrolysis, laser pyrolysis, and atomic/molecular condensation. Chemical methods have a lot of limitations in getting the desired shape and size. These include environmental stability, lack of fundamental understanding of the mechanism, toxicity, extensive analysis, skilled operators, devices involved, and reduce/recycle/reuse. With the advancement of technology and the need for an eco-friendly approach, green synthesis of nanoparticles has revolutionized the world. This has caught attention in modern science and technology for nanomaterial synthesis. Green synthesis has an answer to many fundamental questions like minimization of waste, pollution reduction, and the use of safer solvent for synthesis. Green synthesis reduces the use of unwanted solvent, being sustainable and reliable. To achieve these objectives, a suitable solvent and a natural source are necessary. Green synthesis uses both plant extracts as well as microorganisms (fungi, bacteria, algae) for the production of metal/metal oxide nanoparticles. Green synthesis methods are dependent on parameters like pH, temperature, pressure, and solvent. For all these to be adequate, there is a need for plant extracts that can provide a holistic environment. Plant extracts are a rich source of aldehydes, ketones, flavanones, amines, terpenoids, carboxylic acids, ascorbic acids, and phenols. These components help in the reduction of metals to metal oxide nanoparticles. This has a variety of uses ranging from antimicrobial to diagnostics. In this book chapter, an overview of types of green synthesis followed by their characterization technique is well explored. Further, the insights on nano-application with prospects have been elaborated exploiting the new avenues in nano-life sciences.

SYNTHESIS OF NANOPARTICLES

Nanoparticles are mostly metal derived; the size ranges from 1-100 nanometers. Many novel approaches have been used for the synthesis of nanoparticles. Earlier synthetic approaches were common to derive nanoparticles but had pros and cons. Hence the green synthesis approach has given a new dimension to various studies. Nanoparticles can be produced using chemical synthesis, which requires high radiation, highly toxic reductants, and stabilizing agents, further they might harm both humans and the ecosystem. Nanoparticles have various processes and applications; for example, nanostructured powders by a flame pyrolysis process are used as commercial products, nanoparticle fabrication by precipitation, and surface controlling agents (SCAs), which have a role in size control and agglomeration avoidance. Standard nanoparticles that are chemically synthesized are SiO_2, TiO_2, FeOx, mainly used in *in vitro* tumor cell penetration and hyperthermal treatment [1]. Endosymbionts share a commensal relationship with the host organism. They have an application in nanoparticle synthesis; one among them is silver nanoparticles. A unique property of silver is that it is integrated into antimicrobial applications, biosensor materials, composite fibers, cryogenic super-conducting materials, cosmetic products, and electronic components. The silver nanoparticle was synthesized using endosymbionts *Pseudomonas fluorescens* CA 417 inhabiting *Coffea arabica* L. further characterized using spectroscopic techniques like UV-Vis spectroscopy at maximum absorption of 425nm. The average particle size was determined by dynamic light scattering (DLS) method that revealed the size to be 20.66 nm. These synthesized silver nanoparticles showed antibacterial activity on test pathogens. This also led to the feasibility study on both hydrophilic and hydrophobic substances [2].

To overcome all these problems, green synthesis of nanoparticles using plants and microorganisms makes it eco-friendly, cost-effective, with reduced use of organic solvent, averting the use of waste, and leading to reduction of pollution. "Green synthesis" aims to achieve the goal of eliminating hazardous substances if not entirely at least to the extent that it does not cause any harm to the environment by using ideal solvent systems and making the most use of natural resources. The synthesis of metallic nanoparticles through the biological precursor method depends on several factors such as pressure, temperature, solvent, and pH conditions. The synthesis of nanoparticles can be through bacteria, fungi, yeast, plants, and solvent-based systems.

Bacterial Mediated Synthesis

Bacterial species are mainly used in industrial and biotechnological applications such as bioleaching, genetic engineering, and bioremediation [3]. Bacteria can reduce metal ions and play a significant role in nanoparticle preparation [4]. For the synthesis of metal/metal oxide nanoparticles, several different bacterial species are utilized; the most used microorganisms are prokaryotes and actinomycetes. Bacterial synthesis of nanoparticles is preferred because of the ease of manipulating the bacteria [5]. Some bacterial strains that are enormously used for the synthesis of silver nanoparticles that are bio-reduced with different shape/size include *Escherichia coli*, Enterobacter cloacae, Lactobacillus casei, Bacillus cereus, Aeromonas sp. SH10 Phaeocystis antarctica, Shewanella oneidensis, Bacillus amyloliquefaciens, Bacillus indicus, Geobacter spp., Arthrobacter gangotriensis, Corynebacterium sp. SH09, Pseudomonas proteolytica, and *Bacillus cecembensis*. Some bacteria that are used for the synthesis of gold nanoparticles include *Plectonema boryanum UTEX 485, Desulfovibrio desulfuricans, Bacillus subtilis 168, Shewanella alga, Rhodopseudomonas capsulate, E. coli DH5a,* and *Bacillus megaterium D01.*

Fungi Mediated Synthesis

Fungi mediated synthesis of metal/metal oxide nanoparticles is effective in getting the desired shape and size. This is possible due to various intracellular enzymes present in fungi [6]. Fungi are found to synthesize an enormous amount of nanoparticles when compared to bacteria [7]. As compared to other organisms fungi have better activity due to the presence of proteins, reducing components, and enzymes on their cell surfaces [8]. The metallic nanoparticles are synthesized by enzymatic reduction (reductase) that takes place in the cell wall/cell of the fungus. Silver-tolerant yeast strain *Saccharomyces cerevisiae* broth is reported to biosynthesize silver and gold nanoparticles.

Plant Extract Synthesis

Plant's ability to accumulate heavy metal in their parts makes them a better candidate for nanoparticle synthesis. Biosynthesis of nanoparticles using plant extracts is advised for its simplicity, feasibility, and effectiveness. A variety of plants can be used to synthesize nanoparticles through the "one-pot" process and can be used to stabilize and reduce the metallic nanoparticles. Components of the plant include biomolecules like coenzymes, carbohydrates, and proteins with the ability to reduce metal salt into nanoparticles. Plant-assisted synthesis of nanoparticles was first investigated on gold and silver metal nanoparticles. Several plants were used to synthesize gold and silver metallic nanoparticles, including *Aloe barbadensis* Miller (aloe vera), *Coriandrum sativum* (coriander), *Azadirachta indica* (neem), *Cymbopogon flexuosus* (lemongrass), *Osimum sanctum* (tulsi) and *Citrus limon* (lemon). *Ex vivo* synthesis of nanoparticles is intensively researched, whereas the metallic nanoparticles are synthesized mediated through plants (*in vivo*) by reducing the metal salt ions absorbed as salts [9]. Plant leaf extracts like *Coriandrum sativum* (coriander) [10], *Acalypha indica* (copper leaf) [11], and *Aloe barbadensis* Miller (Aloe leaf broth extract) [12] were used to synthesize zinc oxide nanoparticles.

Solvent for Synthesis

Solvent system-based green synthesis is one of the fundamental components in synthesis processes. Water is considered as one of the best suitable ideal solvent systems, as it is cheapest and universal. According to Sheldon, "The best solvent is no solvent, and if a solvent is desirable, then water is ideal" [13]. Partial oxidation of the synthesized gold nanoparticles takes place due to oxygen present in the water that increases the chemical reactivity and plays a major role in its growth [14]. Green synthesis consists of two major routes: a natural extract/source is used as the main component for synthesis, and water is used as the solvent system. Ionic liquids are used for the synthesis of nanoparticles; they act as both protective and as a reductant. Due to the nature of the cations and anions, ionic liquids can either be hydrophilic or hydrophobic. The advantages of using ionic liquids than other solvents include: (a) polar organic compounds, gases, and metal catalysts can easily dissolve in ionic liquids to support biocatalysts, (b) Ionic liquids have a broad range of thermal stability; therefore, they decompose above 300-400°C and melt below room temperature. Ionic liquids are not accepted for the synthesis process due to the problems with its biodegradability. To overcome the problems associated with biodegradability, benign ionic liquids have been established with maximum biodegradation efficiency [15]. Many typical solvents can be used by changing the temperature and pressure above the critical point. The most available supercritical, inert solvent that is non-hazardous, is found to be carbon-di-oxide [16]. Water has a critical temperature of 646K and a pressure of 22.1MPa; therefore, water can serve as a suitable solvent system for many reactions [17].

Mechanism of Synthesis

Green synthesis of metallic nanoparticles through a microorganism based process involves the capturing of the metal ions into the microbial cells; these captured ions are then reduced to metallic nanoparticles through the involvement of enzymes [18]. Silver and gold nanoparticles were synthesized using *Verticillium* sp. and algal biomass by trapping the silver and gold nanoparticles onto the fungal cells through electrostatic interactions. These silver and gold ions were converted into silver and gold nuclei that later grew. The primary requirement for the synthesis of these nanoparticles is NADH and NADH-dependent nitrate reductase. The mechanism of bioreduction results in metal salt ions, and in turn, metallic nanoparticles remain unexplored [19]. Green synthesis of metallic nanoparticles through plant leaf extracts involves metal precursor solution mixed with the leaf extract at different conditions [20]. The conditions include the phytochemical concentration, the type of phytochemicals, pH, the concentration of the metal salt, and temperature. These conditions enhance the yield, stability, and control the rate of formation of nanoparticles [21]. Compared to bacteria and fungi, the phytomolecules present in the plants are found to reduce metal ions with less time and without any incubation period [22]; due to this property, plant extract is considered to be the best source for metal and metal oxides nanoparticles. Plant extracts act as both stabilizing and as reducing agents in the synthesis of nanoparticles and enhance the synthesis process [23]. The key components present in the plant that are involved in the bioreduction process include terpenoids, aldehydes, ketones, flavones, sugars, amides, carboxylic acids [24]. The functional groups present in flavonoids enhance the capability to reduce metal ions; enol-form is converted into keto-form by releasing the hydrogen atom, this phenomenon is called as tautomerism. Plant extracts consist of sugars like glucose and fructose that are involved in the formation of metallic nanoparticles. The major role of glucose in the synthesis of nanoparticles is involved with different sizes and shapes. The fructose-mediated synthesis of gold and silver nanoparticles is mono-disperse in nature [25]. Synthesized nanoparticles that are mediated through plant extract were found to be associated with proteins when confirmed through FTIR analysis [26]; amino acids also have different mechanisms of reducing the metal ions. Arginine, lysine, methionine, and cysteine are dexterous in binding with silver ions [27]. Over the last decade, green synthesis of metal and metal oxide nanoparticles has become the most attractive area of research. Various kinds of natural extracts, including bacteria, fungi, yeasts, and plant extracts have been used as a proficient resource for the production of nanoparticles [28]. The mechanism of synthesis of the nanoparticles, the role of the solvents, and the existing problems associated with the synthesis of nanoparticles have been explained in detail, referring to the available literature (Fig. **1**) and various species-mediated conversion Table **1**.

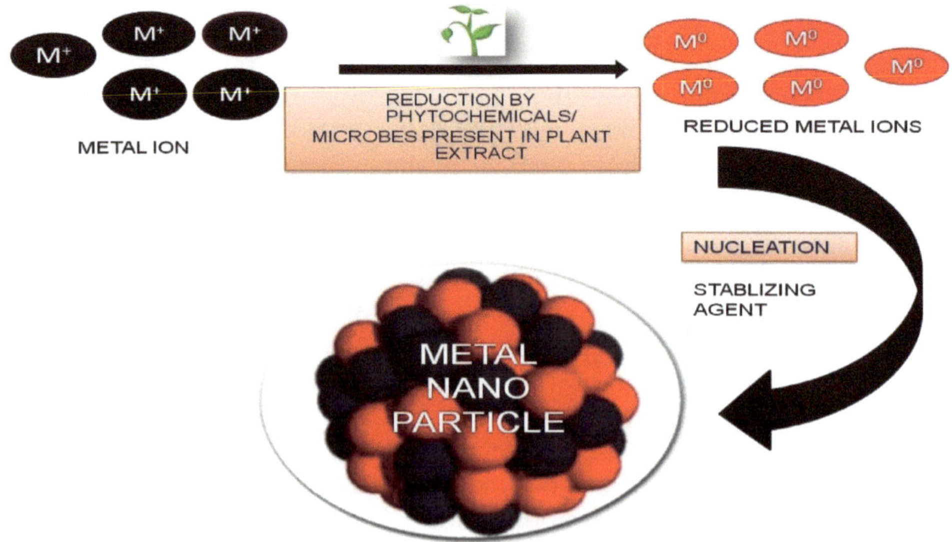

Fig. (1). Procedure for the synthesis of metal and metal oxide nanoparticles using plant and microbe extract.

Table 1. Green synthesis of nanoparticles from microbe and plant extracts.

Sl. No	Species	Nanoparticle	Size (nm)	References
Bacteria				
1	*Bacillus cereus*	Silver	20-40	[29]
2	*Pseudomonas proteolytica, Bacillus cecembensis*	Silver	6-13	[30]
3	*Bacillus megaterium* D01	Gold	<2.5	[31]
4	*Plectonema boryanum* UTEX 485	Gold	<10-25	[32]
5	*Magnetospirillum magnetotacticum*	Iron oxide	47	[33]
6	*Aquaspirillum magnetotacticum*	Iron oxide	40-50	[34]
7	*Klebsiella aerogenes*	Cadmium sulfide	20-200	[35]
8	*E. coli*	Cadmium sulfide	2-5	[36]
Fungus				
9	*Rhizopus nigricans*	Silver	35-40	[37]
10	*Verticillium*	Silver	21-25	[38]
11	Thermophilic filamentous fungi	Gold	6-40	[39]
12	*Trichothecium sp.*	Gold	10-25	[40]
13	*Aspergillus terreus*	Zinc oxide	8	[41]
14	*Aspergillus flavus* TFR7	Titanium dioxide	12-15	[42]
Yeast				

(Table 1) cont.....

Sl. No	Species	Nanoparticle	Size (nm)	References
15	*MKY3*	Silver	2-5	[43]
16	*Saccharomyces cerevisiae broth*	Gold	4-15	[44]
Plant Origin				
17	*Brassica juncea* (mustard)	Silver	2-35	[45]
18	*Carica papaya* (papaya)	Silver	60-80	[46]
19	*Citrus limon* (lemon)	Silver	<50	[47]
20	*Cycas sp.* (cycas)	Silver	2-6	[48]
21	*Eucalyptus citriodora* (neelagiri)	Silver	20	[49]
22	*Avena sativa* (oat)	Gold	5-20	[50]
23	*Coriandrum sativum* (coriander)	Gold	7-58	[51]
24	*Cymbopogon flexuosus* (lemongrass)	Gold	200-500	[52]
25	*Syzygium aromaticum* (clove buds)	Gold	5-100	[53]
26	*Medicago sativa* (alfalfa)	Gold	2-40	[54]
27	*Sedum alfredii Hance*	Zinc oxide	53.7	[55]
28	*Gardenia jasminoides Ellis* (gardenia)	Palladium	3-5	[56]

CHARACTERIZATION OF PLANT MEDIATED NANOPARTICLES HAVING MICROBIAL ACTIVITY

General Characterization

Nanoparticles exist in a nanometer-scale possessing unique physical and chemical properties. They are majorly aerosols, suspensions, or emulsions. The characterization of nanoparticles is broadly described as nanometrology, which deals with the characterization of the physical and chemical properties of nanoparticles. This contributes to studying nanotoxicology, health, and safety hazards. A wide range of instruments characterize the synthesized nanoparticles, which involve UV-visible spectroscopy, X-ray diffraction, transmission electron microscopy, scanning electron microscopy, Fourier transformed infrared, and dynamic light scattering (Fig. **2**).

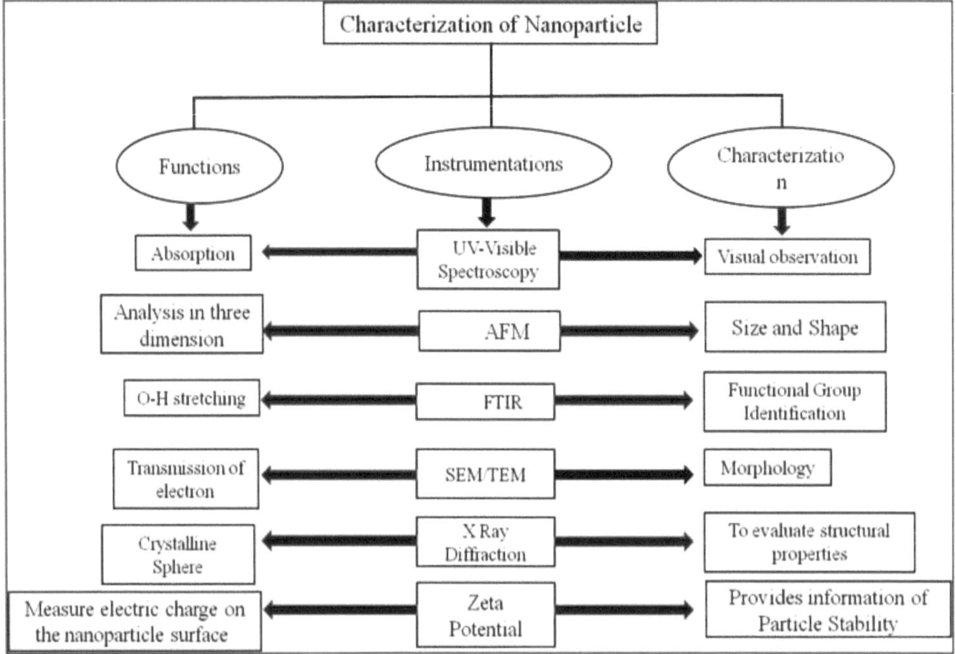

Fig. (2). Account of instruments and their applications in nanotechnology.

UV- Visible Spectroscopy

UV- visible spectroscopy is a widely used method to determine the concentration of an analyte in solution (*e.g.*: organic compounds). A ray of light from a visible or UV light source is separated into its component wavelengths by a prism or diffraction grating. Each monochromatic (single wavelength) beam is split into two equal intensity beams by a half-mirrored device. The sample beam passes the solution in the sample. The other beam called the reference passes the solvent. The intensities of these light beams are then measured by electronic detectors and are compared. The ultraviolet (UV) region scanned usually is from 200 to 400 nm, and the visible portion is from 400 to 800 nm. Visible light and ultraviolet light are used to analyze the chemical structure of a substance at 200-400 nm [57].

X-ray Diffraction

X-ray diffraction is a non-destructive technique for characterizing crystalline material. X-ray diffraction is the adaptable scattering of x-ray photons by atoms in a periodic lattice. It provides information on structures, preferred crystal orientations, and other parameters, such as average grain size, crystallinity, strain, and crystal defects. X-ray diffraction peaks are formed by a monochromatic beam of X-rays scattered through constructive interference in a sample at specific angles from each set of lattice planes. The peak intensities are found by the atomic positions within the lattice planes [57].

Transmission Electron Microscopy

TEM is one of the most frequently used tools for the atomic-scale characterization of atomic and electron structure. TEM forms an image from the interaction of the electrons with the sample as the beam is transmitted through the specimen, and electrons are scattered. The advanced system of electromagnetic lenses focuses on the distributed electrons into a diffraction pattern or image depending on the mode of operation [58].

Fourier Transformed Infrared

FTIR is a tool used to obtain an infrared spectrum of absorption or emission of the sample (solid, liquid, or gas). It is used to characterize organic, polymeric, and inorganic materials. It scans the test sample and collects the data of its chemical properties. Fourier transformed infrared spectroscopy (FTIR) uses discrete energy levels to study functional groups based on their vibrations on the surface of materials. The functional groups in the material absorb light that is transmitted through the sample with specific intensity. This happens when the frequency of vibrations and the frequency of incoming light correspond to bonds between the atoms. Chemical environment, mass, and the type of vibrations are the factors that influence vibration energy. The functional groups that are present on the material can be determined by scanning over a range of wavelengths (400-4000 cm^{-1}) and recording the amount of transmitted light for each wavelength [59].

Dynamic Light Scattering

Dynamic light scattering measures the intensity of laser light when dispersed through the molecules in a sample solution. This helps in characterizing the aggregation phenomena in the protein sample. The light source from laser light irradiates the sample in the cell. The dispersed light signal is collected with one of two detectors, either at a 90 degree (right angle) or 173 degrees (back angle) scattering angle. The specification of both detectors allows more flexibility in choosing measurement conditions. Particles get dispersed in a variety of liquids. Only liquid refractive index and viscosity need to be known for interpreting the measurement results. The obtained optical signal shows random changes due to the randomly changing relative position of the particles, and the graphs are generated [59].

CHARACTERIZATION OF SILVER NANOPARTICLE (AGNPS)

Synthesized AgNPs using the flower extract of *C. epicheirema* were characterized using diverse spectral analysis

a). *UV-Visible Spectrophotometer*

The initial synthesis of AgNPs was confirmed using a UV-Vis absorption spectrophotometer. The solution absorbed in 350-400 range operated at 10 nm interval results in a reduction of Ag+ ions. The influence of various parameters such as boiling time, concentration, incubating reaction mixture was observed [60].

b). *FTIR Analysis*

The functional group involved in the stabilization was studied by FTIR. The FTIR spectrum recorded in the range of 400-4000 cm^{-1} gives modes of vibration, which are identified and utilized in determining the functional groups [60].

c). *XRD Analysis*

XRD helps in analyzing the structure and composition of synthesized AgNPs operating at a voltage of 40 kV and a current of 30 mA with Cu-Ka radiation in h-2h configurations. The structure of the crystallite sphere is intended from the width of the XRD peaks [60].

d). *Thermogravimetric Analysis*

DTG-60H detects the thermal stability and surface weight loss of AgNPs by evaluating the sample under a nitrogen gas flow of 100.0 ml/min and heating rate of 108°C/min to 1000.8°C [60].

e). *TEM Analysis*

TEM analysis is performed to assess the diameter of biologically synthesized AgNPs and to visualize the shape. Double distilled water is used to disperse the sample. A drop of thin dispersion is sited on a staining mat. Carbon coated copper grid is implanted into the drop with the coated side upwards. After about 10 min, the grid is detached, air-dried, and screened in a transmission Electron microscope [60].

f). FTIR Analysis

The decline in the silver ions to silver nanoparticles is due to the functional group present in it, which is exposed by FTIR analysis. The FTIR spectrum is recorded in the range of 500–4000 cm [60].

Characterization of Gold Nanoparticles (AuNPs)

a). UV- Vis Spectroscopy

Preliminary synthesis of AuNPs was confirmed by the visual observation of forming nanoparticle in the range between 300–800 nm. UV-Vis absorption was carried out, and position of the maxima of localized surface plasmon resonance (LSPR) band was considered, and the peak was observed at 528 nm that is characteristic to AuNPs and which clearly indicated the formation of gold nanoparticles by the color change of the reaction mixture from brown to ruby red and SPR band centered at 525 nm which confirmed the formation of Au nanoparticles. The LSPR absorption band of AuNPs exhibited characteristic bands maximum between 520-580 nm. A wide plasmonic band was observed in the samples and is indicative of spherical shaped AuNPs [61].

b). FTIR

The functional groups and other biomolecules concerned in the formation of gold nanoparticles *via* the reduction of chloroauric acid were illuminated by the FTIR analysis. The FTIR illustrated a broad peak at 3409 cm^{-1} corresponding to the overlapping of stretching vibrations of -OH and -NH$_2$ group, assigned to water and *M. indica* seed extract molecules. The stretching vibration of the aromatic ring appears at 1449 cm$^{-1,}$ and O-H scissoring deformation of an aromatic ring is observed at 1326 cm^{-1}. The band at 1360 cm^{-1} is attributed to C-H stretching. The characteristic bands of C=O aromatic stretching and C-O-C asymmetric stretching are observed at 1207 cm^{-1} and 1180 cm$^{-1,}$ respectively. O=C=C stretching is observed by a characteristic band at 1043 cm^{-1}. The vibrational bands are observed at 838 cm^{-1} that represent the C-O stretching of alcohol. These observed peaks are mainly contributed by the flavanoids, terpenoids, and tannins present in the seed extract that aids in establishing the functional group involved in nanoparticles [61].

c). SEM

To establish the morphology of the synthesized gold nanoparticles, they were subjected to FE-SEM analysis and TEM that demonstrate a spherical morphology with the formation of aggregates ~50nm, and TEM investigation confirms the size of the nanoparticles to be ~50nm. It was observed that the AuNPs have a spherical and pseudospherical shape with a narrow size distribution. It is possible that short reaction times have a potential role in the formation of spherical shaped nanoparticles [61].

d). X-ray Diffraction

X-ray spectroscopy (EDX) is carried out to investigate the elemental configuration of synthesized AuNPs and encircling. EDX spectrum assesses a strong signal, peaks assigned for metallic gold. The presence of other elemental composition of the extracts was not seen in the EDX spectrum as the samples were thoroughly washed to remove unreacted reactants and plant extracts. EDX spectra confirm the purity of the synthesized gold nanoparticles, similar to a reported study [61].

Characterization of Iron Oxide Nanoparticle

a). UV-Visible Spectroscopy

The formation of iron oxide nanoparticles is mainly due to the presence of two main components: iron salt and phyto-extract. The immediate reaction between iron chloride and plant extract is accountable for the change in color, and iron oxide nanoparticles that have been created. The UV- Visible absorption spectra exhibit a peak around 204nm. These findings display that biomolecules are capping on the surface of iron oxide nanoparticles with the absence of surface Plasmon resonance [61].

b). ATR Spectroscopy

The ATR spectra of *Agrewia optiva* provide that the peak at 1219 cm^{-1} is due to C-F stretching vibrations while the peak at 1363 cm^{-1} may be ascribed to C-C stretching of phenyl groups. The C-O stretching vibrations of amide appear at 1637 cm^{-1}. The CH$_2$ bending and symmetric -COO stretching frequency appear at 1416 and 1485 cm^{-1} respectively, due to C-H stretching of alkanes while the peak at 1634 cm^{-1} is because of C=O stretching of acid anhydrides. The absorption peaks lying in the range 3277-3779 cm^{-1} represents the hydroxyl group present in the plant species extract [62].

c). FT-IR

FT-IR analysis is very cardinal in ascertaining the functional group of the biomolecules responsible for capping and stabilizing during the synthesis of nanoparticles. The FT-IR spectrum of iron oxide nanoparticles using *Agrewia optiva* represents peak appearing at 3313-3209 cm^{-1} due to O-H stretching of phenol and also gives a broad range of 1628-1652 cm^{-1} C=O stretching vibrations while the band at 1036 cm^{-1} is due to C-O stretching, whereas the band at 1377 cm^{-1} is due to C-N stretching vibrations of aromatic amines and 846 cm^{-1} is due to C-H bending of alkenes. The multiple peaks appearing at 484 and 538 cm^{-1} are due to Fe-O in conformity [62].

d). SEM Analysis

The morphological analysis of iron-based nanoparticles derived from *Agrewia optiva* by SEM observed them to be in irregular clusters with rough surfaces, agglomerated, quasi-spherical, and their size ranging from 15-60 nm [62].

e). TEM Analysis

Iron oxide nanoparticles' size and morphology were confirmed by TEM. The TEM micrograph of iron oxide nanoparticles using *Agrewia optiva* exhibits some irregular particles. The micrograph shows that the nanoparticles are agglomerated due to the capping of biomolecules on the surface of nanoparticles. The nanoparticles are small in size, and the average size is 14 and 17 nm [62].

f). X-ray Diffraction

The synthesized iron oxide nanoparticles using *Agrewia optiva* were characterized by powdered X-ray diffraction. The main diffraction peaks of *Agrewia optiva* mediated iron oxide nanoparticles appear at different degrees Celsius. These peaks match with the standard data JCPDS number-75-033. The diffraction peaks represent the cubic spinel structure of (Fe_3O_4). The obtained results showed lower intensity because the biomaterials from the leaf extract were capped on the surface of nanoparticles. Iron oxide nanoparticle's average crystallite size is measured by the Debye-Scherrer equation: D=Kλ/(β.cosθ) [62].

Zinc Oxide Nanoparticles

The green synthesized zinc oxide nanoparticle from the methanolic leaf extract was characterized using the following methods:

a). UV-Visible Spectroscopy

This method was used to inspect the confirmation of the synthesized particles. The zinc oxide particles exhibit an absorbance in the range between 300-400 nm. The ZnO nanoparticles synthesized from the leaf extract of *G. pentaphylla* exhibited a strong absorption peak at 351 nm [63].

b). XRD Analysis

The X-ray diffraction pattern was used to evaluate the structural properties of particles and to confirm the crystalline nature and phase purity of ZnO nanoparticles. XRD Spectrum of ZnO nanoparticles displayed several strong diffraction peaks corresponding to 100, 002, 101, 102, 110, 103, 200, 112, 201 and 004 diffraction lines of hexagonal wurtzite structure of ZnO nanoparticles matched with the JCPDS card number 008, 79–2205 and 05–0664. The crystallite size of the narrow and sharp diffraction peak (101) was 30 nm calculated using Debye Scherrer's formula. The narrow peak was used to confirm for the crystallization of synthesized ZnO nanoparticles [63].

c). FTIR Analysis

FTIR analysis was performed to categorize the possible functional groups involved in the synthesis of ZnO nanoparticles. FT-IR spectra of ZnO nanoparticles were in the range of 500–4000 cm^{-1}. The broad peak at 3442 cm^{-1} indicated the -OH stretching vibrations. The sharp peak present in the range of 2943 cm^{-1} indicates the Alkane-CH stretching while the peak at 2848 cm^{-1} is due to the presence of stretching vibrations of the C-H bond. The band at 1741 cm^{-1} is due to the presence of C=O stretching. The peak at 1455 cm^{-1} is the characteristic absorption of C-H bending, the peak at 1125 cm^{-1} can be ascribed to the typical absorption of C-O stretching, and finally, weak band at 876 cm^{-1} is the result of C=C bending [63].

d). SEM

SEM describes the spherical shape and the diameter range of 32-40 nm of ZnO nanoparticles with images [63].

e). TEM

The TEM image of ZnO nanoparticle recorded at 50 nm resolutions is SAED pattern. The SAED pattern reveals that the prepared ZnO material is of polycrystalline material, and the average particle size of the ZnO nanoparticle was calculated using histogram analysis. The average value of particle size is around 36 nm, which is correlated with crystallite size calculated from XRD analysis [63]. Table **2** determines the plant-mediated synthesis of nanoparticles.

Table 2. Characterization of nanoparticle from various plant-mediated extracts.

Type of Nanoparticle	Plant	Plants Part	Size (nm)	Morphology of Nanoparticle	References
Silver	*Datura metel*	Leaves	16-40	Quasi-linear superstructures	[64]
	Alternanthera dentate	Leaves	50-100	Spherical	[65]
	Acorus calamus	Rhizome	31.83	Spherical	[65]
	Boerhaavia diffusa	Whole plant	25	Spherical	[66]
	Tribulus Terrestris	Leaves	16-28	Spherical	[67]
	Eclipta prostrate	Leaves	30-65	Triangles pentagons hexagons	[68]
Gold	*Mangifera indica*	Seed extract	46.8	Spherical	[69]
	Gymnocladus assamicus	Leaf	4-22	Hexagonal	[70]
	Nerium oleander		2-10	Spherical	[71]
	Solanum nigrum		50	Spherical	[72]
	Galaxaura elongata		3.85-77.13	Spherical	[73]
	Sesbania grandiflora		7-43	Spherical	[74]
Iron oxide	*Agrewia optiva*	Leaf	15-70	Spherical	[62]
Zinc oxide	*Glycosmis pentaphylla*	Leaf	32-36	Spherical	[63]
Titanium dioxide	*Annona squamosal*	Peel	23	Spherical	[75]
	Bauhinia variegate	Leaf	6-20	Irregular	[76]
	Calotropis gigantea	Flower	10.52	Spherical	[77]
	Catharanthus roseus	Leaf	25-110	Irregular	[78]
	Euphorbia heteradena Jaub	Leaf	20	Irregular	[79]

APPLICATION OF NANOPARTICLES

Anti-Fungal Property: A tabular representation is given in Table **3**.

Table 3. Examples of antifungal properties of green synthesis derived nanoparticles.

Sl.no	Fungi	Plant	Dose (LC$_{50}$/LC$_{90}$/ MIC)	Size (nm)	Zone or % of Inhibition	References
		Silver				
1	*Penicillium species* *Candida albicans*	*Sesuvium portulacastrum*	-	5-20	18mm 12mm	[89]
2	*N. parvum*	*Sinapis arvensis*	MIC – 2.5µg/mL	55-90	15%	[90]
		Gold				
1	*Candida albicans*	*Pelargonium graveolens*	MIC – 14.1mg/mL	0.55	-	[91]
2	*Candida albicans* *Aspergillus niger*	*Nepenthes khasiana*	-	50-80	10mm 16mm	[92]
		Zinc oxide				
1	*Candida albicans* *Penicillium notatum*	*Zingiber officinale*	-	23-25	10mm 12mm	[93]
2	*Aspergillus fumigatus* *Aspergillus flavus* *Penicillium sp* *Aspergillus niger*	*Camellia sinensis*	-	16	5.3 2.6 6.6 3.0	[94]
		Copper oxide				
4	*Candida albicans*	*Acalypha indica*	-	26-30	10	[95]
5	*F. oxysporum* *F. graminearum* *F. culmorum*	*Tabernaemontanadivaricate*	- -	10-60	28 23 33	[96]

Silver Nanoparticles

Tropaeolum majus L. commonly known as Garden nasturtium or Indian cress is a herbaceous plant majorly grown in South America. Fresh leaves of the plant were collected and dried; ethanol and aqueous extract of the plant was prepared using soxhlet method. Silver nanoparticles were prepared using the extract of *Tropaeolum majus* and silver nitrate solution. Fungal cultures were collected, and the spore suspension of the fungi was used for anti-fungal studies of ethanol, aqueous extracts, and silver nanoparticles. Antifungal activity was tested against *A. niger, C. albicans, P. notatum, T. viridae,* and *Mucor spp.* Among all the test organisms, *P. notatum* and *Mucor spp.* were inhibited more by AgNPs, followed by the remaining fungi. The MIC of *P. notatum* was found to be 31.2 µg/mL. We can conclude that silver nanoparticles have a productive antifungal activity that can be used in the preparation of medicine [80].

Aloe vera is a type of luscious plant that is grown in the Southwest Arabian Peninsula. Antifungal activity was performed by adding different combinations of 100 µL of AgNPs, leaf extract, and salt solution. Antifungal activity was performed by disc diffusion method wherein the zone of inhibition was observed. Antifungal activity was highest against *Aspergillus spp.* and *Rhizopus spp.* Apart from the zone of inhibition because of nanoparticles, the nanoparticles also caused damage to conidial germination, fungal hyphae, inhibiting normal budding and damaging the structure of the cell membrane. The MIC of AgNPs was found to be 21.8ng/mL, which infers that the AgNPs are effective antifungal agents than the leaf extract [81]. Banana is an herbaceous flowering plant, botanically a berry that is an edible fruit grown all over the world. Pathogenic fungal strains of *C. albicans*, *A. niger,* and *Alternaria alternata* were obtained for the antifungal activity. Antifungal activity was performed using the standard Kirby-Bauer disc diffusion method. Different concentrations of AgNPs - 25, 50, 75, and 100 mg/mL were added to PDA plates containing the fungal strains. Antifungal activity was indicated by the zone of inhibition. Antifungal activity was more for *A. niger* with the zone of inhibition of 13.3 mm. With a low concentration of AgNPs, there was no antifungal activity. Antifungal activity is because of the formation of insoluble compounds by inactivation of sulfhydryl groups in the cell wall of fungus and disruption of membrane-bound enzymes that causes cell lysis. By this, we can infer that the AgNPs were effective against *A. niger* and can be used as an efficient antifungal agent against *A. niger* [82].

Gelidiella acerosa is a type of seaweed that is grown in tropical and subtropical regions. Antifungal activity was performed by well diffusion method. The fungal strains used were - a) *Humicola insolens,* b) *Fusarium dimerum,* c) *Mucor indicus,* and d) *Trichoderma reesei.* The plates were added with 50µL of the nanoparticles along with the control containing 5 mg/mL of the standard drug *i.e.,* clotrimazole. Antifungal activity was indicated by the zone of inhibition. Biosynthesized AgNPs were effective in inhibiting the growth of the fungal strains with the zone of inhibition in mm as follows – a) 19, b) 12, c) 14, and d) 12, respectively that indicated the nanoparticles were potent antifungal agents in comparison with the standard drug Clotrimazole. Hence the AgNPs can be used in the preparation of medicines [83].

Ocimum sanctum is commonly known as Tulasi, holy basil because of its religious importance. It is grown in India and the Indian subcontinent. Tulasi leaves were collected, dried, and powdered by grinding. 10g of the dried powder was dissolved in 90% methanol. After 24 hrs, it was filtered and centrifuged. The supernatant was collected by evaporating the solvent. The crude extract was diluted with 5% DMSO and used for further studies. The AgNPs were prepared by adding 1 mM of Silver nitrate and plant extract. Antifungal activity was performed by well diffusion assay method. It was performed against different fungal strains- a) *C. albicans*, b) *C. kefyr*, c) *A. niger*, d) *C. tropicalis*, e) *A. flavus*, and f) *A.fumigatus*. Antifungal activity was indicated by the zone of inhibition in the plate. Antifungal activity was performed with the nanoparticles and in comparison with the standard drugs ketoconazole and itraconazole. The highest antifungal activity was against the strains b) a) and c) with the zone of inhibition 15mm, 13mm, and 12mm, respectively. The intermediate activity was against d) e) and f) with the zone of inhibition 11mm, 6mm, and 7mm, respectively. These results indicate that the synthesized AgNPs were a potent antifungal agent [84].

Gold Nanoparticles

Abelmoschus esculentus L. commonly known as okra or lady finger is a flowering plant majorly grown in tropical, sub-tropical and warm temperate regions of the world. The seeds were collected, washed with distilled water, dried for 15 days, and the dried seeds were powdered. The prepared seed powder was mixed with ion free water and boiled for 30mins, cooled, filtered, and was used fresh to prepare AuNPs. Gold nanoparticles were prepared using the aqueous extract of the seeds (40mL) and aqueous chloroauric acid. Fungal cultures were isolated from the soil and used for the antifungal study. Antifungal activity was done against *Puccinia graminis, Aspergillus flavus, Aspergillus niger,* and *Candida albicans* using the standard well diffusion method. AuNPs were very effective in inhibiting the growth of *Puccinia graminis* with a zone of inhibition of 17mm, *Candida albicans* with a zone of inhibition of 18mm, *Aspergillus flavus* with the zone of inhibition of 16mm and *A. niger* with the zone of inhibition of 15mm. From these results, we can infer that the biosynthesized AuNPs is an effective antifungal agent, and these AuNPs can be used in the preparation of medicine. AuNPs can be used as an antimicrobial agent, and this can be used in the food industry as preservatives [85].

Terminalia chebula, commonly known as black or *Chebulic myrobalan,* is grown in India, Srilanka, China, and other South Asian countries. *W. bancrofti* is the causal agent for filariasis (elephantiasis) characterized by swelling of leg (elephant leg). The synthesized nanoparticles were subjected to antifilarial assay against *W. bancrofti* and *S. cervi* by the method of MIT assay. LC_{50} was determined by the assay. Percentage inhibitions at different doses were found to be 9.1%, 32.8%, 76.04%, 88.3% and 93.7% for 5µg/mL, 10µg/mL, 20µg/mL, 30µg/mL and 40µg/mL, respectively. LC_{50} of microfilaria of *S.cervi* and adult filariids were found to be 8.27%, 31.3%, 74.8%, 87.2%, and 91.03%, respectively. A slight increase in microfilaricidal activity was observed against *W. bancrofti*. Viability was reduced, and this was found to be 9.47%, 32.8%, 76.38%, 89%, and 93.47%, respectively. LC_{50} and LC_{90} values were determined and are found to be 14.3, and 38 µg/mL, LC_{50} and LC_{90} of microfilaria and adult *S. cervi* were determined to be 13.97 and 35.71µg/mL, respectively. In the case of microfilaria of *W. bancrofti,* a decrease in LC_{50} and LC_{90} was observed as 13.9 and 35.57µg/mL. By the results of MIT assay, it was inferred that the biosynthesized AuNPs is a potent antifilarial agent against both human and bovine filariids [86].

Oxide Nanoparticles

Cissus quadrangularis is commonly known as veldt grape, devil's backbone, and adamant creeper is a perennial plant of the grape family that is grown in India, Srilanka, Bangladesh, and African countries. The leaf powder was obtained from Vellore local market. 10g of leaf powder was added to 300mL of distilled water and boiled for 1hour in a boiling water bath; after the required time, it was filtered, concentrated, and was refrigerated. The CuO nanoparticles were synthesized using 20 mg/mL of the plant extract and 1mM of Copper acetate. The antifungal activity was performed against *A. niger* and *A. flavus*. Antifungal activity was done using the Clinical and Laboratory Standards Institute (CLSI) method. 1 mg/mL of strain and 1 mg/mL of the biosynthesized CuO NPs were added in two concentrations (500 and 1000ppm) to the media (Potato Dextrose Broth), stirred for 1 week; biomass was obtained by filtration and was calculated for the antifungal activity of the two species in comparison with the standard antifungal drug Carbendazim. From the CLSI antifungal study, the CuO NPs had efficient antifungal property in comparison with the standard antifungal Carbendazim. CuO NPs damaged the cytoplasm and led to the apoptosis of the fungus. 500ppm of CuO NPs inhibited the growth of 82% of *A. niger,* 1000ppm of CuO NPs inhibited 88% of *A. niger,* and the standard antifungal inhibited 40% and 43%, respectively. 500ppm of CuO NPs inhibited 82% of the growth of *A. flavus,* and 1000ppm of CuO NPs inhibited 88% of *A. flavus*. These results infer that the green synthesized CuO NPs were potent antifungal agents [87].

Trianthema portulacastrum is commonly known as black pigweed, giant pigweed, and desert horse purslane. It is a weed that is grown in Africa, North America, and South America. Plant biomass was collected from the field, washed with distilled water to separate particulate matters which are adhered to the biomass. Biomass was dried; the powder was prepared by grinding the biomass. The plant extract was prepared by mixing 40g of powder in 100mL distilled water with constant stirring for 3 hours. ZnO NPs were prepared by mixing 10mL of the prepared extract and $ZnSO_4$. Antifungal activity was performed against *Aspergillus niger*, *A. flavus,* and *A. fumigatus.* Antifungal activity was performed by adding the mixture 100 μg/L of nanoparticles and DMSO to the tubes containing Sabaroud's Dextrose Agar with fungi, and the tubes were incubated for 7 days. Inhibition of the mycelial growth with the area of fungal growth was observed and expressed in terms of percentage inhibition. Antifungal activity studies were carried out in comparison with the standard drug Terbinafine. ZnO NPs were efficient in the inhibition of mycelial growth. 45% of the linear growth of *Aspergillus niger*, 41% of linear growth of *A. flavus,* and 51% of linear growth of *A. fumigatus* were inhibited by ZnO NPs. From these results, ZnO NPs have been proven to be effective antifungal agents [88].

Antibacterial Property

Silver nanoparticles: Since ancient times, silver is enormously used as a therapeutic to treat various diseases [97]. Even before antibiotics were used, silver was used to treat burns and wounds [98]. Gram-positive and gram-negative bacteria exhibit antibacterial activity against silver nanoparticles differently; they compete with one another [99]. It is found that gram-negative bacterial strains are more sensitive to AgNPs when compared to gram-positive bacteria or vice-versa [100]. Silver nanoparticles are positively charged, and the bacterial cellular membrane is negatively charged; AgNPs accumulate on the negatively charged bacterial membrane and cause conformational changes in the membrane. This conformational change causes more permeability to the bacterial cell membrane. Transportation of the nanoparticles in and out of the cellular membrane leads to cell death [101]. Silver nanoparticles block transcription and translation by entering the bacterial cell and by binding to its genetic material [102]. Antibacterial activity of nanoparticles is of two types: biocidal action and inhibitory action [103]. The antibacterial activity of nanoparticles depends on several parameters, including temperature, pH, silver nitrate concentration, and types of bacteria Table **4** [104, 105].

Table 4. Illustrations of nanoparticles for their anti-bacterial efficacy.

Bacteria	Nanoparticle	Plant	Dose	Time	Inference	References
E. coli,S. aureus, and B. subtilis	Silver nanoparticle	*Selaginella bryopteris*	1.0 mL	48-72 hrs	The best antibacterial effect was against *E. coli*	[113]

(Table 4) cont.....

Bacteria	Nanoparticle	Plant	Dose	Time	Inference	References
E. coli, S. aureus, and K. pneumoniae	Ferric oxide nanoparticle	*Ruellia tuberosa*	75 µL	24 hrs	The best antibacterial effect was against *E. coli* and *K. pneumoniae*	[114]
S. aureus, B. cereus, S. thyphimurium and *E. coli.*	Silver nanoparticle	*Glutamicum corniculatum* (L.) Curtis	30 µL	16 hrs	*E. coli, S. thyphimurium, S. thyphimurium, and B. cereus* was the increasing order	[115]
E. coli, B. subtilis and *S. aureus.*	Cupric oxide nanoparticle	*Madhuka longifolia*	100 µL	24hrs	Zone of inhibition was 15.67±0.68mmfor *E. coli*	[116]
B. cereus, S. aureus, E. coli, S. typhi, K. pneumoniae, S. aureus, and B. cereus	Zinc oxide nanoparticle	*Albizia lebbeck*	10 µL	48hrs	The best antibacterial activity was seen against *E. coli* and *S. typhi*	[117]
E. coli, S. typhi, S. enterica, and B. subtilis	Silver nanoparticle	*Tithonia diversifolia*	0.2 mL	24hrs	The best antibacterial activity was seen against *B. subtilis*	[118]
E. coli, and B. subtilis	Silver nanoparticle	*Rhazya stricta*	50 µL	24hrs-48hrs	The best antibacterial activity was against *E. coli* than *B. subtilis*	[119]
S. epidermidis and *E. coli*	Gold nanoparticle	*Coleus aromaticus*	0.5 MacFarland	24 hrs	The best antibacterial activity was against *E. coli* than *S. epidermidis*	[120]
A. hydrophila	Platinum nanoparticle	Orange peel extract	0.5 µL	24 hrs	Antibacterial activity was observed	[121]
B. subtilis, S. aureus, P. mirabilis, S. typhi	Zinc oxide nanoparticle	*Pedalium Murex*	100 µL	24 hrs	Antibacterial activity was seen against *P. mirabilis* and *S. typhi*	[122]
E. coli, P. aeruginosa B. subtilis and *S. aureus.*	Gold nanoparticle	thyme	60 µL	24 hrs	Antibacterial activity was seen against all the bacteria	[123]

(Table 4) cont.....

Bacteria	Nanoparticle	Plant	Dose	Time	Inference	References
S. aureus and *E. coli*	Gold nanoparticle	*Mangifera indica*	2.5 µL	24 hrs	Significant growth inhibition was seen for both *E. coli* and *S. aureus*	[61]

Stem bark extract from *Ficus krishnae* was used for the synthesis of silver nanoparticles. The extract was tested against various organisms, including *Salmonella typhimurium* (MTCC98), *Escherichia coli* (MTCC 45), and *Staphylococcus aureus* (ATTC 29122). These silver nanoparticles penetrate the cell membrane and interact with proteins that contain sulfur and with DNA. They target the respiratory chain, and finally, cell division leading to cell death. These nanoparticles release silver ions that enhance the bactericidal activity [106, 107]. The best activity was exhibited by *Staphylococcus aureus* with a zone of inhibition of 12mm with 6mm of the extract followed by *Salmonella typhimurium* and *Escherichia coli* with a zone of inhibition of 13mm and 18mm, respectively.

Gold Nanoparticles

Gold nanoparticles are one of the nano-scaled metallic nanoparticles that have been widely studied because of their tunable surface plasmon resonance (SPR), electronic properties, and optical properties. They are widely used in biomedical sciences that include tumor imaging, photothermal therapy, drug delivery, and bio-labeling [68]. The antibacterial activity of biosynthesized *Nigella arvensis* gold nanoparticles was tested against gram-positive bacterial strains consisting of *Staphylococcus epidermidis* (ATCC 12228), *Pseudomonas aeruginosa* (ATCC27253), *Escherichia coli* (ATCC 25922), *Staphylococcus aureus* (ATCC 43300), *Serratia marcescens* (ATCC 13880), and *Bacillus subtilis* (ATCC 6633). The zone of inhibition was calculated through a well diffusion method along with minimum inhibitory concentration. The best activity was exhibited by *Staphylococcus epidermidis* with a full zone of inhibition at 250 µg/mL of the extract. The mechanism of action of the gold nanoparticles involves binding to the cell membrane and causing conformational changes disrupting the cell membrane leading to degradation and finally cell death. Inside the bacterial cell, they bind to the genetic material of the bacteria and inhibit transcription and translation, leading to growth inhibition and cellular damage [108, 109].

Oxide Nanoparticles

Even ZnO have shown antibacterial properties against *E. coli, P. aeruginosa and S. aureus;* the results obtained were impressive. The particle size ranged from 100-800nm among all three bacteria; better results were obtained against *S.*

aureus. This paves the way for the use of ZnO nanoparticle against skin pathogens. The optimum concentration of 6 mM showed better MIC value against bacteria [110].

The antimicrobial properties of CuO NPs were studied using *Escherichia coli* ATCC 25922 and *Staphylococcus aureus* ATCC 43300 as multidrug-resistant (MDR) bacteria. The anti-bacterial activities of CuO nanoparticles were concluded based on the diameter of the inhibition zone in disk diffusion tests of NPs. The antibacterial effect on *E.coli* 33±0.57 and 6±2 mm, as well as *S. aureus*, shows no growth signs [111].

The antibacterial activity of TiO_2 was studied against *Escherichia coli* (*E. coli*) in an actual food packaging application test under various conditions, including types of light (fluorescent and ultraviolet (UV)) and the length of time the film was exposed to light. The antibacterial activity of TiO_2 was evaluated through two types of experiments under UV irradiation: (I) in a slurry with physiological water (stirred suspension); and (II) in a drop deposited on a glass plate, the significant effect of the nature of the suspension on the photocatalytic disinfection ability was highlighted. The results exhibited significant antibacterial activities after 2 h and 4 h. It is suggested that improving the formulation would increase its efficiency [112].

MEDICINAL APPLICATION

In the preview of human welfare, nanotechnology has a huge role to contribute; a few are illustrated in Table **5** below.

Table 5. Medicinal applications of metal and metal oxide nanoparticles.

Nanoparticles	Plant	Activity	Dose	References
Silver	*Tropaeolum majus*	Anticancer	156 µg/mL -IC_{50}	[80]
Zinc Oxide	*Ziziphus nummularia*	In vitro cytotoxic	200 µg/mL	[124]
Zinc Oxide	*Trianthema Portulacastrum*	Anti-oxidant	500 µg/mL	[88]
Zinc Oxide	*Caulerpa peltate*	Anti-biofilm	-	[125]
Gold	*Terminaliachebula*	Anti-filarial	LC_{50} – 38 µg/mL	[86]
Copper Oxide	*Cissus quadrangularis*	Antifungal	500 ppm	[126]
Silver	*Alternanthera sessilis*	Antioxidant	IC_{50} – 300.6 µg/mL	[127]
Carbon	-	Enhances susceptibility to seizures	-	[128]

Nanoparticles	Plant	Activity	Dose	References
Gold (fluorescent)	-	Growth factor expression study in colorectal cancer	-	[129]
Bimetallic – Silver Platinum nanoparticles	-	Osteopromotive anti-microbial	-	[130]

FUTURE PROSPECTS AND CONCLUSION

Nanotechnology has influenced the world with its uniqueness and applicability but there is still a long way to go to achieve the goal of its applicability [131, 132]. The future of nanotechnology and green synthesis is not very much evident. There are many questions to be answered; the problems need to be assessed and solved at every step of the process. Questions on synthesis majorly lie in the production of metallic nanoparticles (Fig. **3**). There are a lot of plants and microbes from which nanoparticles are being extracted, but the effective ones are not quantified. The stability of nanoparticles is to be explored more. There is a need for understanding the amount of the extract required , what happens when up-scaled, which is the best-suited solvent, which of the nanoparticle shows the better result, and what is the efficacy of the extract?

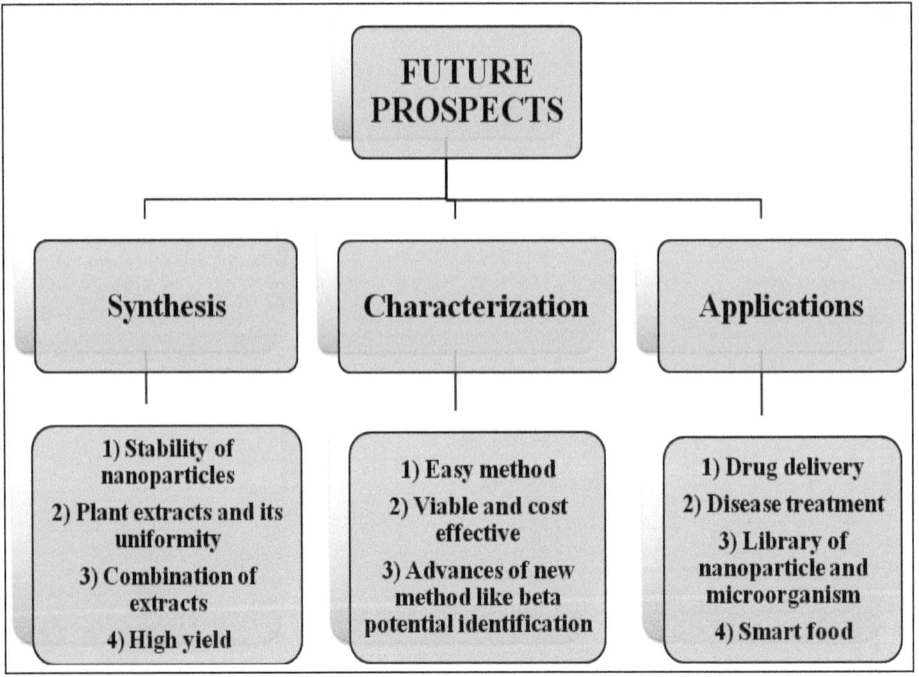

Fig. (3). Prospects of metal and metal oxide green synthesis derived nanoparticle.

These questions pave the way for a better synthesis procedure. The next question is about the characterization of the nanoparticles. The instrumentation involved is tedious and time taking which adds on to the cost and labor. Hence there is a need for better and faster characterization of the nanoparticle. This will reduce the cost and will devote more time to the application of it. The next question is the nanoparticle, and its application; nanoparticles are extracted from various plant and microbial sources. This has been applied to various microbes and disease systems. But the effort should be made to bring out a combination of nanoparticles for a better understanding of the system and as well as its effectiveness. Rather than using various extractions, effort has to be made for a single source and multiple applications.

CONSENT FOR PUBLICATION

Not applicable.

CONFLICT OF INTEREST

The authors declare that no conflict of interest.

ACKNOWLEDGEMENTS

All the authors are thankful to Dr. Shaukath Ara Khanum, Department of Chemistry, Yuvaraja College, University of Mysore, Mysore for the long-term collaboration in understanding the biology of phytochemical molecules. Mr. Pankaj Satapathy would like to thank DST-KSTePS, GoK, for providing DST Ph.D. fellowship (LIF-09-2018-19). Ms. Aishwarya. T. Devi would like to thank the Indian Council of Medical Research (ICMR) for the award of Senior Research Fellow (SRF) Award Letter Number - File no.5/3/8/55/ITR-F/2018-ITR dated 11.6.2018. All authors thank the Hon'ble Vice-Chancellor, JSS Science and Technology University, Principal, SJCE, Mysore for his encouragement and JSS research foundation for their constant inspiration. Mr. Avinash MG would like to thank the Indian Council of Medical Research (ICMR) for the award of Senior Research Fellow (SRF) Award Letter Number - File no. AMR/Fellowship/17/2019 ECD-II dated 28.6.2019. FZ sincerely acknowledges the University Grants Commission (UGC), Govt. of India, New Delhi, for awarding Raman Post-Doctoral Fellowship 2014-15 to USA (Ref No. F.5-97/2014 (IC) FD dairy no: 6725). Further, we extend our gratitude towards the management and office bearers of Dayananda Sagar University, Bengaluru, Karnataka, India, for constant inspiration, motivation, and encouragement to pursue scientific research.

REFERENCES

[1]   Stober W, Fink A, Bohn EJ. Controlled growth of monodisperse silica spheres in the micron size range. J Colloid Interface Sci 1968; 26(1): 62-9.

[2]   Zameer F, Gopal S, Krohne G, Kreft J. Development of a biofilm model for *Listeria monocytogenes.* World J Microbiol Biotechnol 2009; 26(6): 1143-7.
[http://dx.doi.org/10.1007/s11274-009-0271-4]

[3]   Gericke M, Pinches A. Microbial production of gold nanoparticles. Gold Bull 2006; 39(1): 22-8.
[http://dx.doi.org/10.1007/BF03215529]

[4]   Iravani S. Bacteria in nanoparticle synthesis: current status and future prospects. Int Sch Res Notices 2014; 2014: 359316.
[http://dx.doi.org/10.1155/2014/359316] [PMID: 27355054]

[5]   Thakkar KN, Mhatre SS, Parikh RY. Biological synthesis of metallic nanoparticles. Nanomedicine (Lond) 2010; 6(2): 257-62.
[http://dx.doi.org/10.1016/j.nano.2009.07.002] [PMID: 19616126]

[6]   Chen YL, Tuan HY, Tien CW, Lo WH, Liang HC, Hu YC. Augmented biosynthesis of cadmium sulfide nanoparticles by genetically engineered *Escherichia coli.* Biotechnol Prog 2009; 25(5): 1260-6.
[http://dx.doi.org/10.1002/btpr.199] [PMID: 19630084]

[7]   Mohanpuria P, Rana NK, Yadav SK. Biosynthesis of nanoparticles: technological concepts and future applications. J Nanopart Res 2008; 10(3): 507-17.
[http://dx.doi.org/10.1007/s11051-007-9275-x]

[8]   Narayanan KB, Sakthivel N. Synthesis and characterization of nano-gold composite using *Cylindrocladium floridanum* and its heterogeneous catalysis in the degradation of 4-nitrophenol. J Hazard Mater 2011; 189(1-2): 519-25.
[http://dx.doi.org/10.1016/j.jhazmat.2011.02.069] [PMID: 21420237]

[9]   Prasad Ashwini, Baker Syed. Phytogenic synthesis of silver nanobactericides for antibiofilm activity against human pathogen H pylori 2019; 1(4): 341-7.

[10]   Anastas PT. JC Warner Green Chemistry. Theory Pract 1998.

[11]   Gnanasangeetha D, Thambavani DS. Biogenic production of zinc oxide nanoparticles using *Acalypha indica.* J Chem Biol Phys Sci 2013; 4(1): 238.

[12]   Gunalan S, Sivaraj R, Rajendran V. Green synthesized ZnO nanoparticles against bacterial and fungal pathogens. Progress in Natural Science: Materials International 2012; 22(6): 693-700.
[http://dx.doi.org/10.1016/j.pnsc.2012.11.015]

[13]   Shanker U, Jassal V, Rani M, Kaith BS. Towards green synthesis of nanoparticles: from bio-assisted sources to benign solvents. A review. Int J Environ Anal Chem 2016; 96(9): 801-35.

[14]   Sylvestre JP, Poulin S, Kabashin AV, Sacher E, Meunier M, Luong JH. Surface chemistry of gold nanoparticles produced by laser ablation in aqueous media. J Phys Chem B 2004; 108(43): 16864-9.
[http://dx.doi.org/10.1021/jp047134+]

[15]   Bouquillon S, Courant T, Dean D, *et al.* Biodegradable ionic liquids: selected synthetic applications. Aust J Chem 2007; 60(11): 843-7.
[http://dx.doi.org/10.1071/CH07257]

[16]   Wittmann K, Wisniewski W, Mynott R, *et al.* Supercritical carbon dioxide as solvent and temporary protecting group for rhodium-catalyzed hydroaminomethylation. Chemistry 2001; 7(21): 4584-9.
[http://dx.doi.org/10.1002/1521-3765(20011105)7:21<4584::AID-CHEM4584>3.0.CO;2-P] [PMID: 11757649]

[17]   Pollet P, Eckert CA, Liotta CL. Solvents for sustainable chemical processes. WIT Trans Ecol Environ 2011; 154: 21-31.
[http://dx.doi.org/10.2495/CHEM110031]

[18]   Sneha K. Sathish kumar M, Mao J, Kwak IS, Yun YS. *Corynebacterium glutamicum*-mediated crystallization of silver ions through sorption and reduction processes. Chem Eng J 2010; 162(3): 989-96.
[http://dx.doi.org/10.1016/j.cej.2010.07.006]

[19]   Zameer F, Kreft J, Gopal S. Interaction of the dual species biofilms of *Listeria monocytogenes* and *Staphylococcus epidermidis*. J Food Saf 2010; 30(4): 954-68.
[http://dx.doi.org/10.1111/j.1745-4565.2010.00254.x]

[20]   Mittal AK, Chisti Y, Banerjee UC. Synthesis of metallic nanoparticles using plant extracts. Biotechnol Adv 2013; 31(2): 346-56.
[http://dx.doi.org/10.1016/j.biotechadv.2013.01.003] [PMID: 23318667]

[21]   Dwivedi AD, Gopal K. Biosynthesis of silver and gold nanoparticles using *Chenopodium album* leaf extract. Colloids Surf A Physicochem Eng Asp 2010; 369(1-3): 27-33.
[http://dx.doi.org/10.1016/j.colsurfa.2010.07.020]

[22]   Jha AK, Prasad K, Kumar V, Prasad K. Biosynthesis of silver nanoparticles using Eclipta leaf. Biotechnol Prog 2009; 25(5): 1476-9.
[http://dx.doi.org/10.1002/btpr.233] [PMID: 19725113]

[23]   Meghashri. S, Chauhan. JB, Syed. AA and Farhan Zameer. Effect of *Ocimum tenuiflorum* leaf extract against infective endocarditis. Int J Phytomed 2011; 3(4): 470-4.

[24]   Prathna TC, Chandrasekaran N, Raichur AM, Mukherjee A. Biomimetic synthesis of silver nanoparticles by *Citrus limon* (lemon) aqueous extract and theoretical prediction of particle size. Colloids Surf B Biointerfaces 2011; 82(1): 152-9.
[http://dx.doi.org/10.1016/j.colsurfb.2010.08.036] [PMID: 20833002]

[25]   Panigrahi S, Kundu S, Ghosh S, Nath S, Pal T. General method of synthesis for metal nanoparticles. J Nanopart Res 2004; 6(4): 411-4.
[http://dx.doi.org/10.1007/s11051-004-6575-2]

[26]   Ashwini P, Sumana MN, Shilpa U, *et al.* Farhan Zameer, Nagendra Prasad M.N. A review on *Helicobacter pylori*: its biology, complications and management. Int J Pharm Pharm Sci 2014; 7(1): 14-20.

[27]   Tan YN, Lee JY, Wang DI. Uncovering the design rules for peptide synthesis of metal nanoparticles. J Am Chem Soc 2010; 132(16): 5677-86.
[http://dx.doi.org/10.1021/ja907454f] [PMID: 20355728]

[28]   Singh J, Dutta T, Kim K-H, Rawat M, Samddar P, Kumar P. 'Green' synthesis of metals and their oxide nanoparticles: applications for environmental remediation. J Nanobiotechnology 2018; 16(1): 84.
[http://dx.doi.org/10.1186/s12951-018-0408-4] [PMID: 30373622]

[29]   Zameer F, Rukmangada MS, Chauhan JB, *et al.* Evaluation of adhesive and anti-adhesive properties of *Pseudomonas aeruginosa* biofilms and its inhibition by herbal plants. Iran J Microbiol 2016; 8(2): 108-19.
[PMID: 27307976]

[30]   Shivaji S, Madhu S, Singh S. Extracellular synthesis of antibacterial silver nanoparticles using psychrophilic bacteria. Process Biochem 2011; 46: 1800-7.
[http://dx.doi.org/10.1016/j.procbio.2011.06.008]

[31]   Wen L, Lin Z, Gu P, *et al.* Extracellular biosynthesis of monodispersed gold nanoparticles by a SAM capping route. J Nanopart Res 2009; 11(2): 279-88.
[http://dx.doi.org/10.1007/s11051-008-9378-z]

[32]   Lengke MF, Fleet ME, Southam G. Morphology of gold nanoparticles synthesized by filamentous cyanobacteria from gold(I)-thiosulfate and gold(III)--chloride complexes. Langmuir 2006; 22(6): 2780-7.

[http://dx.doi.org/10.1021/la052652c] [PMID: 16519482]

[33]   Philipse AP, Maas D. Magnetic colloids from magnetotactic bacteria: chain formation and colloidal stability. Langmuir 2002; 18(25): 9977-84.
[http://dx.doi.org/10.1021/la0205811]

[34]   Mann S. Structure, morphology, and crystal growth of bacterial magnetite.Magnetite biomineralization and magnetoreception in organisms. Boston, MA: Springer 1985; pp. 311-32.
[http://dx.doi.org/10.1007/978-1-4613-0313-8_15]

[35]   Holmes JD, Smith PR, Evans-Gowing R, Richardson DJ, Russell DA, Sodeau JR. Energy-dispersive X-ray analysis of the extracellular cadmium sulfide crystallites of *Klebsiella aerogenes.* Arch Microbiol 1995; 163(2): 143-7.
[http://dx.doi.org/10.1007/BF00381789] [PMID: 7710328]

[36]   Beulah KC, Aishwarya T. Devi, Waseem K, Meghashri S, Hedgekatte R, Nagendra Prasad MN, Dhananjaya BL, Zameer F. Phyto-Antiquorumones: An Herbal Approach for Blocking Bacterial Trafficking and Pathogenesis. Int J Pharm Pharm Sci 2015; 7(1): 29-34.

[37]   Ravindra BK, Rajasab AH. A comparative study on biosynthesis of silver nanoparticles using four different fungal species. Int J Pharm 2014; 6(1): 372-6.

[38]   Soni N, Prakash S. Fungal-mediated nano silver: an effective adulticide against mosquito. Parasitol Res 2012; 111(5): 2091-8.
[http://dx.doi.org/10.1007/s00436-012-3056-x] [PMID: 22864863]

[39]   Molnár Z, Bódai V, Szakacs G, *et al.* Green synthesis of gold nanoparticles by thermophilic filamentous fungi. Sci Rep 2018; 8(1): 3943.
[http://dx.doi.org/10.1038/s41598-018-22112-3] [PMID: 29500365]

[40]   Ahmad A, Senapati S, Khan MI, Kumar R, Sastry M. Extra-/intracellular biosynthesis of gold nanoparticles by an alkalotolerant fungus, Trichothecium sp. J Biomed Nanotechnol 2005; 1(1): 47-53.
[http://dx.doi.org/10.1166/jbn.2005.012]

[41]   Raliya R, Tarafdar JC. Biosynthesis and characterization of zinc, magnesium and titanium nanoparticles: an eco-friendly approach. Int Nano Lett 2014; 4(1): 93.
[http://dx.doi.org/10.1007/s40089-014-0093-8]

[42]   Raliya R, Biswas P, Tarafdar JC. TiO_2 nanoparticle biosynthesis and its physiological effect on mung bean (*Vigna radiata* L.). Biotechnol Rep (Amst) 2014; 5: 22-6.
[http://dx.doi.org/10.1016/j.btre.2014.10.009] [PMID: 28626678]

[43]   Kowshik M, Ashtaputre S, Kharrazi S, *et al.* Extracellular synthesis of silver nanoparticles by a silver-tolerant yeast strain MKY3. Nanotechnology 2002; 14(1): 95.
[http://dx.doi.org/10.1088/0957-4484/14/1/321]

[44]   Mourato A, Gadanho M, Lino AR, Tenreiro R. Biosynthesis of crystalline silver and gold nanoparticles by extremophilic yeasts. Bioinorg Chem Appl 2011; 2011: 546074.
[http://dx.doi.org/10.1155/2011/546074] [PMID: 21912532]

[45]   Haverkamp RG, Marshall AT. The mechanism of metal nanoparticle formation in plants: limits on accumulation. J Nanopart Res 2009; 11(6): 1453-63.
[http://dx.doi.org/10.1007/s11051-008-9533-6]

[46]   Mude N, Ingle A, Gade A, Rai M. Synthesis of silver nanoparticles using callus extract of *Carica papaya*-a first report. J Plant Biochem Biotechnol 2009; 18(1): 83-6.
[http://dx.doi.org/10.1007/BF03263300]

[47]   Najimu Nisha S, Aysha OS, Syed Nasar Rahaman J, *et al.* Lemon peels mediated synthesis of silver nanoparticles and its antidermatophytic activity. Spectrochim Acta A Mol Biomol Spectrosc 2014; 124: 194-8.
[http://dx.doi.org/10.1016/j.saa.2013.12.019] [PMID: 24486863]

[48]   Jha AK, Prasad K. Green synthesis of silver nanoparticles using Cycas leaf. International Journal of Green Nanotechnology: Physics and Chemistry 2010; 1(2): 110-7.
[http://dx.doi.org/10.1080/19430871003684572]

[49]   Ravindra S, Mohan YM, Reddy NN, Raju KM. Fabrication of antibacterial cotton fibres loaded with silver nanoparticles via "Green Approach". Colloids Surf A Physicochem Eng Asp 2010; 367(1-3): 31-40.
[http://dx.doi.org/10.1016/j.colsurfa.2010.06.013]

[50]   Armendariz V, Herrera I, Jose-yacaman M, Troiani H, Santiago P, Gardea-Torresdey JL. Size controlled gold nanoparticle formation by *Avena sativa* biomass: use of plants in nanobiotechnology. J Nanopart Res 2004; 6(4): 377-82.
[http://dx.doi.org/10.1007/s11051-004-0741-4]

[51]   Narayanan KB, Sakthivel N. Coriander leaf mediated biosynthesis of gold nanoparticles. Mater Lett 2008; 62(30): 4588-90.
[http://dx.doi.org/10.1016/j.matlet.2008.08.044]

[52]   Shankar SS, Rai A, Ahmad A, Sastry M. Controlling the optical properties of lemongrass extract synthesized gold nanotriangles and potential application in infrared-absorbing optical coatings. Chem Mater 2005; 17(3): 566-72.
[http://dx.doi.org/10.1021/cm048292g]

[53]   Raghunandan D, Bedre MD, Basavaraja S, Sawle B, Manjunath SY, Venkataraman A. Rapid biosynthesis of irregular shaped gold nanoparticles from macerated aqueous extracellular dried clove buds (*Syzygium aromaticum*) solution. Colloids Surf B Biointerfaces 2010; 79(1): 235-40.
[http://dx.doi.org/10.1016/j.colsurfb.2010.04.003] [PMID: 20451362]

[54]   Gardea-Torresdey JL, Gomez E, Peralta-Videa JR, Parsons JG, Troiani H, Jose-Yacaman M. *Alfalfa* sprouts: a natural source for the synthesis of silver nanoparticles. Langmuir 2003; 19(4): 1357-61.
[http://dx.doi.org/10.1021/la020835i]

[55]   Qu J, Luo C, Hou J. Synthesis of ZnO nanoparticles from Zn-hyperaccumulator (*Sedum alfredii* Hance) plants. Micro & Nano Lett 2011; 6(3): 174-6.
[http://dx.doi.org/10.1049/mnl.2011.0004]

[56]   Jia L, Zhang Q, Li Q, Song H. The biosynthesis of palladium nanoparticles by antioxidants in *Gardenia jasminoides* Ellis: long lifetime nanocatalysts for p-nitrotoluene hydrogenation. Nanotechnology 2009; 20(38): 385601.
[http://dx.doi.org/10.1088/0957-4484/20/38/385601] [PMID: 19713585]

[57]   Nagendraswamy G, Lakshmi RV, Bushra BA, *et al.* Extraction and evaluation of antimicrobial and antiviral efficacy of *Terminalia Bellirica* fruits. Indo Am j pharm 2013; 3(2): 4262-8.

[58]   Williams DB, Carter CB. The transmission electron microscope.Transmission electron microscopy. Boston, MA: Springer 1996; pp. 3-17.
[http://dx.doi.org/10.1007/978-1-4757-2519-3_1]

[59]   Sulthana R, Taqui SN, Zameer F, Syed UT, Syed AA. Adsorption of ethidium bromide from aqueous solution onto nutraceutical industrial fennel seed spent: Kinetics and thermodynamics modeling studies. Int J Phytoremediation 2018; 20(11): 1075-86.
[http://dx.doi.org/10.1080/15226514.2017.1365331] [PMID: 30156921]

[60]   Prasad Ashwini, Devi Aishwarya Tripurasundari. Phyto-Antibiofilm elicitors as potential inhibitors of *Helicobacter pylori* 3Biotech 2019; 9(53): 1-9.

[61]   Vimalraj S, Ashokkumar T, Saravanan S. Biogenic gold nanoparticles synthesis mediated by Mangifera indica seed aqueous extracts exhibits antibacterial, anticancer and anti-angiogenic properties. Biomed Pharmacother 2018; 105: 440-8.
[http://dx.doi.org/10.1016/j.biopha.2018.05.151] [PMID: 29879628]

[62]   Mirza AU, Kareem A, Nami SAA, *et al.* Biogenic synthesis of iron oxide nanoparticles using *Agrewia*

optiva and *Prunus persica phyto* species: Characterization, antibacterial and antioxidant activity. J Photochem Photobiol B 2018; 185: 262-74.
[http://dx.doi.org/10.1016/j.jphotobiol.2018.06.009] [PMID: 29981488]

[63] Vijayakumar S, Krishnakumar C, Arulmozhi P, Mahadevan S, Parameswari N. Biosynthesis, characterization and antimicrobial activities of zinc oxide nanoparticles from leaf extract of *Glycosmis pentaphylla* (Retz.) DC. Microb Pathog 2018; 116: 44-8.
[http://dx.doi.org/10.1016/j.micpath.2018.01.003] [PMID: 29330059]

[64] Kesharwani J, Yoon KY, Hwang J, Rai M. Phytofabrication of silver nanoparticles by leaf extract of Datura metel: hypothetical mechanism involved in synthesis. J Bionanosci 2009; 3: 39-44.
[http://dx.doi.org/10.1166/jbns.2009.1008]

[65] Nakkala JR, Mata R, Gupta AK, Sadras SR. Biological activities of green silver nanoparticles synthesized with *Acorous calamus* rhizome extract. Eur J Med Chem 2014; 85: 784-94.
[http://dx.doi.org/10.1016/j.ejmech.2014.08.024] [PMID: 25147142]

[66] Suna Q, Cai X, Li J, Zheng M, Chenb Z, Yu CP. Green synthesis of silver nanoparticles using tea leaf extract and evaluation of their stability and antibacterial activity. Colloids Surf A Physicochem Eng Asp 2014; 444: 226-31.
[http://dx.doi.org/10.1016/j.colsurfa.2013.12.065]

[67] Mariselvam R, Ranjitsingh AJA, Usha Raja Nanthini A, Kalirajan K, Padmalatha C, Mosae Selvakumar P. Green synthesis of silver nanoparticles from the extract of the inflorescence of *Cocos nucifera* (Family: Arecaceae) for enhanced antibacterial activity. Spectrochim Acta A Mol Biomol Spectrosc 2014; 129: 537-41.
[http://dx.doi.org/10.1016/j.saa.2014.03.066] [PMID: 24762541]

[68] Rajakumar G, Abdul Rahuman A. Larvicidal activity of synthesized silver nanoparticles using Eclipta prostrata leaf extract against filariasis and malaria vectors. Acta Trop 2011; 118(3): 196-203.

[69] Yang N. WeiHong L, Hao L. Biosynthesis of Au nanoparticles using agricultural waste mango peel extract and its *in vitro* cytotoxic effect on two normal cells. Mater Lett 2014; 134: 67-70.
[http://dx.doi.org/10.1016/j.matlet.2014.07.025]

[70] Tamuly C, Hazarika M, Bordoloi M. Biosynthesis of Au nanoparticles by *Gymnocladus assamicus* and its catalytic activity. Mater Lett 2013; 108: 276-9.
[http://dx.doi.org/10.1016/j.matlet.2013.07.020]

[71] Tahir K, Nazir S, Li B, *et al. Nerium oleander* leaves extract mediated synthesis of gold nanoparticles and its antioxidant activity. Mater Lett 2015; 156: 198-201.
[http://dx.doi.org/10.1016/j.matlet.2015.05.062]

[72] Muthuvel A, Adavallan K, Balamurugan K, Krishnakumar N. Biosynthesis of gold nanoparticles using *Solanum nigrum* leaf extract and screening their free radical scavenging and antibacterial properties. Biomedicine & Preventive Nutrition 2014; 4(2): 325-32.
[http://dx.doi.org/10.1016/j.bionut.2014.03.004]

[73] Abdel-Raouf N, Al-Enazi NM, Ibraheem IB. Green biosynthesis of gold nanoparticles using *Galaxaura elongata* and characterization of their antibacterial activity. Arab J Chem 2017; 10: S3029-39.
[http://dx.doi.org/10.1016/j.arabjc.2013.11.044]

[74] Das J, Velusamy P. Catalytic reduction of methylene blue using biogenic gold nanoparticles from *Sesbania grandiflora* L. Journal of the Taiwan Institute of Chemical Engineers 2014; 45(5): 2280-5.
[http://dx.doi.org/10.1016/j.jtice.2014.04.005]

[75] Madhumitha G, Rajakumar G, Roopan SM, *et al.* Acaricidal, insecticidal, and larvicidal efficacy of fruit peel aqueous extract of *Annona squamosa* and its compounds against blood-feeding parasites. Parasitol Res 2012; 111(5): 2189-99.
[http://dx.doi.org/10.1007/s00436-011-2671-2] [PMID: 22006187]

[76]   Zhu X, Pathakoti K, Hwang HM. Green synthesis of titanium dioxide and zinc oxide nanoparticles and their usage for antimicrobial applications and environmental remediation. In: Shukla AK, Iravani S, Eds. Green Synthesis, Characterization and Applications of Nanoparticles. Elsevier 2019; pp. 223-63.
[http://dx.doi.org/10.1016/B978-0-08-102579-6.00010-1]

[77]   Marimuthu S, Rahuman AA, Jayaseelan C, *et al.* Acaricidal activity of synthesized titanium dioxide nanoparticles using Calotropis gigantea against Rhipicephalus microplus and Haemaphysalis bispinosa. Asian Pac J Trop Med 2013; 6(9): 682-8.
[http://dx.doi.org/10.1016/S1995-7645(13)60118-2] [PMID: 23827143]

[78]   Velayutham K, Rahuman AA, Rajakumar G, *et al.* Evaluation of *Catharanthus roseus* leaf extract-mediated biosynthesis of titanium dioxide nanoparticles against *Hippobosca maculata* and *Bovicola ovis*. Parasitol Res 2012; 111(6): 2329-37.
[http://dx.doi.org/10.1007/s00436-011-2676-x] [PMID: 21987105]

[79]   Nasrollahzadeh M, Atarod M, Sajjadi M, Sajadi SM, Issaabadi Z. Plant-mediated green synthesis of nanostructures: mechanisms, characterization, and applications. Interface Science and Technology. Elsevier 2019; 28: pp. 199-322.

[80]   Valsalam S, Agastian P, Arasu MV, *et al.* Rapid biosynthesis and characterization of silver nanoparticles from the leaf extract of *Tropaeolum majus* L. and its enhanced *in-vitro* antibacterial, antifungal, antioxidant and anticancer properties. J Photochem Photobiol B 2019; 191: 65-74.
[http://dx.doi.org/10.1016/j.jphotobiol.2018.12.010] [PMID: 30594044]

[81]   Medda S, Hajra A, Dey U, Bose P, Mondal NK. Biosynthesis of silver nanoparticles from *Aloe vera* leaf extract and antifungal activity against *Rhizopus* sp. and *Aspergillus* sp. Appl Nanosci 2015; 5(7): 875-80.
[http://dx.doi.org/10.1007/s13204-014-0387-1]

[82]   Das J, Velusamy P. Biogenic synthesis of antifungal silver nanoparticles using aqueous stem extract of banana. Nano Biomed Eng 2013; 5(1): 34-8.
[http://dx.doi.org/10.5101/nbe.v5i1.p34-38]

[83]   Vivek M, Kumar PS, Steffi S, Sudha S. Biogenic silver nanoparticles by *Gelidiella acerosa* extract and their antifungal effects. Avicenna J Med Biotechnol 2011; 3(3): 143-8.
[PMID: 23408653]

[84]   Rout Y, Behera S, Ojha AK, Nayak PL. Green synthesis of silver nanoparticles using *Ocimum sanctum* (Tulashi) and study of their antibacterial and antifungal activities. J Microbiol Antimicrob 2012; 4(6): 103-9.
[http://dx.doi.org/10.5897/JMA11.060]

[85]   Jayaseelan C, Ramkumar R, Rahuman AA, Perumal P. Green synthesis of gold nanoparticles using seed aqueous extract of *Abelmoschus esculentus* and its antifungal activity. Ind Crops Prod 2013; 45: 423-9.
[http://dx.doi.org/10.1016/j.indcrop.2012.12.019]

[86]   Roy P, Saha SK, Gayen P, Chowdhury P, Santi P. Sinha Babu. Exploration of ant filarial activity of gold nanoparticle against human and bovine filarial parasites: A nanomedicinal mechanistic approach. Colloids Surf B Biointerfaces 2017; 7765(17): 30707-5.

[87]   Devipriya D, Roopan SM. *Cissus quadrangularis* mediated ecofriendly synthesis of copper oxide nanoparticles and its antifungal studies against *Aspergillus niger, Aspergillus flavus*. Mater Sci Eng C 2017; 80: 38-44.
[http://dx.doi.org/10.1016/j.msec.2017.05.130] [PMID: 28866178]

[88]   Khan ZUH, Sadiq HM, Shah NS, *et al.* Greener synthesis of zinc oxide nanoparticles using *Trianthema portulacastrum* extract and evaluation of its photocatalytic and biological applications. J Photochem Photobiol B 2019; 192: 147-57.
[http://dx.doi.org/10.1016/j.jphotobiol.2019.01.013] [PMID: 30738346]

[89]   Nabikhan A, Kandasamy K, Raj A, Alikunhi NM. Synthesis of antimicrobial silver nanoparticles by callus and leaf extracts from saltmarsh plant, *Sesuvium portulacastrum* L. Colloids Surf B Biointerfaces 2010; 79(2): 488-93.
[http://dx.doi.org/10.1016/j.colsurfb.2010.05.018] [PMID: 20627485]

[90]   Khatami M, Pourseyedi S, Khatami M, Hamidi H, Zaeifi M, Soltani L. Synthesis of silver nanoparticles using seed exudates of *Sinapis arvensis* as a novel bioresource, and evaluation of their antifungal activity. Bioresour Bioprocess 2015; 2(1): 19.
[http://dx.doi.org/10.1186/s40643-015-0043-y]

[91]   Kumari A, Kumar V, Yadav SK. The Use of Syzygium cumini in Nanotechnology In the Genus Syzygium. CRC Press 2017; pp. 171-94.
[http://dx.doi.org/10.1201/9781315118772-10]

[92]   Bhau BS, Ghosh S, Puri S, Borah B, Sarmah DK, Khan R. Green synthesis of gold nanoparticles from the leaf extract of *Nepenthes khasiana* and antimicrobial assay. Adv Mater Lett 2015; 6(1): 55-8.
[http://dx.doi.org/10.5185/amlett.2015.5609]

[93]   Janaki AC, Sailatha E, Gunasekaran S. Synthesis, characteristics and antimicrobial activity of ZnO nanoparticles. Spectrochim Acta A Mol Biomol Spectrosc 2015; 144: 17-22.
[http://dx.doi.org/10.1016/j.saa.2015.02.041] [PMID: 25748589]

[94]   Senthil kumar SR, Sivakumar T. Green tea (*Camellia sinensis*) mediated synthesis of zinc oxide (ZnO) nanoparticles and studies on their antimicrobial activities. Int J Pharm Pharm Sci 2014; 6(6): 461-5.

[95]   Sivaraj R, Rahman PK, Rajiv P, Narendhran S, Venckatesh R. Biosynthesis and characterization of *Acalypha indica* mediated copper oxide nanoparticles and evaluation of its antimicrobial and anticancer activity. Spectrochim Acta A Mol Biomol Spectrosc 2014; 129: 255-8.
[http://dx.doi.org/10.1016/j.saa.2014.03.027] [PMID: 24747845]

[96]   Shende S, Ingle AP, Gade A, Rai M. Green synthesis of copper nanoparticles by *Citrus medica* Linn. (Idilimbu) juice and its antimicrobial activity. World J Microbiol Biotechnol 2015; 31(6): 865-73.
[http://dx.doi.org/10.1007/s11274-015-1840-3] [PMID: 25761857]

[97]   Cassir N, Rolain JM, Brouqui P. A new strategy to fight antimicrobial resistance: the revival of old antibiotics. Front Microbiol 2014; 5: 551.
[http://dx.doi.org/10.3389/fmicb.2014.00551] [PMID: 25368610]

[98]   Rai M, Yadav A, Gade A. Silver nanoparticles as a new generation of antimicrobials. Biotechnol Adv 2009; 27(1): 76-83.
[http://dx.doi.org/10.1016/j.biotechadv.2008.09.002] [PMID: 18854209]

[99]   Srikar SK, Giri DD, Pal DB, Mishra PK, Upadhyay SN. Green synthesis of silver nanoparticles: a review. Green and Sustainable Chemistry 2016; 6(01): 34.
[http://dx.doi.org/10.4236/gsc.2016.61004]

[100] Dehnavi AS, Raisi A, Aroujalian A. Control size and stability of colloidal silver nanoparticles with antibacterial activity prepared by a green synthesis method. Synth React Inorg Met-Org Nano-Met Chem 2013; 43(5): 543-51.
[http://dx.doi.org/10.1080/15533174.2012.741182]

[101] Chanda S. Silver nanoparticles (medicinal plants mediated): a new generation of antimicrobials to combat microbial pathogens–a review Microbial Pathogens and Strategies for Combating Them: Science Technology and Education. Badajoz, Spain: Formatex Research Center 2014; pp. 1314-23.

[102] Ahmed S, Ahmad M, Swami BL, Ikram S. A review on plants extract mediated synthesis of silver nanoparticles for antimicrobial applications: A green expertise. J Adv Res 2016; 7(1): 17-28.
[http://dx.doi.org/10.1016/j.jare.2015.02.007] [PMID: 26843966]

[103] Perni S, Hakala V, Prokopovich P. Biogenic synthesis of antimicrobial silver nanoparticles capped with L-cysteine. Colloids Surf A Physicochem Eng Asp 2014; 460: 219-24.
[http://dx.doi.org/10.1016/j.colsurfa.2013.09.034]

[104] Marambio-Jones C, Hoek EM. A review of the antibacterial effects of silver nanomaterials and potential implications for human health and the environment. J Nanopart Res 2010; 12(5): 1531-51.
[http://dx.doi.org/10.1007/s11051-010-9900-y]

[105] Rajesh kumar S, Bharath LV. Mechanism of plant-mediated synthesis of silver nanoparticles–a review on biomolecules involved, characterization and antibacterial activity. Chem Biol Interact 2017; 273: 219-27.
[http://dx.doi.org/10.1016/j.cbi.2017.06.019] [PMID: 28647323]

[106] Vasanth N, Melchias G, Kumaravel P. Ficus benghalensis mediates synthesis of silver nanoparticles: the green approach yields NPs that are its anti-bacterial and anti-oxidant. World J Pharm Sci 2016; 4(7): 1-12.
[PMID: 27810096]

[107] Amarvani P. Characterization of phyto-nanoparticles from *Ficus krishnae* for their antibacterial and anticancer activities. Drug Dev Ind Pharm 2018; 44(3): 377-84.
[PMID: 29098876]

[108] Srivastava N, Mukhopadhyay M. Biosynthesis and characterization of gold nanoparticles using zooglearamigera and assessment of its antibacterial property. J Cluster Sci 2015; 26(3): 675-92.
[http://dx.doi.org/10.1007/s10876-014-0726-0]

[109] Chahardoli A, Karimi N, Sadeghi F, Fattahi A. Green approach for synthesis of gold nanoparticles from *Nigella arvensis* leaf extract and evaluation of their antibacterial, antioxidant, cytotoxicity and catalytic activities. Artif Cells Nanomed Biotechnol 2018; 46(3): 579-88.
[PMID: 28541741]

[110] Sirelkhatim A, Mahmud S, Seeni A, *et al.* Review on zinc oxide nanoparticles: antibacterial activity and toxicity mechanism. Nano-Micro Lett 2015; 7(3): 219-42.
[http://dx.doi.org/10.1007/s40820-015-0040-x] [PMID: 30464967]

[111] Taran M, Rad M, Alavi M. Antibacterial activity of copper oxide (CuO) nanoparticles biosynthesized by Bacillus sp. FU4: Optimization of experiment design. Pharm Sci 2017; 23(3): 198-206.
[http://dx.doi.org/10.15171/PS.2017.30]

[112] Transcriptome analysis of thiol disulfide redox metabolism genes in *Listeria monocytogenes* in biofilm and planktonic forms. International Journal of Pure and Applied Sciences 2010; 4(1): 21-7.

[113] S S D, M B M, M N SK, *et al.* Antimicrobial, anticoagulant and antiplatelet activities of green synthesized silver nanoparticles using Selaginella (Sanjeevini) plant extract. Int J Biol Macromol 2019; 131: 787-97.
[http://dx.doi.org/10.1016/j.ijbiomac.2019.01.222] [PMID: 30876901]

[114] Vasantharaj S, Sathiyavimal S, Senthilkumar P, LewisOscar F, Pugazhendhi A. Biosynthesis of iron oxide nanoparticles using leaf extract of Ruellia tuberosa: Antimicrobial properties and their applications in photocatalytic degradation. J Photochem Photobiol B 2019; 192: 74-82.
[http://dx.doi.org/10.1016/j.jphotobiol.2018.12.025] [PMID: 30685586]

[115] Allafchian AR, Jalali SA, Aghaei F, Farhang HR. Green synthesis of silver nanoparticles using Glaucium corniculatum (L.) Curtis extract and evaluation of its antibacterial activity IET nanobiotechnology 122018; (5): 8-574.

[116] Das P, Ghosh S, Ghosh R, Dam S, Baskey M. *Madhuca longifolia* plant mediated green synthesis of cupric oxide nanoparticles: A promising environmentally sustainable material for waste water treatment and efficient antibacterial agent. J Photochem Photobiol B 2018; 189: 66-73.
[http://dx.doi.org/10.1016/j.jphotobiol.2018.09.023] [PMID: 30312922]

[117] Umar H, Kavaz D, Rizaner N. Biosynthesis of zinc oxide nanoparticles using *Albizia lebbeck* stem bark, and evaluation of its antimicrobial, antioxidant, and cytotoxic activities on human breast cancer cell lines. Int J Nanomedicine 2018; 14: 87-100.
[http://dx.doi.org/10.2147/IJN.S186888] [PMID: 30587987]

[118] Dada AO, Inyinbor AA, Idu EI, *et al.* Effect of operational parameters, characterization and antibacterial studies of green synthesis of silver nanoparticles using *Tithonia diversifolia.* PeerJ 2018; 6: e5865.
[http://dx.doi.org/10.7717/peerj.5865] [PMID: 30397553]

[119] Shehzad A, Qureshi M, Jabeen S, *et al.* Synthesis, characterization and antibacterial activity of silver nanoparticles using *Rhazya stricta.* PeerJ 2018; 6: e6086.
[http://dx.doi.org/10.7717/peerj.6086] [PMID: 30588401]

[120] Boomi P, Ganesan RM, Poorani G, Gurumallesh Prabu H, Ravikumar S, Jeyakanthan J. Biological synergy of greener gold nanoparticles by using *Coleus aromaticus* leaf extract. Mater Sci Eng C 2019; 99: 202-10.
[http://dx.doi.org/10.1016/j.msec.2019.01.105] [PMID: 30889692]

[121] Castro L, Blazquez ML, Gonzalez F, Munoz JA, Ballester A. Biosynthesis of silver and platinum nanoparticles using orange peel extract: Characterization and applications. IET Nanobiotechnol 2015; 9(5): 252-8.
[http://dx.doi.org/10.1049/iet-nbt.2014.0063]

[122] Babitha N, Priya LS, Christy SR, *et al.* Enhanced Antibacterial Activity and Photo-Catalytic Properties of ZnO Nanoparticles: *Pedalium Murex* Plant Extract-Assisted Synthesis. J Nanosci Nanotechnol 2019; 19(5): 2888-94.
[http://dx.doi.org/10.1166/jnn.2019.16023] [PMID: 30501796]

[123] Hamelian M, Varmira K, Veisi H. Green synthesis and characterizations of gold nanoparticles using Thyme and survey cytotoxic effect, antibacterial and antioxidant potential. J Photochem Photobiol B 2018; 184: 71-9.
[http://dx.doi.org/10.1016/j.jphotobiol.2018.05.016] [PMID: 29842987]

[124] Padalia H, Chanda S. Characterization, antifungal and cytotoxic evaluation of green synthesized zinc oxide nanoparticles using *Ziziphus nummularia* leaf extract. Artif Cells Nanomed Biotechnol 2017; 45(8): 1751-61.
[http://dx.doi.org/10.1080/21691401.2017.1282868] [PMID: 28140658]

[125] Nagarajan S, Arumugam Kuppusamy K. Extracellular synthesis of zinc oxide nanoparticle using seaweeds of gulf of Mannar, India. J Nanobiotechnology 2013; 11(1): 39.
[http://dx.doi.org/10.1186/1477-3155-11-39] [PMID: 24298944]

[126] Devipriya D, Roopan SM. *Cissus quadrangularis* mediated ecofriendly synthesis of copper oxide nanoparticles and its antifungal studies against *Aspergillus niger, Aspergillus flavus.* Mater Sci Eng C 2017; 80: 38-44.
[http://dx.doi.org/10.1016/j.msec.2017.05.130] [PMID: 28866178]

[127] Niraimathi KL, Sudha V, Lavanya R, Brindha P. Biosynthesis of silver nanoparticles using *Alternanthera sessilis* (Linn.) extract and their antimicrobial, antioxidant activities. Colloids Surf B Biointerfaces 2013; 102: 288-91.
[http://dx.doi.org/10.1016/j.colsurfb.2012.08.041] [PMID: 23006568]

[128] He M, Jiang X, Zou Z, *et al.* Exposure to carbon black nanoparticles increases seizure susceptibility in male mice. Nanotoxicology 2020; 14(5): 595-611.
[http://dx.doi.org/10.1080/17435390.2020.1728412] [PMID: 32091294]

[129] Alagaratnam S, Yang SY, Loizidou M, Fuller B, Ramesh B. Mechano-growth factor expression in colorectal cancer investigated with fluorescent gold nanoparticles. Anticancer Res 2019; 39(4): 1705-10.
[http://dx.doi.org/10.21873/anticanres.13276] [PMID: 30952709]

[130] Breisch M, Grasmik V, Loza K, *et al.* Bimetallic silver-platinum nanoparticles with combined osteo-promotive and antimicrobial activity. Nanotechnology 2019; 30(30): 305101.
[http://dx.doi.org/10.1088/1361-6528/ab172b] [PMID: 30959494]

[131] Kounaina K, Deci AT, Patil AG, *et al.* Synthetic gutomics: Deciphering the microbial code for futuristic diagnosis and personalized medicine. In: Satapathy P, Ed. Methods in Microbiology. Elsevier 2018; 46: pp. 197-225.

[132] Chinnaswamy S, Zameer F, Muthuchelian K. Molecular and Biological Mechanisms of Apoptosis and its Detection Techniques. Journal of Oncological Sciences 2020; 6(1): 49-64.

CHAPTER 8

Aptamers as Anti-Infective Agents

Muhammad Ali Syed[1], Nayab Ali[1], Bushra Jamil[2] and Ammar Ahmed[2]

[1] Department of Microbiology, The University of Haripur, Haripur, Pakistan

[2] Department of Medical Laboratory Sciences, University of Lahore, Islamabad campus, Islamabad, Pakistan

Abstract: Rapidly emerging drug resistance in all classes of pathogenic microorganisms has become a challenging task and a global health issue in recent years. There are very limited alternative options available to cure infectious diseases, as the rate of rise in drug resistance in infectious agents is higher than the arrival of new antimicrobial drugs. There is a dire need to look for new types of anti-infective agents, besides looking for new antibiotics. One of the promising types of antimicrobial agents is aptamers, synthesized through systematic evolution of ligands by exponential enrichment (SELEX) technique. Aptamers hold a significant promise for the treatment of various infectious diseases in the future. In the recent past, a number of successful attempts have been made to select and apply aptamers for the detection and binding of infectious agents and their products for therapeutic purposes. This chapter presents a basic introduction to aptamers and their application as anti-infective agents.

Keywords: Aptamers, Antibiotics, Drug Resistance, Infectious Diseases, Systemic Evolution of Ligands by Exponential Enrichment (SELEX).

INTRODUCTION

Infectious diseases have been a major human enemy on the earth, accounting for millions of illnesses and deaths annually [1, 2]. Throughout human history, infectious diseases have been threatening the existence of the human race from extinction by global pandemics of major infectious diseases such as smallpox, typhoid, malaria, influenza, cholera and many others [3, 4]. The current global COVIC-19 pandemic has emerged as one of the most notable global health crises across the globe, where billions of humans are staying at home as a measure to control the spread of disease and reduce morbidity and mortality rate [5].

* **Corresponding author Muhammad Ali Syed:** Department of Microbiology, The University of Haripur, Hattar Road, Haripur, Khyber Pakhtunkhwa, Pakistan;
Tel: +92-995-615075; Email:syedali@uoh.edu.pk; mirwah2000@yahoo.de

Atta-ur-Rahman and M. Iqbal Choudhary (Eds.)
All rights reserved-© 2020 Bentham Science Publishers

Combating infectious diseases has been a dream of scientists of all the time from the oldest civilization to modern age due to the seriousness of the issue [1]. The advent of antibiotics, vaccines, and several other classes of antimicrobial agents against infections caused by different kinds of microorganisms such as bacteria, fungi, viruses, protozoans as well as microbial toxins has played a key role in reducing the global burden of infectious diseases [6]. The novel concept of selective toxicity and magic bullets introduced by Paul Ehrlich in 1900 was found highly fascinating by the medical community and has been a milestone in the history of anti-infective drug discovery [7]. Soon, humans became capable of curing bacterial infectious diseases using a class of antimicrobial agents called *antibiotics*. Penicillin was the first antibiotic introduced by Sir Alexander Fleming in 1928 followed by a range of natural, semi-synthetic and synthetic antibiotics that made it possible to cure the diseases that humans seemed to be fighting throughout the known history [6].

Drug resistance is a real challenge that humans are facing today, which is being reported in all classes of microorganisms [7, 8]. For instance, antibiotic resistance in bacteria is one of the most serious issue healthcare providers are facing today. The emergence of antibiotic resistant strains of pathogenic bacteria cost millions of lives across the globe annually. Multidrug resistant and extremely drug resistant clones of different bacterial species such as *Staphylococcus aureus*, *Pseudomonas aeruginosa*, *Escherichia coli*, *Salmonella enterica* serovar. Typhi, *Mycobacterium tuberculosis*, *Acinetobacter baumannii* appear to be resistant to the majority of antibiotics. There are very few treatment options available in hand, as there are increasing reports of bacterial resistance to drugs of last resort such as vancomycin, colistin, carbapenems, *etc*. Similar situation is with other types of microorganisms such as viruses, protozoans and fungi [8 - 10].

On one hand, drug discovery efforts are aimed at focusing on new antibiotics, on the other hand, new options for the cure of infectious agents are being seriously considered. One of the alternative options is aptamers [9, 11]. In the last few decades, aptamers have attracted more attention due to their potential applications in therapeutics and diagnostics. This class of biomolecules is also being investigated for potential applications in the cure of infectious diseases [12, 13]. This chapter introduces aptamers, their unique features, methods of synthesis and their potential applications to target infectious agents.

APTAMERS

The word aptamer is derived from a Latin word *aptus* meaning "To Fix". Aptamers are single stranded oligonucleotides (ssDNA or RNA), or peptide sequences that bind their targets very specifically. Target may be may be a biomolecule, toxin, cell, viral particle or even an inorganic substance [14]. These short secondary structures of ssDNA or RNA bind their target with high affinity and specificity [12, 15] (Fig. **1**). Since early experiments, a high number of efforts have been made to select aptamers against a range of targets including different microbial species as well as their products. Attempts to study the binding of RNA sequences with proteins began in 1980s when scientists were studying interaction of human immunodeficiency syndrome virus (HIV) and adenovirus nucleic acids with proteins. It was discovered that these viruses produce small structural RNA sequences that bind viral or host cell proteins with high affinity and specificity [16, 17]. *In vitro* selection of aptamers against specific targets using systematic evolution of ligands by exponential enrichment (SELEX) was introduced by Szostak`s and Gold`s groups in 1990 [18, 19].

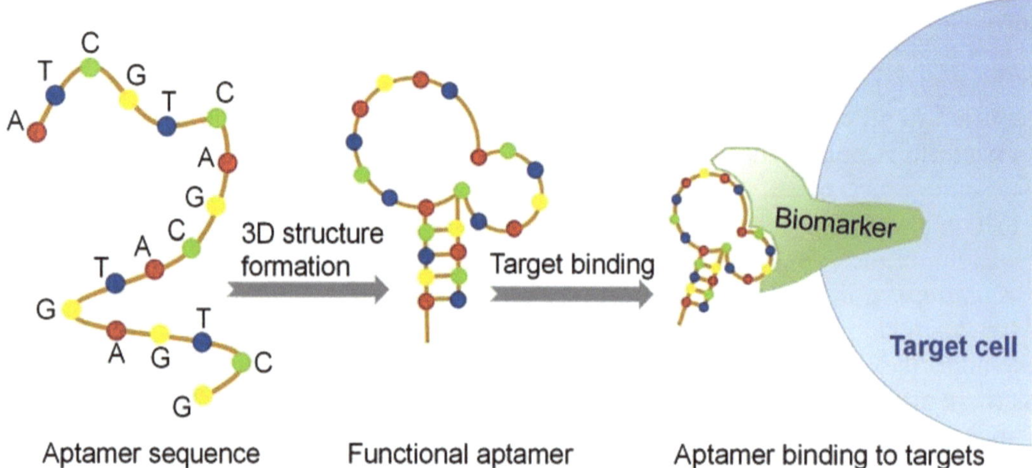

Fig. (1). Schematic diagram of aptamers binding its target. Oligonucleotide sequences first form 3-D structure that binds the target with higher affinity and specificity (Reproduced with permission from [100].

As stated above, aptamers can bind a number of targets. Aptamer binding to their targets rely upon nature of their target as well as flexible nature of aptamers. The short oligonucleotide sequences of ssDNA or RNA aptamers can form a number of three dimensional structures, such as hairpin, pseudoknots, bulges and G-quadruplexes. On the basis of these conformations,

aptamers bind their targets *via* electrostatic interactions, hydrogen bonding, Van der Waals forces and π-π stacking or combination some of these forces [20].

SYSTEMIC EVOLUTION OF LIGANDS BY EXPONENTIAL ENRICHMENT (SELEX)

RNA or DNA aptamers are selected randomly from a pool of oligonucleotide sequences ($\sim 10^{15}$ random sequences) called a library by the process of SELEX [21]. The library is generated by using chemical methods of oligonucleotide synthesis. The complexity of library is important and it may be calculated mathematically.

Each oligonucleotide sequence or probe (ssDNA or RNA) in the library is a short chain of 40-100 nucleotides having random sequence in the middle and fixed sequences in flanking regions. The central or middle region of these oligonucleotides may bind their target in case their secondary structure has high affinity for it. SELEX process comprises of several rounds of selection of oligonucleotide sequences that bind their target. After each round of SELEX, lesser number of binding sequences with higher affinity is selected. Each round of SELEX comprises of three main steps or stages, detail of that is given in following paragraphs (Fig. **2**):

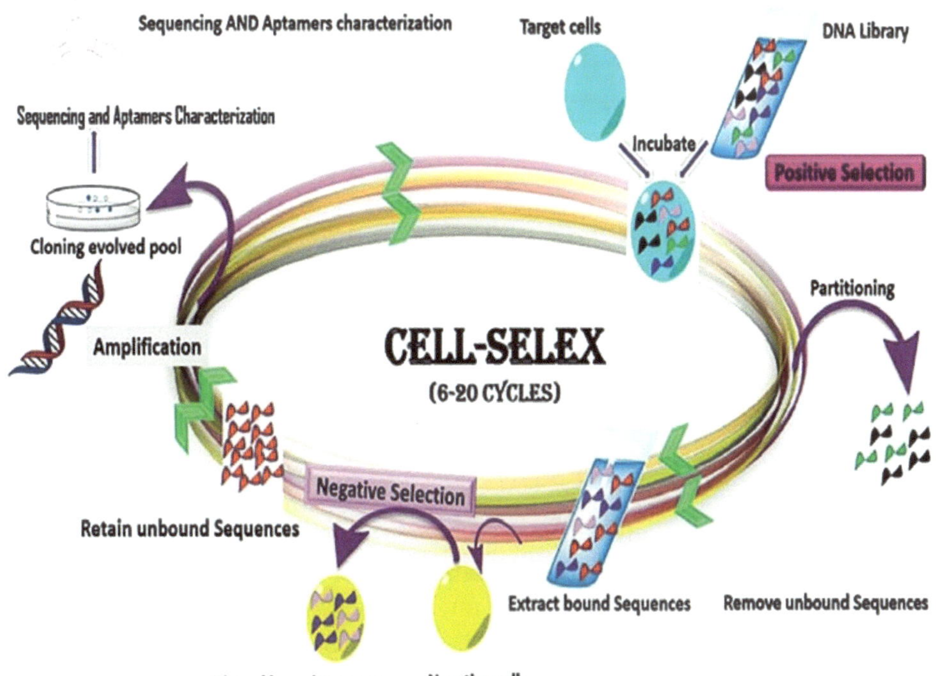

Fig. (2). An overview of different steps of Cell SELEX process. A target microbial cell is exposed to oligonucleotide library. DNA sequences bound to the cell are selected, while the unbound sequences are removed. The oligonucleotide sequences bound to target cell are separated and amplified by PCR and used for next round of SELEX. After several such rounds, selected sequences are PCR amplified and sequenced (Figure reproduced with permission from reference No. 40, https://jbiomedsci.biomedcentral.com/ articles/ 10.1186/s12929-019-0611-0 under creative common licence http://creativecommons.org/ l icenses/ by/4.0/).

I. Incubation of oligonucleotide sequences from a given library or pool ($\sim 100^{15}$ random sequences) with the target molecule or cells. Some of this large pool of oligonucleotide sequences will bind the target with higher affinity. In this step, favorable conditions are provided that aid binding of the nucleic acid probes with their targets.

II. Separation of oligonucleotide-target complexes from unbound oligonucleotide sequences. The unbound sequences are removed and the oligonucleotide sequences bound to the target are selected for next round of SELEX.

III. The oligonucleotides that bound target are separated and amplified by using polymerase chain reaction (PCR). The flanking fixed oligonucleotide sequences serve for binding of PCR primers [21].

IV. The PCR amplification of the selected sequences provides more quantity of probes for next cycle of SELEX [22].

After each round of SELEX, only the oligonucleotide sequences that bind the target with even higher affinity are selected. After several rounds of SELEX, there are only few oligonucleotide sequences left (usually < 10). These oligonucleotide sequences may be sequenced by conventional DNA sequencing methods [22].

Since the development of earlier protocols of SELEX, researchers have made amendments and improvements for better selection of aptamers. Nowadays, a number of different versions of SELEX protocols are available; some of them are just a strategy to improve a selectivity of SELEX or just an additional step. Detail is briefly described in the proceeding paragraphs.

Negative SELEX

In SELEX, the target is attached to immobilization matrix or solid support *i.e.* nitrocellulose membrane or agarose beads. The problem encountered in the process is non-specific selection of aptamers that bind this solid support, hence giving false positive results. These oligonucleotide sequences affect the efficiency of aptamer selection. The problem may be solved by using negative SELEX. In case of negative SELEX, oligonucleotide library is first incubated with the solid support or matrix to which the target is attached. The oligonucleotide sequences binding the solid support are removed from each pool, so that only probes binding the target are selected in each cycle. This strategy has improved the SELEX performance to about 50% [22, 24].

Counter SELEX

Counter SELEX is similar in approach to negative SELEX. The purpose of counter SELEX is to increase the specificity of the selected aptamers. In counter SELEX, oligonucleotide library is incubated with the structures similar to the target. It is especially relevant for the isolation of aptamers against target in a complex matrix, such as membrane proteins or receptors on the surface of the cell. Implementation of counter selection in SELEX enables discrimination between very similar targets. The aptamers binding structurally similar targets are removed, so that aptamers with higher specificity and affinity to the target are selected. This strategy is being applied in a number of SELEX protocols including CELL SELEX [25, 26].

Microfluidic SELEX

Most of the separation protocols work at the interfaces at large scale. They suffer from non-specific binding. Miniaturization of the system enhances surface to volume ratio that increases the stringency of the selection process as well as possibilities of automation, reduces the volume required for the assay and time taken for aptamer selection. In a typical microfluidic system, aptamers may be synthesized to a given target using small volume of targets as well as all other SELEX reagents. Furthermore, these systems are easy to operate requiring lesser expertise, as compared to conventional SELEX protocols. This approach may also be combined in capillary electrophoresis [27].

Capillary Electrophoresis SELEX

Conventional SELEX protocols are labor intensive and time consuming, requiring more than 15 rounds of SELEX for aptamer selection. To overcome this problem, a new type of SELEX was introduced called capillary electrophoresis SELEX (CE SELEX) [28]. It involves separation of bound oligonucleotide sequences from unbound on the basis of difference in their mobility in electrophoresis. CE SELEX is a very fast method of aptamer selection that is completed in few (1–4) rounds. It also aid in reducing non-specific binding and target immobilization is also not required. However, it actually utilizes very expensive equipment and also it is not suitable for small molecules [29, 26].

Cell SELEX

Aptamers may also be selected against molecules on the surface of specific cell types. For example, you may discriminate a particular type of bacteria from bacteria of other species. Aptamers may also be used to discriminate pathogenic and non-pathogenic, antibiotic resistant and susceptible strains of a single bacterial species on the basis of molecular difference in their cell surface. Nevertheless, most of the efforts have been made to select aptamers that selectively bind cancer cells. Counter SELEX may be used to improve the SELEX specificity to remove the aptamers that bind non-specifically (*e.g.* normal cells) [23, 11].

CELL SELEX may utilize a whole live cell as a target for aptamer selection. For this specific type of SELEX, prior knowledge of the target is not required. Aptamers are selected against molecules in their native state. Many potential targets are available on the cell surface. Likewise, protein purification is also not required for this technique. A number of successful attempts have been made to select aptamers against different types of infectious agents such as bacteria, protozoans and yeasts [23, 30].

APTAMERS *VERSUS* ANTIBODIES

Aptamers, also called chemical antibodies, show similarity to antibodies due to their high affinity to their target. Antibodies are classified as high molecular weight whereas the aptamers are classified as the middle molecular weight therapeutic agents and both differ chemically too [31].

Antibodies attract great attention due to their unique features such as higher binding affinity and specificity to their targets. Monoclonal antibodies are in use for several decades for their significant role in diagnostics and therapeutics. They may be synthesized using hybridoma technology and used in a number of applications including research purpose. Larger size of antibodies prevents them from renal filtration. They are stable inside the human body, as they are not degraded by nucleases. Antibodies are massively produced by a number of companies comprising of multi billion global market. In spite of their higher binding affinity, massive production, huge global market and a range of diagnostic and therapeutic as well as research applications, antibodies still suffer from some limitations. Antibody production requires an *in vivo* step, means their production requires a host animal. Furthermore, they are easily denatured at elevated temperatures and cannot be renatured. Being biologically synthesized, their production is difficult to scale up without compromising the product characteristics. In some cases, antibodies may also be immunogenic. Similarly, their larger size limits their bioavailability in some biological compartments [32].

Aptamers may also bind their target with similar affinity and specificity. They can be selected against a single biological or non-biological molecule or entire cell may be used in SELEX for specific aptamer selection against surface molecules. Aptamers have been selected against different drugs, organic compounds as well as different toxins [33]. Some groups have even selected aptamers to metal ions [101]. Furthermore, aptamers are stable molecules that are less vulnerable to degradation at elevated temperatures. Aptamers may re-attain their conformation after denaturation at higher temperatures [33]; therefore, there is a possibility of their reuse in diagnostic applications. Their preparation is facile and economical with very less to no variability [34]. The aptamer selected using SELEX may be sequenced and this sequence information may be used to synthesize aptamers chemically to fulfill future needs. Aptamers offer hence solutions to the problems associated with monoclonal antibodies, *i.e.* reproducibility failures as well as batch to batch variation in diagnostics and therapeutics. Once aptamer sequence is published, it is transferrable and any one can use this information to synthesize aptamer against that particular target [35]. Furthermore, conjugation chemistries of aptamers are orthogonal and functional groups as well as dyes may easily be introduced during their synthesis [32].

Despite many efforts by different groups, aptamers still suffer from some limitations. There are very few aptamers selected against small molecules. In therapeutics and diagnostics, one often needs to target small molecules. Further, they also present a challenge that they are easily cleared by the body due to smaller size or they are degraded by the nucleases inside the body, unless they are chemically modified. Although previous literature [36, 102] claimed low or no immunogenicity of aptamers inside the body, recent work suggests that aptamers may trigger immune response and they should be checked for immunogenicity [103, 104]. In some situations, selecting aptamers is still a challenge, as not every attempt of aptamer selection brings about fruitful results [37]. Furthermore, their pharmacokinetic properties are still unpredictable [32].

Aptamers can be synthesized chemically, making them amenable to all necessary modifications. In order to make aptamers more stable with enhanced specificity and affinity, modifications can be introduced in their structure. For example, RNA aptamers may be made nuclease resistant by introducing some functional groups in their structure such as 2`OH, ` 2NH$_2$ or making their spiegelmers. Furthermore, some groups have attempted to develop multivalent or multidentate aptamers in which more than one aptamers are connected through a linker [37]. Researchers are working on streamlining the methods to cope with the challenges associated with aptamer use. For example, excretion of aptamers from body may be prevented by attaching some biocompatible polymers such as poly ethylene glycol (PEG). PEG conjugated aptamers are retained in the body for several weeks and they are removed very slowly. As stated previously, chemical modifications of aptamers with different functional groups may prevent degradation by nucleases. Aptamers may also be used against intracellular targets such has host cell proteins inside the cells. In such cases, aptamer sequences may be expressed inside the host cells to ensure their accumulation inside the cytoplasm or nucleus Table **1**. Transfection of recombinant expression vector capable of expressing aptamer sequence may produce aptamers inside the cell [39].

APTAMERS AS ANTI-INFECTIVE AGENTS AGAINST PATHOGENIC MICROORGANISMS

Aptamers may be used as therapeutic agents to target microbial cells as well as their products. In a number of studies, aptamers have successfully inhibited or reduced microbial growth. This may be due to binding of aptamers with the bacterial cell surface proteins or cell wall [38].

Both DNA and RNA aptamers may bind bacteria or other microorganisms. RNA aptamers offer complex and stable secondary structures. However, as mentioned before, in case of RNA aptamers nucleotides need to be chemically modified to avoid degradation of RNA aptamers by nucleases. Therefore, RNA aptamers are more expensive to produce than DNA aptamers [39]

Several studies have been carried out to understand aptamer binding, killing or inactivation of microbes. It is understandable that aptamers bind a single or just very few targets on a large microbial cell. The target may vary in different classes of microorganisms as well as in different species or strains of same class of microbes. For example, bacteria have different surface molecules and features than fungi, whereas viruses are quite different than these two [39, 41, 42] (Fig. **3**).

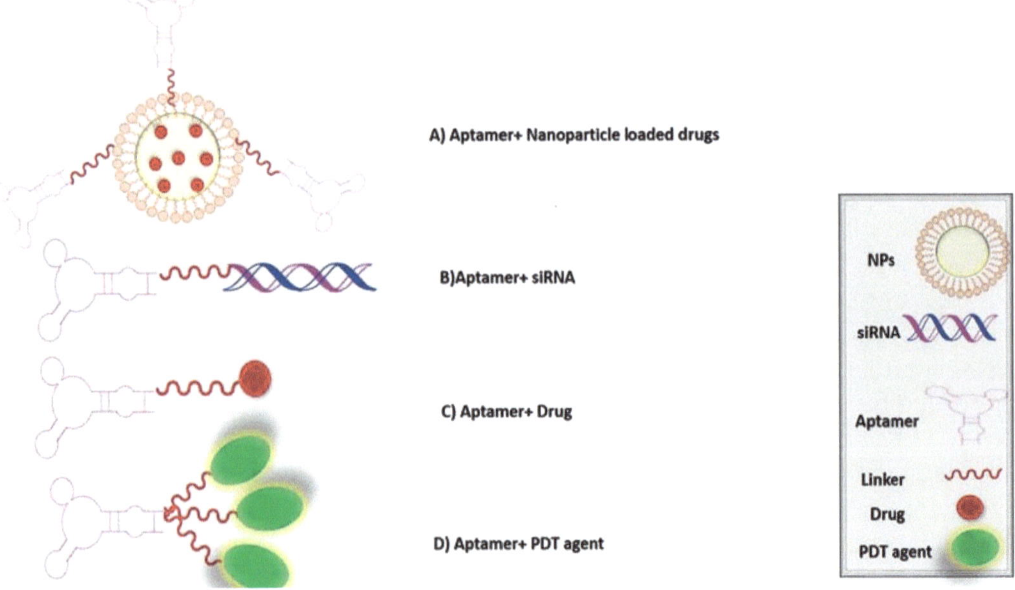

Fig. (3). Schematic representation of therapeutic use aptamers for infectious agents. (Figure reproduced with permission from reference No. 40, https://jbiomedsci.biomedcentral.com/articles/10.1186/s12929-019-0611-0 under creative common licence http://creativecommons.org/licenses/by/4.0/).

A number of studies have been conducted to exactly know the molecular target of aptamers on bacterial surface and killing mechanism. For example, the binding mechanism of DNA aptamers was studied on *Escherichia coli* (*E. coli*) O157H7 [43]. They first selected DNA aptamers against these bacteria and later they treated the bacteria with trypsin and proteinase K. This did not affect aptamer binding on the bacterial surface. They later treated cell with EDTA, which removes bacterial lipopolysaccharide (LPS). It was found that the selected aptamer bound bacterial LPS. Thus, blocking of bacterial surface molecules may result in cell growth inhibition or bacterial binding with host cells. Furthermore, aptamers may also antagonize bacterial surface proteins [42].

Aptamers may also be synthesized against a particular microbial cell or viral surface molecule alone without using entire cell or viruses. Such aptamer may be treated with the microbial cell for killing or inactivation. For example, Choi *et al.* (2011) selected aptamers against haemagglutinin protein of H9N2 Avian flu virus [43]. They cloned the gene encoding H9 and expressed in *E. coli* and then selected DNA aptamers though SELEX. The aptamers not only bound the H9N2 with higher affinity, but they also inhibited viral entry into the host cell due to strong binding to the viral particle. Similar approach has also been applied in the case of bacteria. For example, Pan *et al.* (2005) [44] selected aptamers against type IV fimbriae of *Salmonella enterica* serovar. Typhi. The selected aptamers were able to reduce bacterial invasion into the monocyte cells.

A number of successful attempts have also been made to select aptamers against different types of infectious agents such as bacteria, protozoans, fungi and viruses. It is found that aptamers alone or conjugated with other antimicrobial agents or siRNA can bring about microbial death or inactivation. In *in vivo* studies, aptamers may also be used for targeted drug delivery into the infected cells [40, 42]. Aptamer selection against different types of microorganisms has been discussed in the following sections:

APTAMERS AGAINST PATHOGENIC BACTERIA

Bacteria are the class of microbes that cause highest number of infections among humans and animals. There is a huge list of bacterial pathogens that cause from superficial and opportunistic to serious and life threatening infections. A number of groups have selected aptamers against major disease causing bacterial pathogens after dedicated efforts [40, 11, 13, 45, 46].

Worldwide, tuberculosis exists as a major health problem with increasing morbidity and mortality rate. Annually, 2.0 Million people are infected with TB worldwide and it is one of the top 3 three infectious diseases after HIV and malaria with high mortality rate. A study carried out by Chen *et al.* (2007)

selected DNA aptamers against virulent strain H37Rv of *Mycobacterium tuberculosis* with high binding affinity and specificity. The study showed that the survival rate of the mice challenged with the virulent strain H37Rv prolonged with the single injection of NK$_2$aptamer, suggesting NK$_2$ as a successful anti-tuberculosis agent [47]. Similarly, a study conducted by Rotherham *et al.* suggested that diagnosis of TB in sputum sample is feasible by using culture filtrate protein-10 and early secreted antigen target-6 DNA aptamer (anti- CFP-10.ESAT-6 DNA aptamer) [48].

Treatment of intracellular pathogens like *Salmonella* spp. is a difficult task, because of the poor uptake of antibacterial agents by the infected host cells [49]. Antimicrobial peptides are successful antibacterial compounds, but their applications for intracellular pathogens may be limited due to lower *in vivo* stability of antimicrobial compounds. A study conducted by Yeom *et al.* (2016) showed successful treatment of Hela cell lines infected with *Salmonella enterica* serovar Typhimurium with gold nanoparticles conjugated with DNA aptamer [50].

Staphylococcus aureus (*S. aureus*) is a Gram positive, ubiquitous bacterial species associated with a variety of diseases ranging from superficial dermal infections to life threatening conditions such as endocarditis, pneumonia, toxic shock syndrome leading to multiple organ failure and septicemia [51 - 53]. This pathogen has developed different strategies for antibiotic resistance, making it resistant to a number of antibiotics and therapeutic agents including methicillin. A study conducted by Vivekananda *et al.* (2014) reported that the DNA aptamers synthesized by them successfully neutralized *S. aureus* alpha toxins, a major cause of *S. aureus* cytotoxicity. About 49 aptamers were demonstrated by *in vitro* neutralization assays. Out of these, 4 aptamers AT-27, AT-33, AT-36 and AT-49 were found to inhibit alpha toxin mediated cell death significantly [54].

As stated previously, increasing antibiotic resistance is one of the major hurdles in the treatment of bacterial infections. Bacteria employ various strategies to overcome antibiotic inhibitory effect such as production of beta lactamase enzymes to inhibit the action of beta lactam drugs by *Bacillus cereus*, *S. aureus* and several other bacterial pathogens. To overcome this problem, several β-lactamases inhibitors have been found. But one class of beta lactamases exists against which no beta lactamase inhibitors can work. This class of β-lactamases is known as metalloβ-lactamases [46]. A study conducted by Kim *et al.* (2009) selected ssDNA aptamer against metalo beta lactamase resistant *Bacillus cereus*. The metal ion dependence and inhibition pattern of these aptamers suggest that they can change the metal ion active site. Therefore, their inhibition is highly specific and efficient [55].

APTAMERS AGAINST VIRUSES

Viruses are much smaller in size than bacteria and may cause a variety of infections. The main difference between bacteria and viruses is that viruses are obligate intracellular pathogens and, therefore, they cannot survive without a host cell. In contrast, bacteria can survive at their own. Examples of human viral diseases include AIDS, hepatitis, influenza, polio, rabies, COVID-19 *etc.* [56].

Aptamers have also been reported as therapeutic agents for viral particles. These aptamers inhibit viral replication in their host cell by interfering with different stages of viral replication. Several studies have reported potential application of aptamers in the diagnosis and treatment of viral infections such as hepatitis B virus (HBV), hepatitis C virus (HCV), human immunodeficiency syndrome virus (HIV), herpes simplex virus types 2 (HSV-2) and Ebola *etc.* [57 - 61]. In following paragraph different attempts made to select specific and inhibitory aptamers against different types of viruses are discussed.

Influenza virus is one of the most important types of viruses. In the pathogenesis of influenza A virus, amino acid residues in the N terminus of the polymerase acidic (PA_N) protein plays a key role. Viral RNA promoter binding, protein stability and endonuclease activity is associated with PA domain. Among different subtypes of H5N1 strains, PA domain is conserved making this a suitable target for several therapeutic agents [62]. A study conducted by Yuan *et al.* (2015) reported DNA aptamers against the intact PA protein or PA_N domain of the PA protein. The study selected aptamers against PA_N and 3 aptamers against PA protein. No antiviral efficacy was exhibited by PA selected aptamers, whereas four of the six PA_N selected aptamers exhibited inhibition of both H5N1 virus infection and endonuclease activity [63].

Attempts have also been made to select inhibitory aptamers against hepatitis B virus. Available treatment options against HBV infections have limited efficacy. Interferon alpha induces viral suppression in only about 30 – 40% of HBV infected patients [64]. Recently introduced lamivudine, a nucleoside analogue can significantly suppress viral replication of treated patients. But, lamivudine resistant HBV mutants have been observed with the long term usage of the drug [58, 59]. A study carried out by Butz *et al.* reported C1-1 aptamer against HBV capsid proteins and was found to be effective in inhibition of virus capsid formation. Therefore, this aptamer has the potential to be used as anti HBV agent [65]. A study conducted by Zhang *et al.* (2014) selected DNA aptamers against HBV that could inhibit assembly of nucleocapsid [66]. More recent study by Rashedi *et al.* (2018) have selected DNA aptamers that bind hepatitis B surface antigen [67].

HIV causes one of the most significant viral diseases, accounting for hundreds of thousands of deaths annually. Various antiviral drugs can significantly slow the progression of HIV infection. Highly active antiretroviral therapy (HAART) has gained significant success in combating the disease, but drug resistance and toxicity are still a major issue concerned with HAART. To overcome these problems, development of alternate approaches is essential. One of the alternative approaches to treat HIV infection is the use of combination therapy of small interfering RNA (siRNA) and aptamers. Aptamers will help selective binding of the infected cells expressing viral antigens whereas; siRNA causes inhibition of viral replication. This can successfully inhibit virus replication in the host cell and avoid the emergence of resistant HIV variants [24]. Mufhandi *et al.* (2012) selected an aptamer to target surface glycoprotein gp-120 of HIV virus, thus interfering its entry into the host cell [68]. Similarly, Duclair *et al.* (2015) selected RNA aptamers showing inhibitory action against HIV-1 protease [69]. Likewise, efforts for selecting aptamers to HIV-1 integrase have been made by Rose *et al.* (2019) [79] (Fig. **4**).

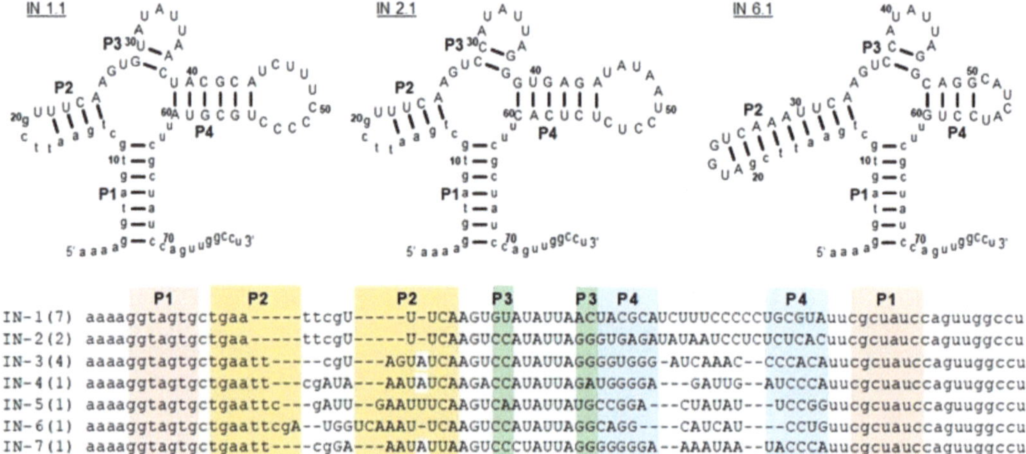

Fig. (**4**). Different aptamers selected to HIV integrase enzyme (Reproduced with permission from 79, https://pubs.acs.org/doi/10.1021/acschembio.9b00237. Note: Further permissions related to the material excerpted should be directed to the ACS).

APTAMERS AGAINST PROTOZOAN PARASITES

Though most of the infectious diseases are caused by bacteria and viruses, but the unicellular parasites are also responsible for some diseases like malaria, toxoplasmosis, giardia, *etc.* [70]. A review by Ospina-Villa *et al.* suggested several RNA and DNA aptamers to treat parasitic infections such as Leishmaniasis, Amoebiasis, and many other parasitic infections affecting the lives of hundreds of thousands of people in both developed as well as underdeveloped world [71]. In following are discussed some studies that selected aptamers against different protozoan species.

Trypanosomiasis, caused by *Trypanosome* species, is a medically significant protozoan disease responsible for high morbidity and mortality in Sub-Saharan Africa and Latin America. *Trypanosome* species possess surface proteins known as variant surface glycoproteins (VSG) that help the parasite to escape from the immune response of the infected cells. Antigenic variation of this protein contributes in protection from the host immune response. Lorger *et al.* (2003) reported RNA aptamers that target the surface proteins of African Trypanosomes. Upon attachment to the target molecules, these aptamers direct antibodies to the surface of trypanosomes thus promoting their elimination [72].

Plasmodium species have also been a point of focus due to the serious human illness caused by them called malaria [73]. Of all plasmodium species, *Plasmodium falciparum* is associated with the severe form of disease in humans. Each year malaria results in about 200-600 million cases and 1 million deaths. To combat the disease, antimalarial agents are available, but drug resistance is a major obstacle. A study conducted by Niles *et al.* (2009 reported use of DNA aptamers to heme binding protein with mode of action similar to chloroquine. Like chloroquine, these aptamers inhibit hemozoin formation *in vitro* [74].

Entamoeba histolyica (*E. histolytica*), causative agent of amoebiasis, is responsible for one of three major causes of parasitic diseases worldwide. According to an estimate, 50 Million people are infected with *E. histolytica* worldwide annually [75]. The cleavage factor *Entamoeba histolytica* cleavage factor Im (EhCFIm25) plays a key role for survival and mobility of *Entamoeba histolytica*. In order to reduce parasite mobility and its capacity to initiate erythrophagocytosis, silencing of EhCFIm25 is needed [76]. Opsina-Villa *et al.* (2018) selected RNA aptamer *via* SELEX that specifically bound to EhCFIm25 of *Entamoeba histolytica,* thus inhibiting its growth and leading to death [77].

FUTURE PERSPECTIVES

To be used as therapeutic agents and in target validation, aptamers serve as promising molecules. As designer drugs, these compounds exhibit several properties like high affinity, specificity and amenability to the required modifications. To facilitate the transition of aptamers from lab conditions to pharmaceuticals, animal and human data is now necessary. The results of studies conducted so far by different groups on use of aptamers as therapeutic agents have shown promising agents. The aptamers may be able to be used to cure infectious diseases and help resolving the issue of microbial drug resistance. Furthermore, aptamers offer an opportunity of targeted drug delivery into the infected cells, since they may be combined with antimicrobial drugs, siRNA/miRNA or nanomaterials [40]. Even aptamers may be selected against living cells. Nevertheless, aptamers still remain largely far from reaching commercialization and market. The list of aptamers in clinical trials is increasing, but most of those in pipeline are for non-infectious diseases [77, 78].

Over the last few years, a number of new methods and improvements in existing SELEX protocols have been introduced. Further, a number of groups are working on improving the stability of aptamers as well as overcome the challenges associated with their use [4]. Though aptamer research is in infancy and lacks set protocols and infrastructure in many institutions, more researchers are being attracted towards it. Moreover, collaboration between academic researchers and industry is essential for development of therapeutic aptamers.

CONCLUSION

Results of the studies conducted so far by different groups on antimicrobial efficacy of DNA and RNA aptamers are promising. Aptamers provide a valuable platform in pharmaceuticals to overcome the ever increasing challenge of drug resistance. Beside this, aptamers possess several advantages, such as low manufacturing cost, stability over a wide temperature range, high efficiency and specificity. Despite so many advantages, very limited aptamers are available as therapeutic agents commercially. Most of the current research on aptamers involves animal models and cell culture. More research is needed in order to evaluate and develop aptamers as therapeutic agents to treat different infections.

CONSENT FOR PUBLICATION

Not applicable.

CONFLICT OF INTEREST

The authors confirm that this chapter content has no conflict of interest.

ACKNOWLEDGEMENTS

Declared none.

REFERENCES

[1]   Bloom DE, Cadarette D. Infectious disease threats in the twenty-first century: strengthening the global response. Front Immunol 2019; 10: 549.
        [http://dx.doi.org/10.3389/fimmu.2019.00549] [PMID: 30984169]

[2]   Brachman PS. Infectious diseases--past, present, and future. Int J Epidemiol 2003; 32(5): 684-6.
        [http://dx.doi.org/10.1093/ije/dyg282] [PMID: 14559728]

[3]   Casanova JL, Abel L. The genetic theory of infectious diseases: a brief history and selected

illustrations. Annu Rev Genomics Hum Genet 2013; 14: 215-43.
[http://dx.doi.org/10.1146/annurev genom 091212-153448] [PMID: 23724903]

[4]   Davydova A, Vorobjeva M, Pyshnyi D, Altman S, Vlassov V, Venyaminova A. Aptamers against pathogenic microorganisms. Crit Rev Microbiol 2016; 42(6): 847-65.
[http://dx.doi.org/10.3109/1040841X.2015.1070115] [PMID: 26258445]

[5]   Chowell G, Mizumoto K. The COVID-19 pandemic in the USA: what might we expect? Lancet 2020; 395(10230): 1093-4.
[http://dx.doi.org/10.1016/S0140-6736(20)30743-1] [PMID: 32247381]

[6]   Ventola CL. The antibiotic resistance crisis: part 1: causes and threats. P&T 2015; 40(4): 277-83.
[PMID: 25859123]

[7]   Tan SY, Grimes S. Paul Ehrlich (1854-1915): man with the magic bullet. Singapore Med J 2010; 51(11): 842-3.
[PMID: 21140107]

[8]   Berman and Krysan. Drug resistance and tolerance in fungi. Nat Rev Microbiol 2020; 20: 1-13.

[9]   Nikaido H. Multidrug resistance in bacteria. Annu Rev Biochem 2009; 78: 119-46.
[http://dx.doi.org/10.1146/annurev.biochem.78.082907.145923] [PMID: 19231985]

[10]   Strasfeld L, Chou S. Antiviral drug resistance: mechanisms and clinical implications. Infect Dis Clin North Am 2010; 24(3): 809-33.
[http://dx.doi.org/10.1016/j.idc.2010.07.001] [PMID: 20674805]

[11]   Syed MA, Jamil B. Aptamers and aptasensors as novel approach for microbial detection and identification: An appraisal. Curr Drug Targets 2018; 19(13): 1560-72.
[http://dx.doi.org/10.2174/1389450119666180105115429] [PMID: 29303077]

[12]   Syed MA, Pervaiz S. Advances in aptamers. Oligonucleotides 2010; 20(5): 215-24.
[http://dx.doi.org/10.1089/oli.2010.0234] [PMID: 20677985]

[13]   Syed MA, Ali N. Nanomaterials for selective targeting of intracellular pathogens. Published in Nanotheranostics: applications and limitations 2019; 1: 115-336.
[http://dx.doi.org/10.1007/978-3-030-29768-8_6]

[14]   Jing M, Bowser MT. Methods for measuring aptamer-protein equilibria: a review. Anal Chim Acta 2011; 686(1-2): 9-18.
[http://dx.doi.org/10.1016/j.aca.2010.10.032] [PMID: 21237304]

[15]   Nimjee SM, White RR, Becker RC, Sullenger BA. Aptamers as therapeutics. Annu Rev Pharmacol Toxicol 2017; 57: 61-79.
[http://dx.doi.org/10.1146/annurev-pharmtox-010716-104558] [PMID: 28061688]

[16]   Dollins CM, Nair S, Sullenger BA. Aptamers in immunotherapy. Hum Gene Ther 2008; 19(5): 443-50.
[http://dx.doi.org/10.1089/hum.2008.045] [PMID: 18473674]

[17]   Song KM, Lee S, Ban C. Aptamers and their biological applications. Sensors (Basel) 2012; 12(1): 612-31.
[http://dx.doi.org/10.3390/s120100612] [PMID: 22368488]

[18]   Tuerk C, Gold L. Systematic evolution of ligands by exponential enrichment: RNA ligands to bacteriophage T4 DNA polymerase. Science 1990; 249(4968): 505-10.
[http://dx.doi.org/10.1126/science.2200121] [PMID: 2200121]

[19]   Ellington AD, Szostak JW. *In vitro* selection of RNA molecules that bind specific ligands. Nature 1990; 346(6287): 818-22.
[http://dx.doi.org/10.1038/346818a0] [PMID: 1697402]

[20]   Cai S, Yan J, Xiong H, Liu Y, Peng D, Liu Z. Investigations on the interface of nucleic acid aptamers and binding targets. Analyst (Lond) 2018; 143(22): 5317-38.

[http://dx.doi.org/10.1039/C8AN01467A] [PMID: 30357118]

[21]   Zhang Y, Lai BS, Juhas M. Recent advances in aptamer discovery and applications. Molecules 2019; 24(5): 941.
[http://dx.doi.org/10.3390/molecules24050941] [PMID: 30866536]

[22]   Sampson T. Aptamers and SELEX: The technology. World Pat Inf 2003; 25(2): 123-9.
[http://dx.doi.org/10.1016/S0172-2190(03)00035-8]

[23]   Ohuchi S. Cell-SELEX technology. BioResearch Open Access 2012; 1(6): 265-75.
[http://dx.doi.org/10.1089/biores.2012.0253]

[24]   Zhou J, Li H, Li S, Zaia J, Rossi JJ. Novel dual inhibitory function aptamer-siRNA delivery system for HIV-1 therapy. Mol Ther 2008; 16(8): 1481-9.
[http://dx.doi.org/10.1038/mt.2008.92] [PMID: 18461053]

[25]   Mercier MC, Dontenwill M, Choulier L. Selection of nucleic acid aptamers targeting tumor cell-surface protein biomarkers. Cancers (Basel) 2017; 9(6): 1-33.
[PMID: 28635657]

[26]   Zhuo Z, Yu Y, Wang M, *et al.* Recent advances in SELEX technology and aptamer applications in biomedicine. Int J Mol Sci 2017; 18(10): 2142.
[http://dx.doi.org/10.3390/ijms18102142] [PMID: 29036890]

[27]   Demobowski SK, Bowser MT. Microfluidic methods for aptamer selection and characterization. Analyst (Lond) 2018; 143(1): 21-32.
[http://dx.doi.org/10.1039/C7AN01046J]

[28]   Mendonsa SD, Bowser MT. *In vitro* evolution of functional DNA using capillary electrophoresis. J Am Chem Soc 2004; 126(1): 20-1.
[http://dx.doi.org/10.1021/ja037832s] [PMID: 14709039]

[29]   Zhu C, Yang G, Ghulam M, Li L, Qu F. Evolution of multi-functional capillary electrophoresis for high-efficiency selection of aptamers. Biotechnol Adv 2019; 37(8): 107432.
[http://dx.doi.org/10.1016/j.biotechadv.2019.107432] [PMID: 31437572]

[30]   Sefah K, Shangguan D, Xiong X, O'Donoghue MB, Tan W. Development of DNA aptamers using Cell-SELEX. Nat Protoc 2010; 5(6): 1169-85.
[http://dx.doi.org/10.1038/nprot.2010.66] [PMID: 20539292]

[31]   Nakamura Y. Aptamers as therapeutic middle molecules. Biochimie 2018; 145: 22-33.
[http://dx.doi.org/10.1016/j.biochi.2017.10.006] [PMID: 29050945]

[32]   Keefe AD, Pai S, Ellington A. Aptamers as therapeutics. Nat Rev Drug Discov 2010; 9(7): 537-50.
[http://dx.doi.org/10.1038/nrd3141] [PMID: 20592747]

[33]   Mascini M. Aptamers and their applications. Anal Bioanal Chem 2008; 390(4): 987-8.
[http://dx.doi.org/10.1007/s00216-007-1769-y] [PMID: 18193207]

[34]   Dhiman A, Kalra P, Bansal V, Bruno JG, Sharma TK. Aptamer-based point-of-care diagnostic platforms. Sens Actuators B Chem 2017; 246: 535-53.
[http://dx.doi.org/10.1016/j.snb.2017.02.060]

[35]   Bauer M, Strom M, Hammond DS, Shigdar S. Anything You Can Do, I Can Do Better: Can Aptamers Replace Antibodies in Clinical Diagnostic Applications? Molecules 2019; 24(23): 4377.
[http://dx.doi.org/10.3390/molecules24234377] [PMID: 31801185]

[36]   Ireson CR, Kelland LR. Discovery and development of anticancer aptamers. Mol Cancer Ther 2006; 5(12): 2957-62.
[http://dx.doi.org/10.1158/1535-7163.MCT-06-0172] [PMID: 17172400]

[37]   Bruno JG. Predicting the uncertain future of aptamer-based diagnostics and therapeutics. Molecules 2015; 20(4): 6866-87.
[http://dx.doi.org/10.3390/molecules20046866] [PMID: 25913927]

[38]   Ali MH, Elsherbiny ME, Emara M. Updates on aptamer research. Int J Mol Sci 2019; 20(10): 2511.
[http://dx.doi.org/10.3390/ijms20102511] [PMID: 31117311]

[39]   Lakhin AV, Tarantul VZ, Gening LV. Aptamers: problems, solutions and prospects. Acta Naturae 2013; 5(4): 34-43.
[http://dx.doi.org/10.32607/20758251-2013-5-4-34-43] [PMID: 24455181]

[40]   Afrasiabi S, Pourhajibagher M, Raoofian R, Tabarzad M, Bahador A. Therapeutic applications of nucleic acid aptamers in microbial infections. J Biomed Sci 2020; 27(1): 6.
[http://dx.doi.org/10.1186/s12929-019-0611-0] [PMID: 31900238]

[41]   Zou Y, Duan N, Wu S, Shen M, Wang Z. Selection, identification, and binding mechanism studies of an ssDNA aptamer targeted to different stages of E. coli O157: H7. J Agric Food Chem 2018; 66(22): 5677-82.
[http://dx.doi.org/10.1021/acs.jafc.8b01006] [PMID: 29756774]

[42]   Özalp VC, Bilecen K, Kavruk M, Öktem HA. Antimicrobial aptamers for detection and inhibition of microbial pathogen growth. Future Microbiol 2013; 8(3): 387-401.
[http://dx.doi.org/10.2217/fmb.12.149] [PMID: 23464374]

[43]   Choi SK, Lee C, Lee KS, *et al.* DNA aptamers against the receptor binding region of hemagglutinin prevent avian influenza viral infection. Mol Cells 2011; 32(6): 527-33.
[http://dx.doi.org/10.1007/s10059-011-0156-x] [PMID: 22058017]

[44]   Pan Q, Zhang XL, Wu HY, *et al.* Aptamers that preferentially bind type IVB pili and inhibit human monocytic-cell invasion by *Salmonella enterica* serovar typhi. Antimicrob Agents Chemother 2005; 49(10): 4052-60.
[http://dx.doi.org/10.1128/AAC.49.10.4052-4060.2005] [PMID: 16189080]

[45]   Hamula CLA, Zhang H, Li F, Wang Z, Chris Le X, Li XF. Selection and analytical applications of aptamers binding microbial pathogens. Trends Analyt Chem 2011; 30(10): 1587-97.
[http://dx.doi.org/10.1016/j.trac.2011.08.006] [PMID: 32287535]

[46]   Schlesinger SR, Lahousse MJ, Foster TO, Kim SK. Metallo-β-lactamases and aptamer-based inhibition. J Pharm (Cairo) 2011; 4(2): 419-28.

[47]   Chen F, Zhou J, Luo F, Mohammed AB, Zhang XL. Aptamer from whole-bacterium SELEX as new therapeutic reagent against virulent *Mycobacterium tuberculosis.* Biochem Biophys Res Commun 2007; 357(3): 743-8.
[http://dx.doi.org/10.1016/j.bbrc.2007.04.007] [PMID: 17442275]

[48]   Rotherham LS, Maserumule C, Dheda K, Theron J, Khati M. Selection and application of ssDNA aptamers to detect active TB from sputum samples. PLoS One 2012; 7(10): e46862.
[http://dx.doi.org/10.1371/journal.pone.0046862] [PMID: 23056492]

[49]   Prokesch RC, Hand WL. Antibiotic entry into human polymorphonuclear leukocytes. Antimicrob Agents Chemother 1982; 21(3): 373-80.
[http://dx.doi.org/10.1128/AAC.21.3.373] [PMID: 7103442]

[50]   Yeom JH, Lee B, Kim D, *et al.* Gold nanoparticle-DNA aptamer conjugate-assisted delivery of antimicrobial peptide effectively eliminates intracellular *Salmonella enterica* serovar Typhimurium. Biomaterials 2016; 104: 43-51.
[http://dx.doi.org/10.1016/j.biomaterials.2016.07.009] [PMID: 27424215]

[51]   Zetola N, Francis JS, Nuermberger EL, Bishai WR. Community-acquired meticillin-resistant *Staphylococcus aureus*: an emerging threat. Lancet Infect Dis 2005; 5(5): 275-86.
[http://dx.doi.org/10.1016/S1473-3099(05)70112-2] [PMID: 15854883]

[52]   Lowy FD. Antimicrobial resistance: the example of *Staphylococcus aureus.* J Clin Invest 2003; 111(9): 1265-73.
[http://dx.doi.org/10.1172/JCI18535] [PMID: 12727914]

[53]   Bhakdi S, Tranum-Jensen J. Alpha-toxin of *Staphylococcus aureus*. Microbiol Rev 1991; 55(4): 733-51.
[http://dx.doi.org/10.1128/MMBR.55.4.733-751.1991] [PMID: 1779933]

[54]   Vivekananda J, Salgado C, Millenbaugh NJ. DNA aptamers as a novel approach to neutralize *Staphylococcus aureus* α-toxin. Biochem Biophys Res Commun 2014; 444(3): 433-8.
[http://dx.doi.org/10.1016/j.bbrc.2014.01.076] [PMID: 24472539]

[55]   Kim SK, Sims CL, Wozniak SE, Drude SH, Whitson D, Shaw RW. Antibiotic resistance in bacteria: novel metalloenzyme inhibitors. Chem Biol Drug Des 2009; 74(4): 343-8.
[http://dx.doi.org/10.1111/j.1747-0285.2009.00879.x] [PMID: 19751419]

[56]   Forterre P. To be or not to be alive: How recent discoveries challenge the traditional definitions of viruses and life. Stud Hist Philos Biol Biomed Sci 2016; 59: 100-8.
[http://dx.doi.org/10.1016/j.shpsc.2016.02.013] [PMID: 26996409]

[57]   Moore MD, Bunka DHJ, Forzan M, *et al.* Generation of neutralizing aptamers against herpes simplex virus type 2: potential components of multivalent microbicides. J Gen Virol 2011; 92(Pt 7): 1493-9.
[http://dx.doi.org/10.1099/vir.0.030601-0] [PMID: 21471320]

[58]   Wandtke T, Woźniak J, Kopiński P. Aptamers in diagnostics and treatment of viral infections. Viruses 2015; 7(2): 751-80.
[http://dx.doi.org/10.3390/v7020751] [PMID: 25690797]

[59]   Zou X, Wu J, Gu J, Shen L, Mao L. Application of Aptamers in virus detection and antiviral therapy. Front Microbiol 2019; 10: 1462.
[http://dx.doi.org/10.3389/fmicb.2019.01462] [PMID: 31333603]

[60]   Lai CL, Chien RN, Leung NW, *et al.* Asia Hepatitis Lamivudine Study Group. A one-year trial of lamivudine for chronic hepatitis B. N Engl J Med 1998; 339(2): 61-8.
[http://dx.doi.org/10.1056/NEJM199807093390201] [PMID: 9654535]

[61]   Dienstag JL, Schiff ER, Wright TL, *et al.* Lamivudine as initial treatment for chronic hepatitis B in the United States. N Engl J Med 1999; 341(17): 1256-63.
[http://dx.doi.org/10.1056/NEJM199910213411702] [PMID: 10528035]

[62]   Dias A, Bouvier D, Crépin T, *et al.* The cap-snatching endonuclease of influenza virus polymerase resides in the PA subunit. Nature 2009; 458(7240): 914-8.
[http://dx.doi.org/10.1038/nature07745] [PMID: 19194459]

[63]   Yuan S, Zhang N, Singh K, *et al.* Cross-protection of influenza A virus infection by a DNA aptamer targeting the PA endonuclease domain. Antimicrob Agents Chemother 2015; 59(7): 4082-93.
[http://dx.doi.org/10.1128/AAC.00306-15] [PMID: 25918143]

[64]   Wright TL, Lau JY. Clinical aspects of hepatitis B virus infection. Lancet 1993; 342(8883): 1340-4.
[http://dx.doi.org/10.1016/0140-6736(93)92250-W] [PMID: 7694023]

[65]   Butz K, Denk C, Fitscher B, *et al.* Peptide aptamers targeting the hepatitis B virus core protein: a new class of molecules with antiviral activity. Oncogene 2001; 20(45): 6579-86.
[http://dx.doi.org/10.1038/sj.onc.1204805] [PMID: 11641783]

[66]   Zhang Z, Zhang J, Pei X, *et al.* An aptamer targets HBV core protein and suppresses HBV replication in HepG2.2.15 cells. Int J Mol Med 2014; 34(5): 1423-9.
[http://dx.doi.org/10.3892/ijmm.2014.1908] [PMID: 25174447]

[67]   Rashedi H, Arjmand S, Ranaei Siadat SO, Pouryaqubi M. Detection of DNA Aptamer with High Affinity against Hepatitis B Surface Antigen by Systematic Evolution of Ligands by Exponential Enrichment. Modares J Biotechnol 2018; 9(3): 317-23.

[68]   Mufhandu HT, Gray ES, Madiga MC, *et al.* UCLA1, a synthetic derivative of a gp120 RNA aptamer, inhibits entry of human immunodeficiency virus type 1 subtype C. J Virol 2012; 86(9): 4989-99.
[http://dx.doi.org/10.1128/JVI.06893-11] [PMID: 22379083]

[69]   Duclair S, Gautam A, Ellington A, Prasad VR. High-affinity RNA aptamers against the HIV-1 protease inhibit both *in vitro* protease activity and late events of viral replication. Mol Ther Nucleic Acids 2015; 4: e228.
       [http://dx.doi.org/10.1038/mtna.2015.1] [PMID: 25689224]

[70]   Solomons NW, Keusch GT. Nutritional implications of parasitic infections. Nutr Rev 1981; 39(4): 149-61.
       [http://dx.doi.org/10.1111/j.1753-4887.1981.tb06762.x] [PMID: 7029357]

[71]   Ospina-Villa JD, López-Camarillo C, Castañón-Sánchez CA, Soto-Sánchez J, Ramírez-Moreno E, Marchat LA. Advances on aptamers against protozoan parasites. Genes (Basel) 2018; 9(12): 584.
       [http://dx.doi.org/10.3390/genes9120584] [PMID: 30487456]

[72]   Lorger M, Engstler M, Homann M, Göringer HU. Targeting the variable surface of African trypanosomes with variant surface glycoprotein-specific, serum-stable RNA aptamers. Eukaryot Cell 2003; 2(1): 84-94.
       [http://dx.doi.org/10.1128/EC.2.1.84-94.2003] [PMID: 12582125]

[73]   Cowman AF, Healer J, Marapana D, Marsh K. Malaria: Biology and Disease. Cell 2016; 167(3): 610-24.
       [http://dx.doi.org/10.1016/j.cell.2016.07.055] [PMID: 27768886]

[74]   Niles JC, Derisi JL, Marletta MA. Inhibiting Plasmodium falciparum growth and heme detoxification pathway using heme-binding DNA aptamers. Proc Natl Acad Sci USA 2009; 106(32): 13266-71.
       [http://dx.doi.org/10.1073/pnas.0906370106] [PMID: 19633187]

[75]   Kantor M, Abrantes A, Estevez A, *et al.* Ochner C·Entamoeba histolytica: Updates in clinical manifestation, pathogenesis, and vaccine development. Can J Gastroenterol Hepatol 2018; 2018: 4601420.
       [http://dx.doi.org/10.1155/2018/4601420] [PMID: 30631758]

[76]   Yang Q, Gilmartin GM, Doublié S. Structural basis of UGUA recognition by the Nudix protein CFI(m)25 and implications for a regulatory role in mRNA 3′ processing. Proc Natl Acad Sci USA 2010; 107(22): 10062-7.
       [http://dx.doi.org/10.1073/pnas.1000848107] [PMID: 20479262]

[77]   Ospina-Villa JD, Dufour A, Weber C, *et al.* Targeting the polyadenylation factor EhCFIm25 with RNA aptamers controls survival in *Entamoeba histolytica*. Sci Rep 2018; 8(1): 5720.
       [http://dx.doi.org/10.1038/s41598-018-23997-w] [PMID: 29632392]

[78]   Ozalp VC, Eyidogan F, Oktem HA. Aptamer-gated nanoparticles for smart drug delivery. J Pharm (Cairo) 2011; 4(8): 1137-57.

[79]   Rose KM, Alves Ferreira-Bravo I, Li M, *et al.* Selection of 2′-deoxy-2′-fluoroarabino nucleic acid (FANA) aptamers that bind HIV-1 integrase with picomolar affinity. ACS Chem Biol 2019; 14(10): 2166-75. https://pubs.acs.org/doi/ 10.1021/ acschembio.9b00237
       [http://dx.doi.org/10.1021/acschembio.9b00237] [PMID: 31560515]

[80]   Bayraç AT, Donmez SI. Selection of DNA aptamers to Streptococcus pneumonia and fabrication of graphene oxide based fluorescent assay. Anal Biochem 2018; 556: 91-8.
       [http://dx.doi.org/10.1016/j.ab.2018.06.024] [PMID: 29964028]

[81]   Frohnmeyer E, Frisch F, Falke S, Betzel C, Fischer M. Highly affine and selective aptamers against cholera toxin as capture elements in magnetic bead-based sandwich ELAA. J Biotechnol 2018; 269: 35-42.
       [http://dx.doi.org/10.1016/j.jbiotec.2018.01.012] [PMID: 29408200]

[82]   Kolovskaya OS, Savitskaya AG, Zamay TN, *et al.* Development of bacteriostatic DNA aptamers for salmonella. J Med Chem 2013; 56(4): 1564-72.
       [http://dx.doi.org/10.1021/jm301856j] [PMID: 23387511]

[83]   DeGrasse JA. A single-stranded DNA aptamer that selectively binds to *Staphylococcus aureus*

enterotoxin B PLOSONE 2012; 7(3): e33410.

[84] Duan N, Ding X, He L, Wu S, Wei Y, Wang Z. Selection, identification and application of a DNA aptamer against *Listeria monocytogenes.* Food Control 2013; 33(1): 239-43.
[http://dx.doi.org/10.1016/j.foodcont.2013.03.011]

[85] Lavu PSR, Mondal B, Ramlal S, Murali HS, Batra HV. Selection and characterization of aptamers using a modified whole cell bacterium SELEX for the detection of *Salmonella enterica* serovar Typhimurium. ACS Comb Sci 2016; 18(6): 292-301.
[http://dx.doi.org/10.1021/acscombsci.5b00123] [PMID: 27070414]

[86] Lijuan C, Xing Y, Minxi W, Wenkai L, Le D. Development of an aptamer-ampicillin conjugate for treating biofilms. Biochem Biophys Res Commun 2017; 483(2): 847-54.
[http://dx.doi.org/10.1016/j.bbrc.2017.01.016] [PMID: 28069377]

[87] Lahousse M, Park H-C, Lee S-C, *et al.* Inhibition of anthrax lethal factor by ssDNA aptamers. Arch Biochem Biophys 2018; 646: 16-23.
[http://dx.doi.org/10.1016/j.abb.2018.03.028] [PMID: 29580944]

[88] Chang TW, Janardhanan P, Mello CM, Singh BR, Cai S. Selection of RNA aptamers against botulinum neurotoxin type A light chain through a non-radioactive approach. Appl Biochem Biotechnol 2016; 180(1): 10-25.
[http://dx.doi.org/10.1007/s12010-016-2081-0] [PMID: 27085355]

[89] Bayramoglu G, Ozalp VC, Oztekin M, Arica MY. Rapid and label-free detection of *Brucella melitensis* in milk and milk products using an aptasensor. Talanta 2019; 200: 263-71.
[http://dx.doi.org/10.1016/j.talanta.2019.03.048] [PMID: 31036183]

[90] Yan W, Gu L, Ren W, *et al.* Recognition of *Helicobacter pylori* by protein-targeting aptamers 2019; 24(3): e12577.

[91] Huang Y, Chen X, Duan N, *et al.* Selection and characterization of DNA aptamers against *Staphylococcus aureus* enterotoxin C1. Food Chem 2015; 166: 623-9.
[http://dx.doi.org/10.1016/j.foodchem.2014.06.039] [PMID: 25053102]

[92] Toscano-Garibay JD, Benítez-Hess ML, Alvarez-Salas LM. Isolation and characterization of an RNA aptamer for the HPV-16 E7 oncoprotein. Arch Med Res 2011; 42(2): 88-96.
[http://dx.doi.org/10.1016/j.arcmed.2011.02.005] [PMID: 21565620]

[93] Escudero-Abarca BI, Suh SH, Moore MD, Dwivedi HP, Jaykus L-A. Selection, characterization and application of nucleic acid aptamers for the capture and detection of human norovirus strains. PLoS One 2014; 9(9): e106805.
[http://dx.doi.org/10.1371/journal.pone.0106805] [PMID: 25192421]

[94] Li W, Feng X, Yan X, Liu K, Deng L. A DNA Aptamer Against Influenza A Virus: An Effective Inhibitor to the Hemagglutinin-Glycan Interactions. Nucleic Acid Ther 2016; 26(3): 166-72.
[http://dx.doi.org/10.1089/nat.2015.0564] [PMID: 26904922]

[95] Joseph DF, Nakamoto JA, Garcia Ruiz OA, *et al.* DNA aptamers for the recognition of HMGB1 from Plasmodium falciparum. PLoS One 2019; 14(4): e0211756.
[http://dx.doi.org/10.1371/journal.pone.0211756] [PMID: 30964875]

[96] Vargas-Montes M, Cardona N, Moncada DM, Molina DA, Zhang Y, Gómez-Marín JE. Enzyme-linked aptamer assay (ELAA) for detection of toxoplasma ROP18 protein in human serum. Front Cell Infect Microbiol 2019; 9: 386.
[http://dx.doi.org/10.3389/fcimb.2019.00386] [PMID: 31799213]

[97] Guerra-Pérez N, Ramos E, García-Hernández M, *et al.* Molecular and Functional Characterization of ssDNA Aptamers that Specifically Bind Leishmania infantum PABP. PLoS One 2015; 10(10): e0140048.
[http://dx.doi.org/10.1371/journal.pone.0140048] [PMID: 26457419]

[98] Bachtiar BM, Srisawat C, Bachtiar EW. RNA aptamers selected against yeast cells inhibit *Candida*

albicans biofilm formation *in vitro*. MicrobiologyOpen 2019; 8(8): e00812.
[http://dx.doi.org/10.1002/mbo3.812] [PMID: 30779315]

[99]　Malhotra S, Pandey AK, Rajput YS, Sharma R. Selection of aptamers for aflatoxin M1 and their characterization. J Mol Recognit 2014; 27(8): 493-500.
[http://dx.doi.org/10.1002/jmr.2370] [PMID: 24984866]

[100]　Yang S, Li H, Xu L, *et al.* Oligonucleotide aptamer-mediated precision therapy of hematological malignancies. Mol Ther Nucleic Acids 2018; 13: 164-75.
[http://dx.doi.org/10.1016/j.omtn.2018.08.023] [PMID: 30292138]

[101]　Qu H, Csordas AT, Wang J, Oh SS, Eisenstein MS, Soh HT. Rapid and label-free strategy to isolate aptamers for metal ions. ACS Nano 2016; 10(8): 7558-65.
[http://dx.doi.org/10.1021/acsnano.6b02558] [PMID: 27399153]

[102]　Eyetech Study Group. Preclinical and phase 1A clinical evaluation of an anti-VEGF pegylated aptamer (EYE001) for the treatment of exudative age-related macular degeneration. Retina 2002; 22(2): 143-52.
[http://dx.doi.org/10.1097/00006982-200204000-00002] [PMID: 11927845]

[103]　Avci-Adali M, Steinle H, Michel T, Schlensak C, Wendel HP. Potential capacity of aptamers to trigger immune activation in human blood. PLoS One 2013; 8(7): e68810.
[http://dx.doi.org/10.1371/journal.pone.0068810] [PMID: 23935890]

[104]　Avci-Adali M, Hann L, Michel T, *et al.* In vitro test system for evaluation of immune activation potential of new single-stranded DNA-based therapeutics. Drug Test Anal 2015; 7(4): 300-8.
[http://dx.doi.org/10.1002/dta.1670] [PMID: 24817283]

SUBJECT INDEX

A

Acids 102, 106, 116, 123, 128, 130, 198, 201, 234
  ascorbic 198
  carboxylic 198, 201
  fatty 102, 106
  gastric 128
  nucleic 116, 123, 130, 234
Actinomycetes 199
Actinomycin 165
Action, biocidal 216
Activity 36, 38, 41, 42, 44, 46, 50, 51, 57, 63, 65, 66, 74, 75, 78, 79, 107, 122, 127, 132, 160, 165, 172, 219, 243
  anti-bacterial 219
  antibiotic 165
  anti-cancer 160
  antimycobacterial 107
  catalytic 57
  cytotoxic 172
  endonuclease 243
  enzymatic 41
  hydrolase 127
  macrophages 132
Acyl carrier protein synthase 162
Acyl-CoA substrate 162
Affinity energies 43, 49, 64
Agents 75, 80, 104, 107, 126, 213, 214, 216
  anti-parasitic 107
  broad-spectrum antiviral 80
  diarrheal 126
  effective antifungal 213, 214, 216
American digestive disease 3
Amino acid residues, hydrophobic 54
Amino acids 57, 148, 161, 162, 163, 165, 201
  hydrophobic 57
  methylated 162
Analogs 35, 48, 49, 50, 52, 53, 54, 55, 56
  fleximers 54
  isatin 49
  peptidomimetic 53
Analysis 144, 209, 211

histogram 211
  molecular docking 144
  morphological 209
Antibacterial 46, 91, 92, 96, 99, 103, 104, 109, 167, 168, 172, 176, 197, 216, 217, 218, 219
  activity 96, 103, 109, 168, 216, 217, 218
  agents, broad-spectrum 104
  drug targets 99
  effect 219
Antibiotic 175
  thienamycin 175
Antifungal 167, 172, 197, 213, 214, 215, 216, 219
  activity 213, 214, 215, 216
    productive 213
Antimicrobial 20, 26, 124, 131, 161, 167, 170, 178, 214, 232, 233, 241, 242
  activities 131, 161, 167
  agents 124, 170, 214, 232, 233, 241
  biosynthetic pathways 178
  peptides 242
  resistance 20, 26
Antimicrobials 91, 114, 115, 123, 159, 165, 167, 169, 171, 176, 178, 179, 180
  microbial 165
  novel 178, 180
  synthesize 176
Aptamers, inhibitory 243
Arthrobacter gangotriensis 199
Aspergillus 202, 212, 214, 216
  flavus 214
  fumigatus 212
  niger 212, 214, 216
  terreus 202
ATP 99, 100, 102, 103, 116
  binding site 100, 103
  -dependent carboxyl group transfer 102
  hydrolysis 100
  native substrate 99
ATPase 100, 130
  activity 100
ATR spectroscopy 208

B

Bacillus 175, 199, 202, 218, 242
  amyloliquefaciens 199
  cecembensis 199
  cereus 199, 202, 242
  indicus 199
  subtilis 175, 199, 218
Bacterial 99, 114, 115, 130, 241
  endonucleases 130
  infections, antibiotic-resistant 114, 115
  invasion 241
  topoisomerases 99
Bacteriophages 114, 115, 116, 118, 121, 124, 126, 127, 128, 129, 131, 132, 134
  anti-staphylococcal 132
Binding pocket 56, 95, 97, 105, 107
  distinct 97
  non-druggable 97
Biocompatible polymers 239
Bioinformatic 145, 159, 169, 177, 178, 180
  analysis 169
  tools 159, 177, 178, 180
    innovative 145
Biosynthesis 102, 104, 123, 153, 161, 171, 175
  fatty acid 104
  lipopolysaccharide 153
  tryptophan 153
Biosynthetic gene cluster (BGCs) 161, 168, 171, 172, 173, 174, 176, 179, 180, 181
Biotin carboxylase (BC) 97, 102, 103
  homodimeric 102

C

Campylobacter jejuni 126, 127
Cancer 2, 133, 220
  colorectal 220
  gastric 2
Candida albicans 212, 214
Candidate proteins 144
Catastrophic proportions 36
Cell 122, 133, 168, 213, 218
  activity 133
  division 218
  lysis 122, 168, 213
Cellular infiltration 132
Cephalosporins 98

Chain 56, 57, 65, 66, 125, 163, 215, 218, 235
  elongating polyketide 163
  food industry production 125
  respiratory 218
  short 235
Characterization of 203, 205, 207, 208
  gold nanoparticles 207
  iron oxide nanoparticle 208
  plant mediated nanoparticles 203
  silver nanoparticle 205
Chicken skin 126
  serotype enteritidis 126
Chikungunya 41
Chloroauric acid 207
Clarithromycin 1, 2, 3, 12, 15, 19, 20, 21, 22, 23, 24, 25, 26, 27
  cure 21
  isolated 22
  resistance 20, 21, 26, 27
Clones 167, 170, 233
  resistant 233
  targeted 170
Clostridium 115, 117, 147, 148
  botulinum 115, 147, 148
  difficile 117
Combination therapy 244
Complexes 53, 99, 102, 236
  biotin-dependent 102
  enzyme-inhibitor 53
  oligonucleotide-target 236
Computational 55, 56, 57, 145
  biology 145
  modeling 56
  techniques 55, 56, 57
Concomitant regimen 1, 2, 3, 4, 13, 14, 16, 17, 18, 20, 21, 22, 23, 24, 25, 26
  non-bismuth quadruple 24
  optimized 24
Concomitant therapy 2, 3, 14, 15, 18, 19, 20, 21, 22, 23, 24, 25, 26, 27
  efficacy of 3, 20, 26
  limitation of 22, 27
  optimized 25
  standard 24
Coronaviruses 35, 37, 38
Cough 38
  dry 38
Cryogenic electron microscopy 107
Cryptotanshinone 43
Cysteine proteases 56